MRI of the LUMBAR SPINE

A Practical Approach to Image Interpretation

MRI of the LUMBAR SPINE

A Practical Approach to Image Interpretation

Neil D Steinmetz, MD

SLACK Incorporated, 6900 Grove Road, Thorofare, NJ 08086

Printed in the United States of America

Library of Congress Catalog Card Number: 86-42942

ISBN: 1-55642-009-9

Published by: SLACK Incorporated
6900 Grove Rd.
Thorofare, NJ 08086

Last digit is print number: 10 9 8 7 6 5 4 3 2 1

Dedication

To Dr. Harry Zachary Mellins, *Clinician*

"Seeing is done with the mind. The camera does not see; it records. The radiologist perceives a shadow, sees a lesion, and imagines the man. The bedside physician sees the man, perceives the signs, and imagines the lesion. They practice from the outside in, and we practice from the inside out. Both are clinicians, for in truth there is no other kind of doctor worthy of the name. The decisive test for all is finally and always at the bedside. This, then, is one concept of the radiologist—with a film on the viewbox, but the bedside on his mind."

Harry Z. Mellins, 1953

Contents

Preface *ix*

Acknowledgements *xi*

1. Introduction *1*
2. The Physics of Magnetic Resonance Imaging *13*
3. Technique of Routine Lumbar Spine Exam *31*
4. Approach to Image Interpretation *49*
5. Normal Anatomy *65*
6. Congenital Variations and Abnormalities *89*
7. Intervertebral Disc Disease *115*
8. Spinal Stenosis *151*
9. Miscellaneous Conditions *181*
10. Pitfalls; Artifacts and Limitations;
 Legal Implications; Future Directions *213*

Appendix A—Screening Forms *239*

Appendix B—Specific Techniques *243*

Appendix C—Reporting Worksheet *247*

Appendix D—Sample Normal Report *249*

Appendix E—Conduct of Depositions *250*

Bibliography *255*

Index *259*

Preface

In February 1986, I presented an informal seminar on interpretation of lumbar spine MRI as part of a continuing medical education program (Palm Beach MRI Update, West Palm Beach, Florida, February 1986). A survey of course attendees revealed that the majority rated the informal image interpretation seminars as the most valuable portion of the program. I interpret the results of this survey as indicating the need for a simple, practical guide to interpretation of lumbar MR images. This book, including and expanding on material presented at that seminar, is an effort to fill that need.

Between May 1985 and August 1986, I have evaluated approximately 750 patients referred for magnetic resonance scanning of the lumbar spine. These studies, using a prototype investigational "surface coil" (now FDA approved), were performed on a 0.6T mobile superconducting magnetic resonance scanner at a community hospital. Except as otherwise noted, images in this monograph have been obtained on this scanner, and represent a sampling of routine clinical work.

Based on this experience, I am now convinced that high resolution MR scanning is the imaging method of choice for most patients with back pain and sciatica. Utilizing surface coils and steep gradients, MR is able to provide spatial resolution approaching that of CT scanning, with contrast resolution far in excess of CT. Sagittal images are obtained directly, with resolution equal to axial sections, without need for reformatting. No injections are necessary to obtain myelogram-like pictures. No harmful biologic effects are known.

Evaluation of the capabilities of lumbar MRI must be carried out against the background of a rapidly evolving technology. When we first received our prototype surface coil (May 1985), we were amazed by the quality of the transverse images. Now these same images are regarded as routine, although no less diagnostic than they were last year. I expect that images next year will be better still.

In this book, I have attempted to relate the findings on MR

studies to the anatomy and pathophysiology familiar to most physicians from conventional radiographs, myelograms, and CT scans. Because MR is a new way of studying the lumbar spine, it may yield some new insights into the subject. Many findings of uncertain clinical significance on lumbar MR scans, such as those related to disc hydration, require further investigation.

Optimal lumbar magnetic resonance imaging is critically dependent on the system capabilities, acquisition protocols, and interpretive standards discussed in Chapters 1 through 4. Studies performed on older generation equipment, or with abbreviated protocols, or interpreted by those with limited interest in and knowledge of lumbar MRI will only serve to give the method a bad name.

This book is intended for those involved in the care and evaluation of patients with low back pain. Although primarily directed toward radiologists, orthopedic surgeons, neurosurgeons, neurologists, and other physicians involved in the diagnosis and care of these patients, it may also be of interest to technologists performing MR studies. Attorneys involved with the extensive litigation associated with back injuries may also find this material of interest.

This book is not intended as an encyclopedic catalogue of back disorders. Rather, it is a personal approach to the practical, day to day interpretation of clinical images.

Neil Steinmetz, M.D.
Atlantis, Florida
August 1986

Acknowledgments

I wish to gratefully acknowledge the contributions of the many individuals without whom this book could not have been written. My partners, William S. Merrell, M.D. and N. Henry Pevsner, M.D. shared the risk of introducing the first mobile MR scanner in the country. They and Dr. Nancy Lawhon participated in the clinical interpretation of the cases presented.

I appreciate the support of the many Palm Beach County physicians who have referred their patients for the magnetic resonance imaging studies which provided the basis for this monograph.

Many technologists have been involved in the acquisition of the images presented here. Particular thanks are due to Russell Khoury, R.T., our Chief MR Technologist who has helped develop the techniques described here, and also helped with photography of the images.

The members of the technical and clerical staff of the Imaging Department at JFK Hospital that have helped by filing and retrieving cases and copying films; this assistance is much appreciated.

Special thanks are due to my secretary, Evelyn Lyman, who has typed the manuscript and seen it through numerous revisions, and to Sidney Solomon who has helped with the drawings.

Finally thanks are due to my family, to my sons Paul, Adam and Jonathan for sharing their father with "The Book," and to my wife Ruth for moral support and for proofreading the manuscript.

CHAPTER 1

Introduction

Back Pain and Sciatica Magnitude of the Problem

Backache ranks high as a cause of lost work days among Americans (Table 1-1). Each year approximately 500,000 workers in the United States sustain back injuries leading to lost time from work and financial compensation. Health care costs, disability payments, and lost productivity related to low back pain syndrome is estimated at some 20 billion dollars annually, making this among the most costly of medical disorders. Eight million Americans are estimated to suffer from chronic low back pain.

From an individual viewpoint the costs are just as staggering. In monetary terms the medical costs, disability payments, and legal settlements related to a single back injury frequently total hundreds of thousands of dollars, and occasionally in excess of one million dollars. The human cost in terms of pain and suffering, lost productivity, and chronic disability is even greater.

Need for Precise Diagnosis

It is axiomatic that rational treatment ot low back pain and sciatica requires a precise understanding of the underlying pathophysiology in the individual patient.

Fortunately, most episodes of low back pain and sciatica resolve spontaneously. Thus when initial history and physical examination suggest limited injury or abnormality, without significant neurological deficit, an initial trial of empirically based conservative treatment is warranted.

Patients with neurological deficit, and those not responding to conservative measures, require additional evaluation. The choice

Table 1-1
The High Cost of Pain

Complaint	Lost Work Days (Millions)
Headaches	156.9
Backaches	88.8
Muscle Pains	58.2
Joint Pains	107.8
Stomach Pains	98.7
Menstrual Pains	14.5
Dental Pains	15.1

Source: Newsweek December 2, 1985

between continued conservative care and surgical intervention rests on a precise understanding of a patient's anatomic abnormalities as they relate to his functional deficit. Rational planning of the type and extent of surgery, if any, clearly depends on correlation of the precise anatomic data available with modern imaging methods to the patient's clinical situation.

Over 50 years have passed since the pioneering work of Mixter and Barr (1933) on the role of disc herniation in low back pain and sciatica. Today physicians and patients alike frequently equate sciatica with a *slipped disc*. This has resulted in what has been called a "disc dynasty" (Finneson 1973). The resulting tunnel vision, with focus on disc abnormalities to the exclusion of all others, has frequently led to inappropriate or incomplete surgery. The most common cause of failed back surgery syndrome is an incomplete or inappropriate initial operation. Often this can be related to a preoperative lack of appreciation of the full extent of anatomic abnormality present, further stressing the requirement for precise diagnosis.

Why Magnetic Resonance Imaging?

The advent of water soluble myelography and computed tomography in the past ten years have accelerated our understanding of the anatomic and pathophysiologic abnormalities underlying low back pain syndrome. Nonetheless, even the advent of high resolution computed tomography with multiplanar *reformatting* and computed tomographic myelography with water soluble agents has not fully satisfied the need for a completely safe, non-invasive, widely accepted test for the health of the low back. I believe that magnetic resonance represents such a test.

Although most early predictions were quite skeptical of the ability of magnetic resonance imaging to evaluate musculoskeletal disease, more recent experience has proven them incorrect. The varying signal pattern of structures surrounding cortical bone (which itself produces no signal) allows precise assessment of both osseous and soft tissue structures. This lack of MR signal from cortical bone actually represents an advantage as compared to x-ray methods in which surrounding dense bone interferes with precise evaluation of structures contained within the spinal canal. The ability of magnetic resonance to directly image anatomy in multiple planes represents an additional advantage.

Approach to the Patient With Low Back Pain

Evaluation of low back pain begins with history and physical examination. Analysis of the pain distribution, sensory and motor dysfunction, reflex changes, and response to straight leg raising helps in differentiating the involved levels (Table 1-2).

Plain film radiography is generally the initial imaging study performed in patients with back pain and sciatica. This is helpful in evaluation of spinal alignment and gross bony abnormalities, although the amount of information present is limited. The role of dynamic radiology (bending films) remains controversial.

We generally perform a high-resolution, detailed (see Chapter 3) magnetic resonance scan as the next imaging procedure following plain films when definitive evaluation is required. This study, carefully performed on modern equipment (Section 1-5) and properly interpreted and correlated to clinical diagnosis, provides a definitive diagnosis in most patients with low back pain with or without sciatica. Disc disease and spinal stenosis are accurately depicted as are inflammatory or neoplastic processes. All information needed for surgical planning is generally present. A normal study excludes significant anatomic abnormality with a high degree of confidence. When the findings on magnetic resonance imaging explain the clinical presentation, further imaging studies are rarely necessary.

Table 1-2
Differentiation of Involved Levels

Disc Level	Area of Pain	Sensory Dysfunction (Subjective & Objective)	Motor Dysfunction	Reflex Changes	Straight Leg Raising Test
L5-S1	Low back Buttock Sciatic distribution extending to lateral aspect of foot	Lateral aspect foot	Minimal plantar flexion foot	Diminished or absent Achilles reflex	Positive
L4-5	Low back Buttock Sciatic distribution extending over dorsum of foot toward big toe	Dorsum of foot	Extensor weakness big toe and foot	None	Positive
L3-4	Low back lateral buttock and hip. Posterolateral aspect of thigh and anterior tibial area.	Posterolateral thigh and anterior tibial area, rarely below upper third of leg	Quadriceps weakness	Diminished patellar reflex	Patients positive 50%

Modified from Finneson

If the magnetic resonance imaging study is technically inadequate, or fails to explain clinical findings, computed tomography is generally our next recommendation. We perform these studies without contrast material, reserving the use of intravenous contrast for evaluation of post-surgical cases or inflammatory disease, and the use of water soluble intrathecal contrast for those patients having conventional myelography or in whom arachnoiditis is suspected. We perform most of our CT studies utilizing gantry angulation through the disc spaces, reserving the use of sagittal and coronal reformatting for specific indications, most commonly evaluation of spinal fusion. High resolution CT remains an excellent method of spinal evaluation when magnetic resonance is not available.

Although Magnetic Resonance Imaging appears to be more

sensitive than nuclear bone scanning for marrow abnormalities (Daffner et al., 1986), the whole body bone scan remains a practical and less expensive method of performing a total skeletal evaluation in patients with suspected metastatic disease. Magnetic resonance imaging is superior to either nuclear bone scan or Gallium scan in evaluation of discitis and osteomyelitis. Plain film tomography is still of occasional use in evaluation of the lumbar spine such as for traumatic abnormalities. Discography and epidural venography we now regard as of historic interest only.

Scanner Requirements

In general the spatial resolution required of an imaging modality is determined by the size of the anatomic structures and abnormalities to be imaged. Thus it is not surprising that the technical capabilities required for high resolution Magnetic Resonance Imaging of the lumbar spine are quite similar to the widely accepted requirements for high resolution CT scanning. Based on physical principles to be discussed in Chapter 2 the following generalizations apply.

As with CT, the optimal slice thickness is in the range of 3 to 5 millimeters; thinner sections obtained in reasonable times are too grainy, and thicker sections suffer from partial volume artifact. The gap between slices should be as small as possible. Receiver coil and system electronics should be optimized to maximize the signal to noise ratio and contrast obtained. Pulse sequences must be chosen to discriminate among various tissues. Imaging in the axial plane is essential; as with CT, this can be obtained either parallel to the intervertebral discs or in a true axial plane. Technical factors must be chosen so as to provide in-plane resolution on the order of 1 mm. Unlike CT, sagittal images are obtained directly rather than by reconstruction, and thus have equivalent resolution to the axial images. These requirements, although quite stringent, are now within the capabilities of most commercially available MR scanners.

Early comparative studies showed lumbar spine MR at a slight relative disadvantage compared to CT. These studies, done on early generation MR equipment, utilized MR slices of 1 cm or greater and were done without surface coils. Studies such as these do not accurately reflect the current capabilities of spinal MRI. In our recent experience, spinal MRI performed on equipment meeting the technical requirements discussed above is a superior study.

The Magnetic Resonance Imaging Examination

Most patients are able to undergo a magnetic resonance imaging study without difficulty. We have imaged patients as young as a few months of age and as old as 85 years. Contraindications are few (Table 1-3).

At this time, the presence of a cardiac pacemaker represents an absolute contraindication to magnetic resonance imaging based upon the interaction of the magnetic field with the pacemaker reed switch. Other electronic implants such as cochlear implants or spinal cord stimulators likewise represent contraindications to MR.

Cerebral aneurysm clips represent a contraindication because of the risk of the magnetic field creating torque on the clip with resultant dislodgement. This applies specifically to cerebral aneurysm clips; other types of surgical clips including those about previously resected abdominal aneurysms do not represent a contraindication.

Other metallic surgical implants do not contraindicate MR scanning although they may cause some local artifact by distortion of the magnetic field about the implant. We have successfully scanned several patients with indwelling hip prostheses, for example.

Table 1-3
Contraindications to MRI

Contraindications to MRI
Absolute
Electronic Implant, Especially Cardiac Pacemaker
Cerebral Aneurysm Clip
Intraocular Iron Foreign Body
Relative
Pregnancy
Inability to Cooperate
Life Support Apparatus

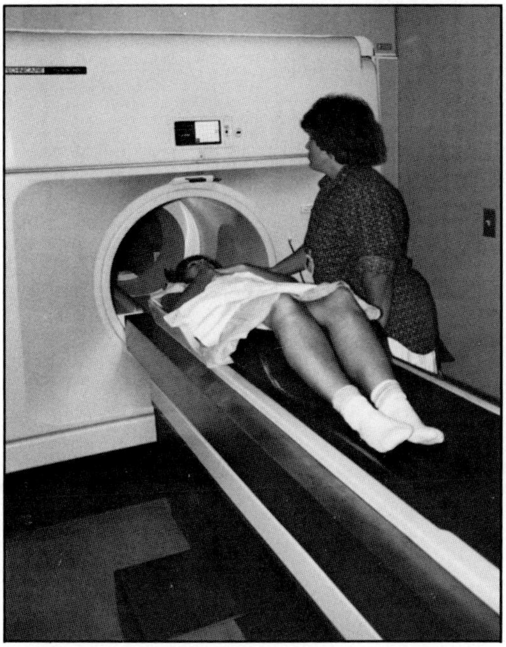

Figure 1-1A: Patient about to be placed into the scanner. Note the knees flexed over a cushion and the arms placed comfortably on the chest.

Although surgical metallic implants of stainless steel or other materials are only weakly magnetic and present no hazard, iron foreign bodies may represent a difficulty. We have had one patient who wished to terminate an examination because of the unpleasant sensation of the magnet "tugging" on a piece of shrapnel in his arm, although no injury resulted. A case of ocular injury due to a small intraocular iron foreign body in a former machinist has been reported (Kelly et al., 1986). Patients requiring complex life support and/or monitoring equipment are not candidates for magnetic resonance imaging at this time with most available scanners. These restrictions rarely apply to patients evaluated for low back pain. Patients must be able to cooperate or be adequately sedated to remain still for the duration of the examination.

Prior to MR examination, a patient screening form is completed for all patients, and a brief history obtained (Appendix A). The scanning procedure is explained to the patient in detail, and the patient is given an opportunity to have his questions answered. Although no special preparation is required, patients are asked to empty their bladder prior to the start of the study. The patient is placed on the scanning couch in the supine position with his knees

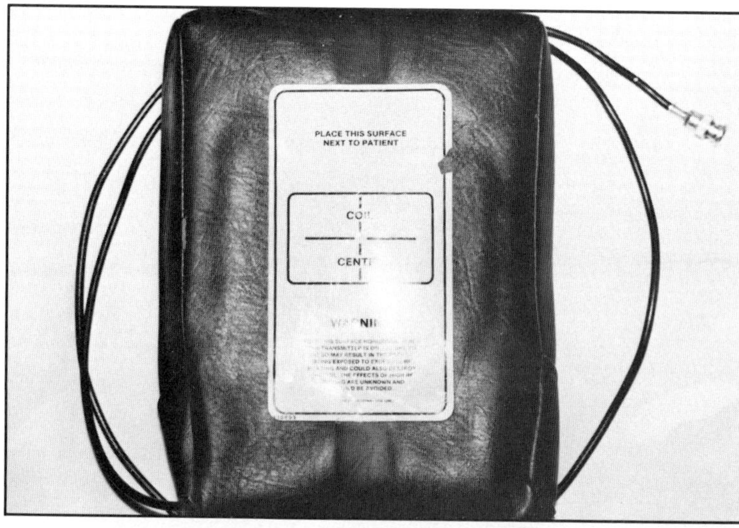

Figure 1-1B: Lumbar surface coil. The metallic coil is encased within a padded pouch. Note the coaxial connector. Coil is placed beneath the lumbar spine for patient studies.

Table 1-4
Claustrophobia

Problem	Solution
Feeling of Confinement	Open-face coils, Mirrors, Close eyes
Lack of Communication	Intercom, Friend or Parent in Room
Lack of Ventilation	Air conditioning with Air Flow
Noise	Music, Earplugs
Immobility	Scheduling, Wiggling, Breaks, W.C.
Apprehension	Explanation, (Sedation)

flexed and placed into the scanner (Figure 1-1). The scanning protocol is designed so that the relatively longer acquisitions take place first, while the patient is still fresh, with shorter acquisitions at the end. Between acquisitions the patient is allowed to rest and stretch. Although occasional patients may require sedation or pain medication, we have found that the majority of patients tolerate the examination procedure easily if it is carefully explained.

A small number of patients will have difficulty completing the examination because of claustrophobia. Causes of this problem include not only the feeling of confinement induced by the surrounding equipment, but also lack of communication and ventilation, noise of the gradient coils, prolonged immobility, and apprehension. Solutions directed at various aspects of this problem (Table 1-4) allow most patients to complete the study. Manufacturer provided hardware modifications include open-faced coils, mirrors in the scanning tunnel, intercom facility for patients, and adequate air-conditioning. Simple maneuvers such as having the patient close his eyes or providing ear plugs are sometimes helpful. A friend, technologist, or parent in the scan room itself may help allay apprehension.

Absolute, statuelike immobility for an extended period is difficult for most patients. Although MR studies are quite sensitive to motion, only the part of the body being studied need remain absolutely still. For example, a patient previously unable to cooperate may complete a study with ease after he is informed that slight wiggling of his fingers and toes will not interfere with his lumbar spine examination.

CHAPTER 2

The Physics of Magnetic Resonance Imaging

The Physics of Magnetic Resonance Imaging

Introduction

The physical basis of magnetic resonance imaging is complex. Fortunately, only a limited knowledge of basic physics is required for the practical clinical interpretation of magnetic resonance images of the lumbar spine. This chapter will discuss physical principles with particular emphasis on the user selectable variables which influence the quality and appearance of the images obtained. Readers interested in a more detailed explanation are referred to the works of Wolf and Popp (1985) and of Bradley (1985).

The formation of the MR image depends on the ability of certain atomic nuclei, particularly hydrogen, to absorb and re-emit radio frequency energy when placed in a magnetic field. The frequency at which energy is absorbed and re-emitted, known as the resonant or *Larmor* frequently, is proportional to the strength of the magnetic field.

Like x-ray CT, MR is a tomographic, computer based, digital imaging modality. Unlike CT, MR is capable of obtaining images directly in any desired plane. X-ray CT images display the variation of a single variable, electron density, in the tissue examined. The corresponding variable in MR is signal intensity (amplitude), which in turn represents a complex function of proton (hydrogen) density, relaxation parameters, and motion. The interrelationship of these tissue parameters with the user selectable imaging factors (pulse sequence) accounts for the sensitivity and complexity of the MR images.

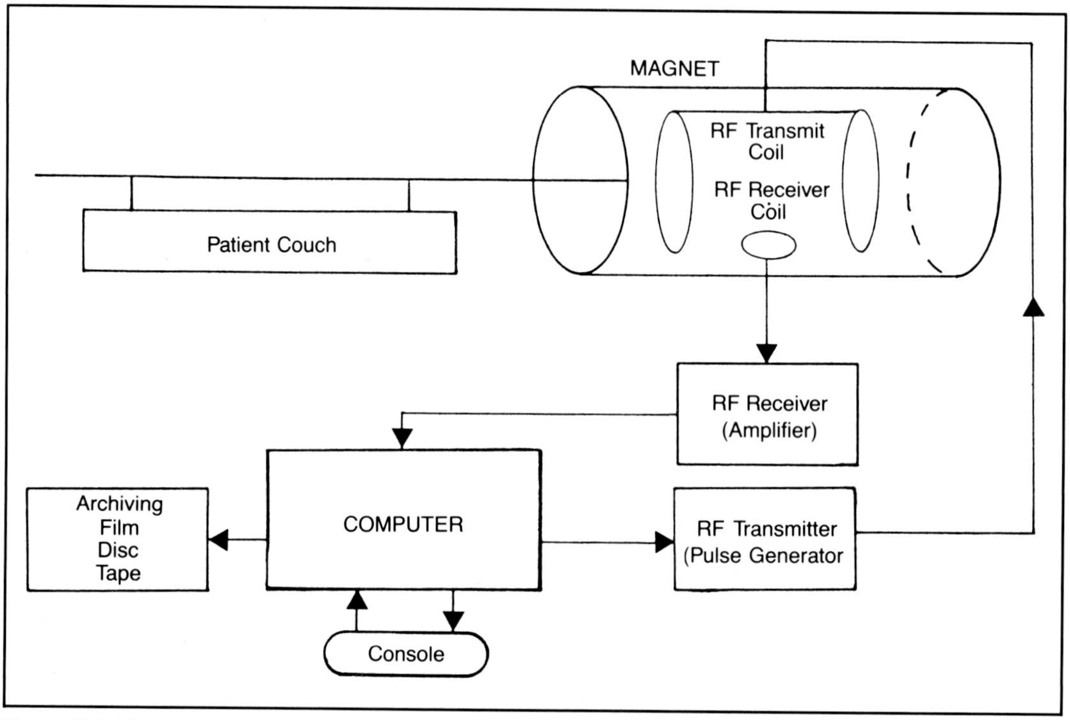

Figure 2-1: Major components of an MR system.

System Description

A complete Magnetic Resonance Imaging system (Figure 2-1) includes a suitable magnet, patient handling subsystem, gradient coils and electronics, radio frequency transmitting and receiving electronics and coils, image processing and control computers, and a display and archiving system.

Magnet

Clinical MR imaging requires a magnetic field in the range of 3,000 to 40,000 times the earth's magnetic field (0.15T - 2T). Typically the magnet producing this field is large enough to surround the patient's body, and has a uniformity on the order of 5 - 50 parts per million over the imaging region of interest.

A variety of magnet types including permanent magnets, resistive electromagnets, iron core electromagnets, and superconducting (cryogenic) electromagnets have been utilized to produce the magnetic field. Although there has been great controversy about magnet type and field strength, excellent spinal images have been obtained with each of these types of magnets, and throughout the range of field strengths discussed. The images in this book have been obtained utilizing a 0.6T superconducting magnet.

Patient Handling

The patient handling system consists of a moveable couch of non-magnetic materials on which the patient lies and is placed within the bore of the magnet. A well designed couch allows for patient comfort and for rapid removal of the patient from the magnet in an emergency. Also included in the patient handling package should be provision for ventilation, noise suppression, and other patient comfort factors.

Gradient System

The ability to form an *image* utilizing magnetic resonance (spatial localization) depends on the introduction of a small known variation (gradient) in the magnetic field. This known variation in magnetic field strength permits us to assign the correct point of origin of the magnetic resonance signal based upon the frequency. This is analogous to our ability to determine which key has been struck on a piano by listening to the frequency of the tone produced.

In actual practice the gradient subsystem consists of coils of wire appropriately placed within the main magnet so as to produce the desired gradients in the X, Y and Z planes, along with the control electronics.

Radio Frequency Subsystem

The radio frequency (RF) system includes the RF pulse generator, transmitting and receiving antennae (coils), and radio receiver electronics. High quality MR images depend to a great degree on the ability of the pulse generator to produce RF pulses of carefully controlled power, frequency, and duration, and on the sensitivity of the receiving coils and electronics to the very low voltage signals produced by the body. Signal transmission and reception may either be by the same or separate coils. Receiver coils are divided into *body* coils which are sensitive to the whole body, and closely coupled or *surface* coils which have a smaller sensitive region but improved signal to noise response within that region.

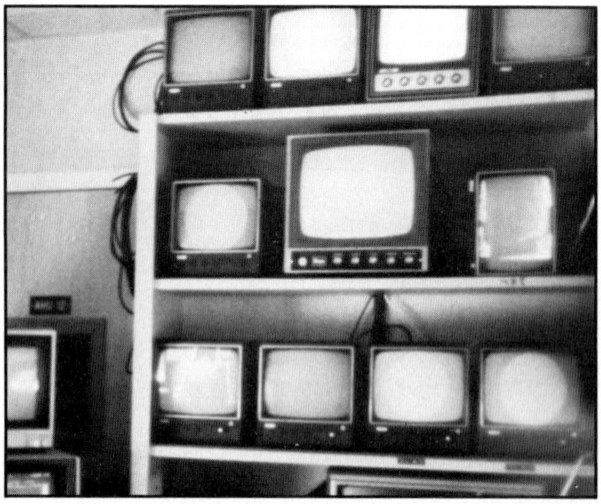

Figure 2-2: Remote video monitor in the radiology reading room is connected to the mobile MR system outside the hospital.

Computer

The computer system is responsible for controlling and coordinating the functions of the other subsystems and processing and displaying the images. Thus the computer should be capable of performing multiple tasks simultaneously, and have adequate speed and memory so as not to slow down the overall imaging process. Fast, flexible, easily used software is desirable.

Display and Archiving

The images are displayed on a monitor at the console, and may also be displayed remotely (Figure 2-2). Short term storage such as computer disc is required, and archiving to magnetic tape or other media may be helpful, although we do not save tapes permanently. Studies are filmed by technologists utilizing a standard multiformat camera, and most studies are interpreted from the hard copy rather than at the console.

Relaxation Parameters

The net magnetization vector of an object is the sum of the magnetizations of the individual protons (spins). Outside a magnetic field these sum to zero. When the object is placed in a magnetic field, a new equilibrium is reached, with a slight excess of magnetizations aligned with the field. This occurs as an exponential process with a time constant denoted as T1, also called the spin lattice or longitudinal relaxation time. The same time con-

Table 2-1
T1 and T2 Values Obtained From Normal Tissue

Tissue	T1 (MSEC + S.D.)	T2 (MSEC + S.D.)
Muscle	541 ± 141	35 ± 6
Subcutaneous Fat	218 ± 68	61 ± 18
Vertebral Marrow	420 ± 112	50 ± 12
Nucleus Pulposus	1078 ± 396	65 ± 17
Ligament/tendon	864 ± 206	107 ± 16

Modified from Richardson

stant governs the re-equilibration of the spins with the main magnet field following perturbation by an RF pulse.

MR imaging equipment is designed to detect radio frequency signals in the transverse (X-Y) plane, where the direction of the main magnetic field is denoted as the longitudinal (Z) axis. A burst of RF energy at the Larmor frequency of carefully defined length and intensity to tip the net magnetization from the Z axis to the X-Y plane is denoted as a 90° pulse. Following application of such a pulse, a signal (voltage) is detected by the receiver coil. This signal decays by two different mechanisms. T1 relaxation (spin lattice) represents the re-equilibration of the magnetization vector along the longitudinal (Z) axis as discussed above. This is characterized by the T1 relaxation time.

Signal also decays due to loss of coherence (dephasing) of the individual spins in the X-Y plane. This is caused by local variations in magnetic field strength, both those related to non-homogeneity of the main magnetic field and those related to the local chemical environment of the protons. Those protons experiencing a greater than average magnetic field will spin (precess) at slightly greater than average frequency, and those in a weaker than average field at a correspondingly lower frequency. This loss of signal due to dephasing is also an exponential process. The dephasing due to the local chemical environment is irreversible and is characterized by a time constant T2, hence the term T2 relaxation. This may also be denoted as transverse or spin-spin relaxation time.

The physical and chemical factors which determine the values of T1 and T2 are complex and controversial and will not be discussed here. In general T1 is always greater than or equal to

Figure 2-3: Timing diagram for a spin-echo pulse sequence. The 180° pulse follows the 90° pulse by a time equal to TE/2. The echo is formed at time TE. The sequence is repeated following the repetition time TR.

T2, with representative values presented in Table 2-1. Note that these values are a function of magnetic field strength so that the importance of the actual measured values is limited.

The Spin Echo Pulse Sequence

A pulse sequence may be regarded as a prescription specifying the type and timing of the excitations to be used in obtaining an MR measurement, and the time interval allowed for equilibration between measurements. The most commonly used excitations are the 90° and the 180° pulse; these are the only ones to be discussed here.

A 90° pulse signifies an excitation with the proper amount of energy to tip the magnetization from the longitudinal to the transverse plane or vice versa. The 180° pulse tips magnetization from the plus Z to the minus Z axis. Spins in the X-Y plane are also inverted. This inversion of spins in the X-Y plane permits a rephasing of the MR signal, cancelling out field inhomogeneities.

In a spin-echo imaging sequence (Figure 2-3) a 90° RF pulse is followed (at a time TE/2) by a 180° pulse. At time TE, the signal which had become dephased will once again become coherent producing a "spin echo." A commonly used analogy to explain this phenomenon is that of a race. Following the firing of the starter's gun the contestants will be separated along the track. If the starter fires his gun again and the contestants reverse direction but maintain the same speed, they will once again arrive at the finish line together. In the case of the MR experiment rephasing will compensate for the field non-homogeneities, but there will be some loss of signal related to the true T2 relaxation reflecting the physical-chemical state of the protons. The sensitivity of this

Table 2-2
The Effect of TR and TE on Image Weighting

TR	TE	Weighting
Short	Short	T1
Long	Long	T2
Long	Short	Proton Density

sequence to the value of T2 depends upon the choice of TE as discussed below.

The second timing parameter defining a spin echo pulse sequence is TR, the repetition time. This is the time between one 90° pulse and the next. This interval is required to allow the sample to re-equilibrate along the X axis. If TR is greater than 5 times the T1 value of the sample equilibration is for all practical purposes complete. Shorter TR allows only partial re-equilibration (partial saturation), with the degree of equilibration dependent upon T1.

At this point, it is appropriate to introduce the concept of the *weighted image*. Although signal intensity with the spin echo sequence is a function of proton density, T1, and T2, the timing parameters (TR and TE) can be chosen so that any of these factors dominates the appearance of the image (Table 2-2). Choosing a long TR decreases dependence on T1, since all tissues present have time to fully re-equilibrate. Conversely, short TR introduces T1 dependence by allowing substances with short T1 to re-equilibrate whereas those with long T1 only partially re-equilibrate.

Short TE suppresses T2 dependence by allowing little time for dephasing. Longer TE allows those substances with short T2 to dephase disproportionately to those with long T2, hence the dependence on T2 or "T2-weighting." Use of long TR and short TE suppresses dependence on either relaxation parameter and thus yields an image dependant primarily on the proton density distribution.

Although there are many other pulse sequences available, the spin echo technique is the most widely used at the current time. All of the MR images in this book have been obtained with this technique. Other methods including inversion recovery imaging,

Table 2-3
The MR Gray Scale

	T1W	T2W
Brighter	Fat	Water
↑	Marrow	Fat
	Muscle	Marrow
	Water	Muscle
	Ligaments and Tendons	Ligaments and Tendons
	Rapidly Flowing Blood	Rapidly Flowing Blood
	Cortical Bone	Cortical Bone
Darker	Air	Air

Table 2-4
The Effects of T1, T2 and Proton Density on MR Signal Intensity

	T1	T2	Proton Density
Brighter	Short	Long	High
Darker	Long	Short	Low

chemical shift imaging, and a variety of more rapid imaging methods utilizing pulses less than 90° and gradient reversals are regarded as experimental at this time and will not be discussed here.

Following the initial 180° rephasing pulse of a spin echo sequence one or more additional echoes may be obtained by applying additional 180° pulses. Such a multi-echo technique allows one to obtain both short TE and long TE images during a single acquisition.

The MR Gray Scale

MR images are usually presented as maps of signal intensity, with the brightness of each pixel proportionate to the total signal received from the voxel (volume element) it represents. Because

Table 2-5
Signal Intensity of Musculoskeletal Tissues

High
Fat
Marrow
Very Low
Air
Cortical Bone
Ligaments and Tendons
Fibrocartilage
Low to Intermediate
Muscle
Hyaline Articular Cartilage
Variable
(Low Intensity With T1 Weighting, High Intensity with T2 Weighting)
Fluid
Inflammatory or edematous tissue
Neoplastic tissue
Hematoma (intensity varies with age)

After Richardson

of the complex dependence of the MR signal on the relaxation parameters and sequence parameters, the relative brightness of various tissues is not constant. Table 2-3 presents a relative brightness scale for typical substances on T1 and T2 weighted images. Table 2-4 shows the relative brightness as a function of T1, T2, and mobile protons.

Although these relationships are complex, the relative brightness of many musculoskeletal tissues remains constant for a variety of clinically useful pulse sequences (Table 2-5). Thus subcutaneous and marrow fat tend to have high intensity; muscle and hyaline articular cartilage low to medium intensity; and air, cortical bone, ligaments, tendons and fibrocartilage very low intensity. The notable exceptions to this pattern involve structures with high water content, which have low intensity on T1 weighting and high intensity on T2 weighting. Examples would include fluid filled structures such as cysts, effusions, or the thecal sac; inflammatory or edematous tissue; and neoplastic tissue. Signal intensity of hematomas also varies, depending on age of the hematoma and strength of the magnetic field.

Gradient and Phase Encoding

Of the numerous techniques described for obtaining MR images, the most widely utilized today involves a mathematical technique known as two-dimensional Fourier transform (2DFT). Details of this method are beyond the scope of this chapter but certain practical consequences need to be mentioned.

With the 2DFT method information in one direction (gradient encoded) is obtained utilizing a linear magnetic field gradient and the Larmor relationship, whereas information along the perpendicular axis (phase encoded) is obtained utilizing phase information. Thus a full line of information in the gradient encoded direction may be acquired with a single excitation, whereas each line of data along the phase encoded direction requires a separate excitation. Because of this MR images are frequently obtained with unequal numbers of pixels in the X and Y directions, typically with 256 pixels in the gradient encoded direction and anywhere from 128 to 256 pixels in the phase encoded direction.

A second consequence of the 2DFT method relates to motion sensitivity. Because motion artifact tends to be propagated in the phase encoded direction, the proper choice of phase encoded and gradient encoded axes may reduce the motion artifact in a region of interest.

Multislice Imaging

Magnetic resonance is generally performed as a tomographic imaging method. This requires selection of an appropriate slice thickness based upon the anatomy examined. Other factors being equal, the thick slices produce more signal and thin slices produce less signal. However, thick slices tend to include differing structures and tissues within the same voxel (partial volume effect), and are thus limited in their ability to examine structures significantly smaller than the slice thickness. The trade-off here is very much analagous to that in x-ray CT. Not surprisingly, the optimal slice thickness for lumbar examinations seems to be in the range of 3-5mm, just as for CT.

Although single slice imaging offers slightly superior resolution, multislice techniques are utilized because of practical time constraints. With spin echo pulse sequences TR is usually much longer than TE; with multislice techniques the waiting time is

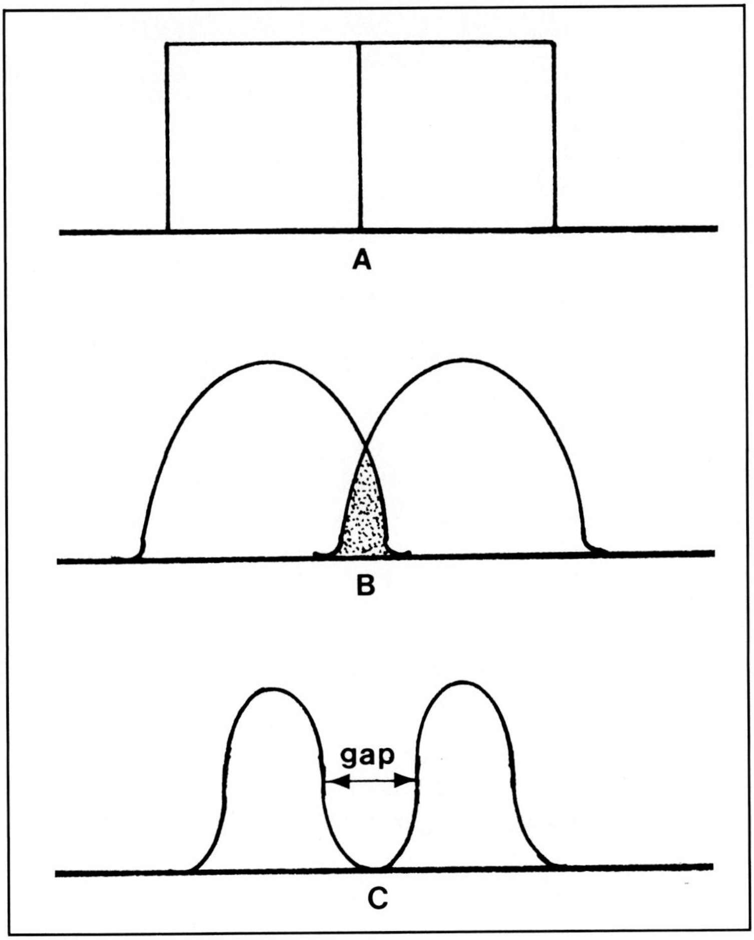

Figure 2-4: Slice profiles. Ideal slice selective pulses are represented by square waves (A). Real pulses more closely resemble modified sine waves, so that slices either overlap (B), causing loss of detail, or are separated by gaps (C).

utilized to obtain information about additional slices.

Slice selective pulses (Figure 2-4) are not perfect square waves, but rather imperfect approximations. Because of this we are left with a choice of either attempting to obtain contiguous slices, in which case there will be some interference between slices (cross talk), or alternatively of leaving a gap between slices. For lumbar scanning with 4mm thick slices a 1mm gap seems an acceptable compromise.

Table 2-6
Acquisition Time for Typical Sequences

TR (msec)	TE (msec)	NEX	Ny	AT (min)	Slices
300	30	2	128	1	7
500	40	2	128	2	9
500	40	4	160	5	9
500	30	4	192	6	11
500	40	6	256	13	9
950	40	6	128	12	17
2000	40	3	128	13	36
2000	120	2	128	9	15
2000	120	4	128	17	15
2000	120	4	256	34	15

Imaging Time

With 2DFT imaging three user selectable variables determine the amount of time required to obtain a series of images. The repetition time (TR) and the number of lines of data in the phase encoding (Y) direction (N_y) have already been discussed. The third factor is the number of excitations (N_{ex}).

Because the MR signal is so weak, the overall statistical quality of the image (signal to noise ratio) can be improved utilizing signal averaging. In typical clinical applications each line of data may be acquired anywhere from one to ten or more times, and then signal averaged.

The product of these three factors represents the acquisition time (A.T.) for an imaging experiment. Thus:

$$\text{A.T.} = \text{TR X } N_y \text{ X } N_{ex}.$$

Note that with multislice methods multiple slices are obtained within this time period. Table 2-6 presents some examples.

Theoretically, the number of slices available in a multislice sequence is TR over TE. In practice, because of lag time in the electronics, the actual maximum number of slices available is somewhat less, approximately TR/(TE+15) for our system.

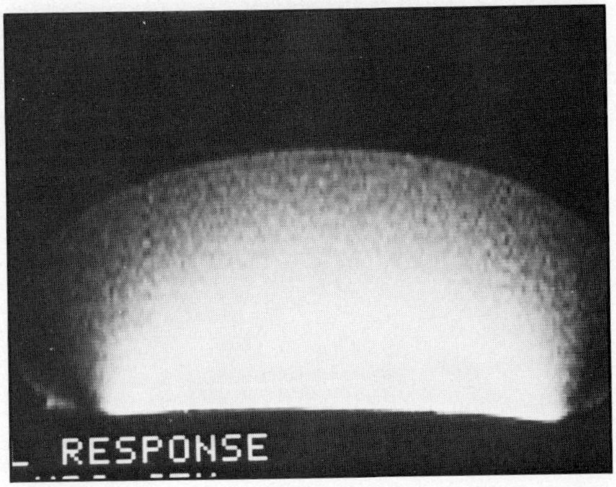

Figure 2-5: Sensitivity pattern of our surface coil. Scanning of a water phantom shows the drop in sensitivity as distance from the coil increases.

Effects of Surface Coil Response on Images

With most MR systems available today, high resolution spine imaging is optimized by the use of closely coupled receiver coils, commonly but not always correctly referred to as "surface coils." These special purpose coils improve image quality in a region of interest primarily because of their decreased sensitivity to noise from outside the region of interest. As usual, there is a trade-off. Surface coils generally examine a smaller field of view than do body coils and also have a non-uniform sensitivity pattern (Figure 2-5). This non-uniform response requires the interpreter to exercise caution when commenting on the significance of intensity variations in surface coil images. Computer software to correct for this intensity variation is theoretically possible, but not generally available.

In a digital image, each pixel in the image equals a dimension in the patient equal to the field of view divided by the matrix size. For example, if the field of view were 25.6cm and the matrix size were 256×256, then each image pixel would represent 1mm in the patient. Because surface coil images generally have a smaller field of view than body coil images, they provide greater spatial resolution assuming equal matrix size. In order to take advantage of this theoretically greater spatial resolution, steeper magnetic field gradients are required. This type of magnification may be referred to as *gradient zoom*.

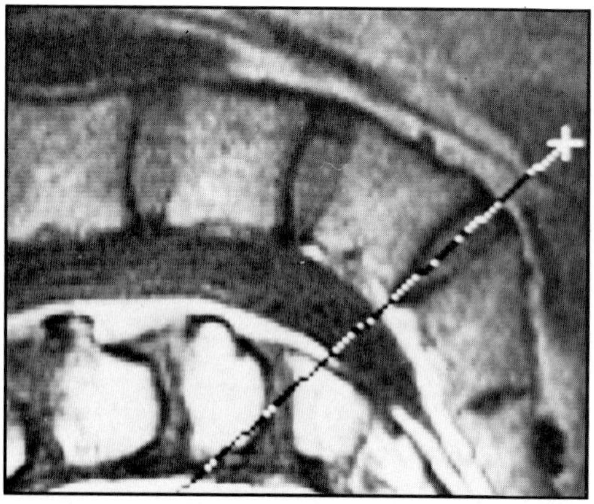

Figure 2-6A: Sagittal scout with indicator line marking the plane of the axial section through the angled L5-S1 disc space.

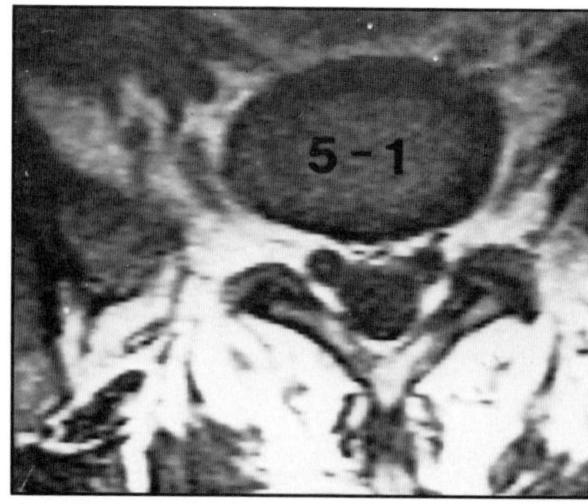

Figure 2-6B: "Angled axial" image through the L5-S1 disc space indicated in A.

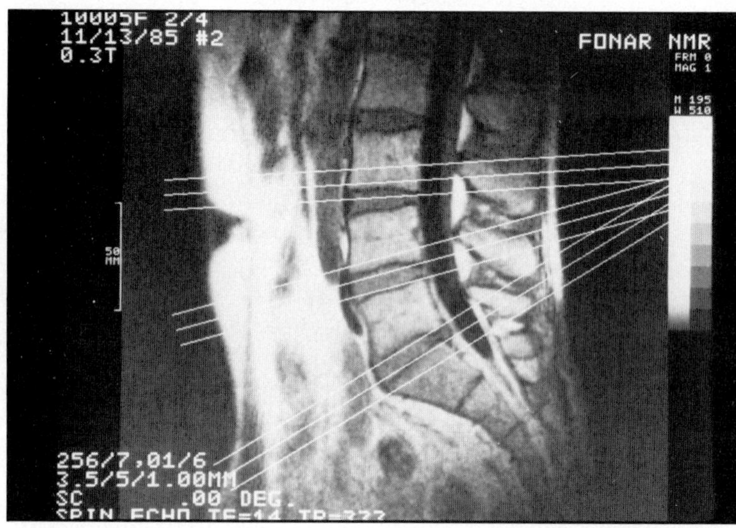

Figure 2-7: A multislice acquisition arranged with angled axial slices passing through disc spaces at *varying* angles. This has been termed multiply angled, variable internal orthogonal ("MAVIN") imaging. (Courtesy of Fonar Corp).

Angled and Oblique Imaging Planes

In addition to the standard coronal, sagittal, and axial planes, MR permits electronic selection of angled, oblique, and compound angled imaging planes.

In the lumbar spine, angled axial images are routinely obtained

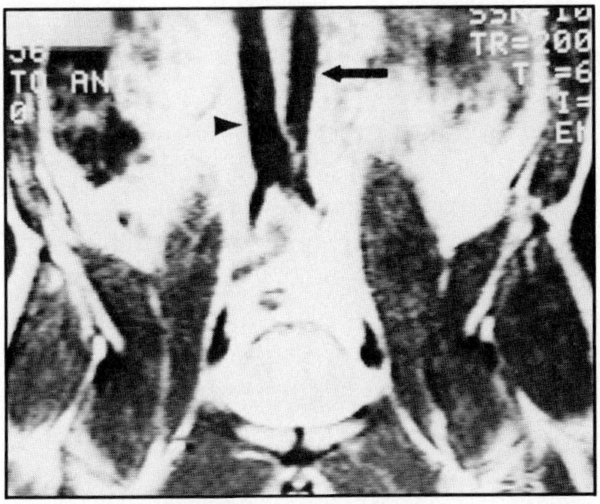

Figure 2-8: Rapidly flowing blood has low signal. Note absence of signal in the aorta (arrow) and inferior vena cava (arrowhead).

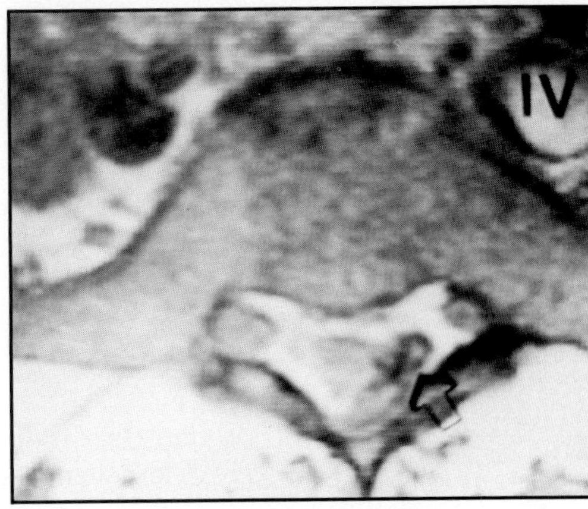

Figure 2-9: Paradoxical enhancement. In a multislice sequence, slowly flowing blood entering the region examined has increased signal due to fully saturated protons. Note the bright signal in the left iliac vein (IV).

in a plane parallel to the disc spaces (Figure 2-6). The ability to obtain multiple slices at different angles (Figure 2-7) is now available from several manufacturers.

Flow Effects

Effects of flow on MR imaging are complex. Fortunately they are rarely important to the understanding of lumbar MR studies. In general, rapidly flowing blood causes a loss of MR signal ("flow void"), so that major vessels appear dark on MR images (Figure 2-8). With multislice techniques slowly flowing blood entering a slice may produce an area of bright signal known as paradoxical enhancement (Figure 2-9). Flow effects with multi-echo imaging are even more complex.

Safety

The safety of Magnetic Resonance Imaging has been carefully studied; within the range of magnetic fields, gradients, and RF power deposition in clinical use no harmful effects are known.

The important safety considerations in MR imaging relate to electronic implants and ferromagnetic objects. Patients and personnel with cardiac pacemakers must be excluded from the magnetic environment. Most surgical implants are minimally ferromagnetic and do not represent contraindication to MR scanning; the notable exceptions are cerebral aneurysm clips which, although only weakly ferromagnetic, represent a contraindication to MR scanning because of their critical location. The presence of an intraocular ferromagnetic foreign body contraindicates MR scanning.

Ferromagnetic stretchers, oxygen bottles, scissors, etc. have the potential to become lethal missiles and must be excluded from the scan room. Provision must be made for patient monitoring, and rapid patient evacuation from the scanner in the event of emergency.

In summary, MR scanning has no known harmful biological effects. Safety depends on careful patient screening and scan area security as described above.

CHAPTER 3

Technique of Lumbar Spine Examination

Technique of Lumbar Spine Examination

A complete magnetic resonance imaging examination of the lumbar spine consists of a series of acquisitions designed to solve a clinical problem. Selection of the parameters defining an individual acquisition, and of the acquisitions comprising an imaging protocol, requires a compromise between imaging time, image quality, imaging plane, and field of view.

Choices to be made in defining an individual acquisition include receiver coil, patient positioning, imaging plane, thickness and number of slices and interslice gaps, pulse sequence parameters, and photographic format. We use the term *MR Protocol* to denote a series of acquisitions frequently used together to solve a particular clinical question. The term *MR Patient Protocol* is used to define the sequence of acquisitions for a particular patient, which may include a routine protocol, routine protocol with additional acquisitions, or a customized protocol. Appendix B includes examples of completed *MR Prescription* forms for a patient examined with the routine lumbar protocol.

Imaging Planes

The *sagittal* plane is utilized in all spine cases. This provides a radiographic type survey of the vertebrae, intervertebral discs, and spinal canal, and permits assessment of multiple levels on a single image. Our 5½ inch square prototype surface coil includes a field of view from approximately L1-2 to the mid-sacrum in most patients; if pathology at the thoracolumbar junction level is suspected, we obtain additional sagittal images centered higher, or a survey sagittal view with the body coil. Our routine lumbar protocol includes a multislice sagittal acquisition with T1) weighting (Figure 3-1) as well as a single slice midline sagittal acquisition with

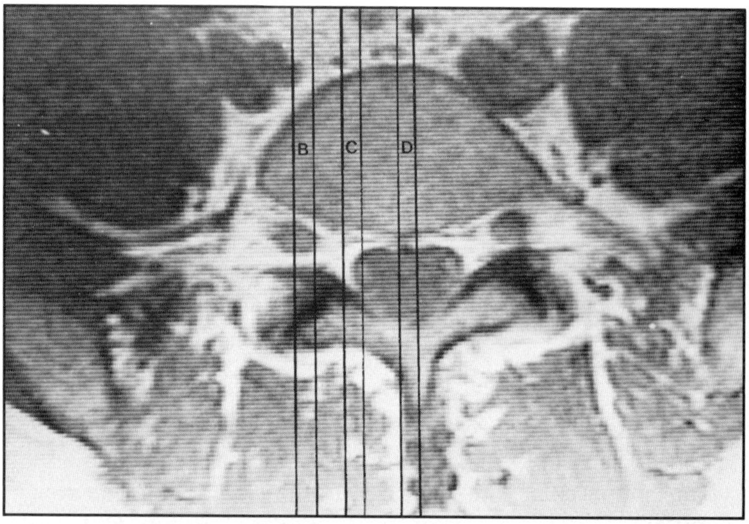

Figure 3-1A: Transverse reference image indicating the key planes for evaluation in sagittal view.

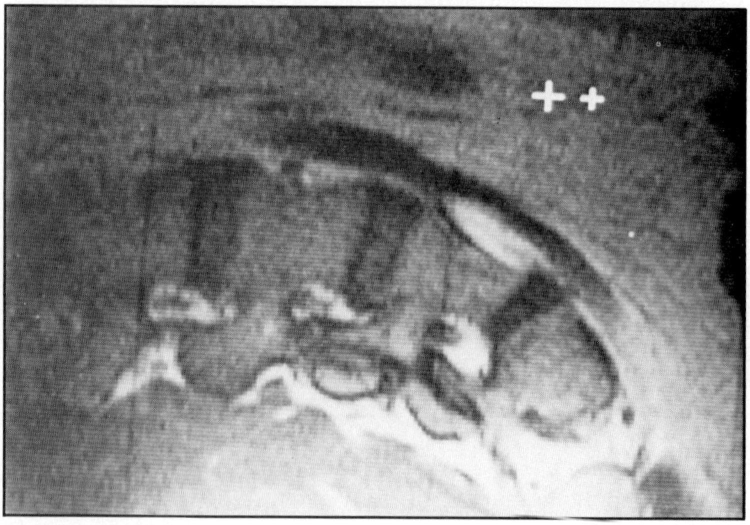

Figure 3-1B: Section through the intervertebral canals.

a long TR and multiple (usually 8) echoes to provide varying degrees of proton density and T2 weighting (Figure 3-2).

A set of images in an angled *axial* plane (Figure 3-3) is routinely obtained in most cases, including all cases of suspected disc herniation or spinal stenosis. Angulation of the sections is chosen so as to approximately parallel the intervertebral discs (Figure

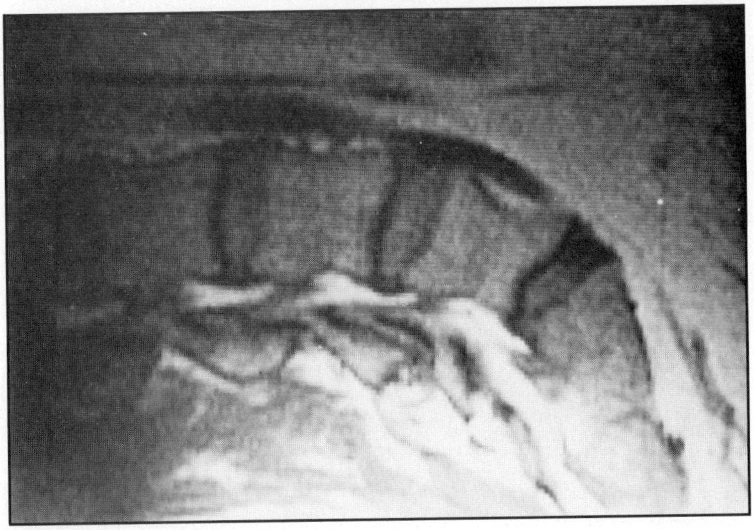

Figure 3-1C: Sagittal section through the lateral recess. The medial margin of the pedicles is partially included.

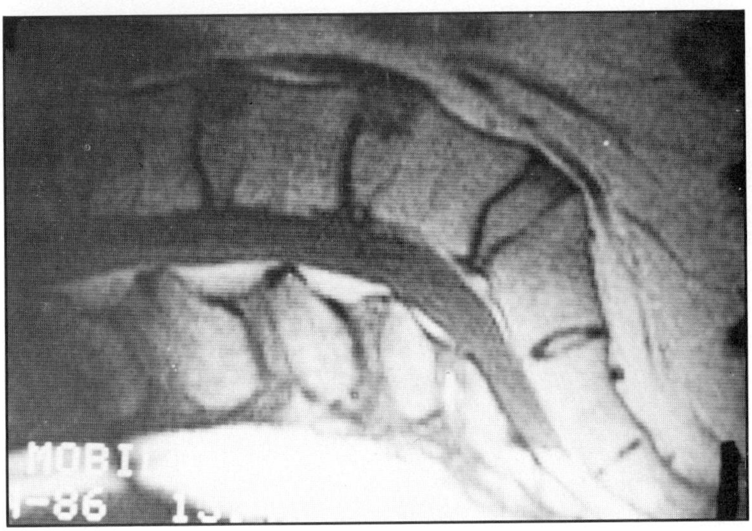

Figure 3-1D: Midline sagittal plane.

3-3a), and the sections are obtained with relative T1-weighting. This generally permits examination from the mid-vertebral body of L4 down into the sacrum in a single acquisition; if the sagittal sections suggest abnormality at a higher level, an additional axial acquisition centered higher is obtained.

Figure 3-2: Midline sagittal plane, multiecho sequence (8 echoes).

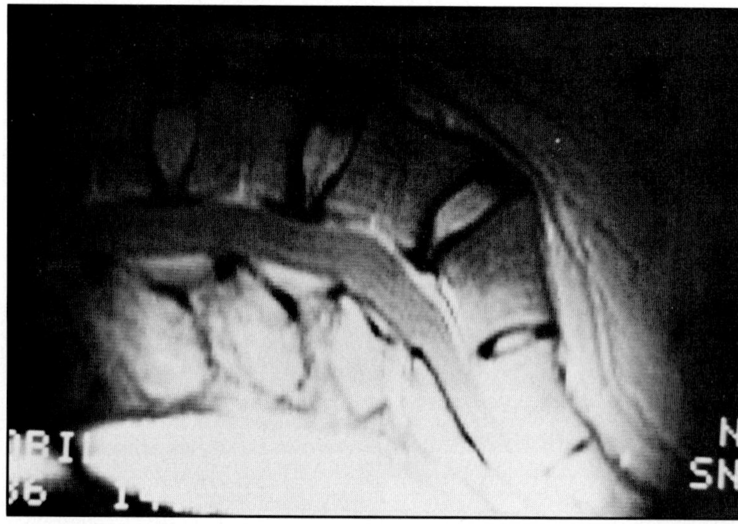

Figure 3-2A: TR2000,TE30

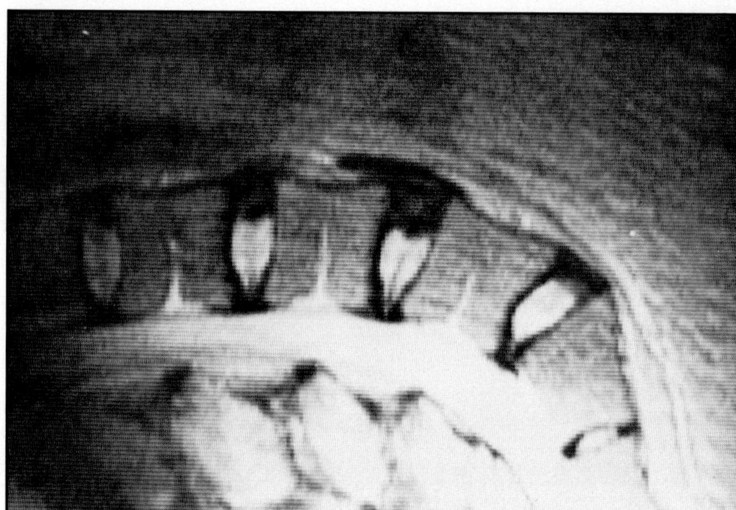

Figure 3-2B: TR2000,TE90

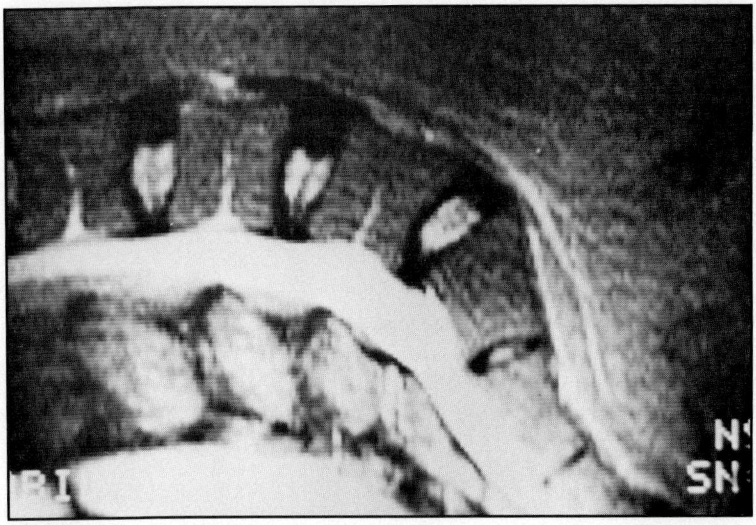

Figure 3-2C: TR2000,TE150

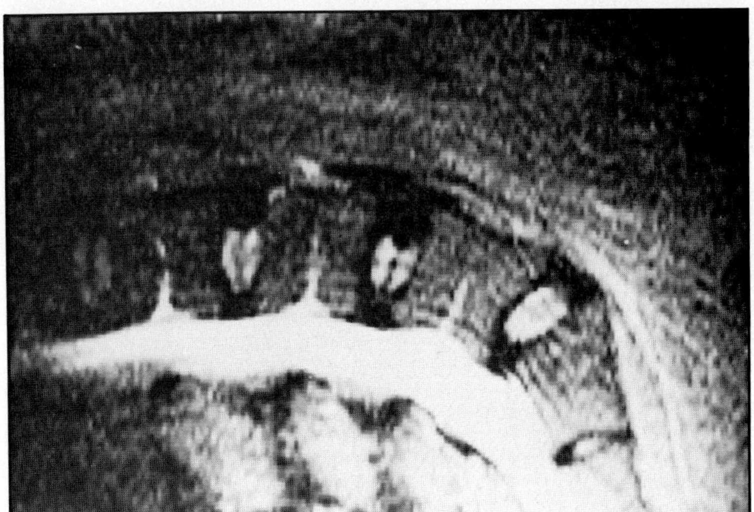

Figure 3-2D: TR2000,TE240

Figure 3-3A: Sagittal scout view indicating plane of the angled axial sections.

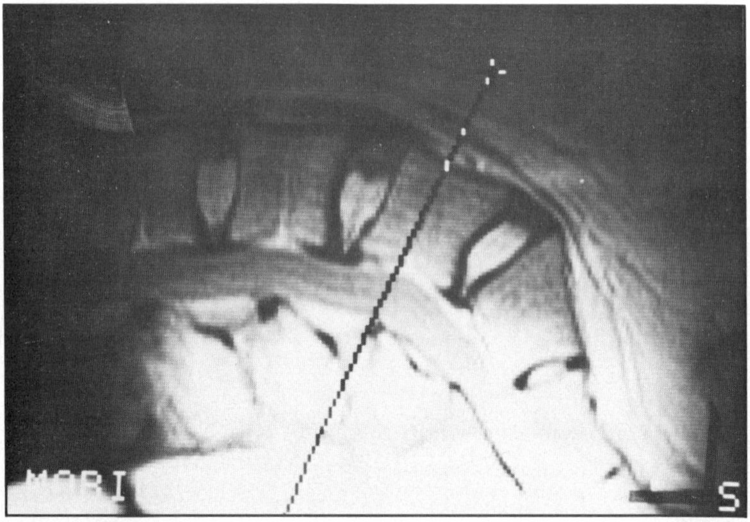

Figure 3-3B: Axial image through the level of the L5 pedicles. The L5 roots are just medial to the pedicles.

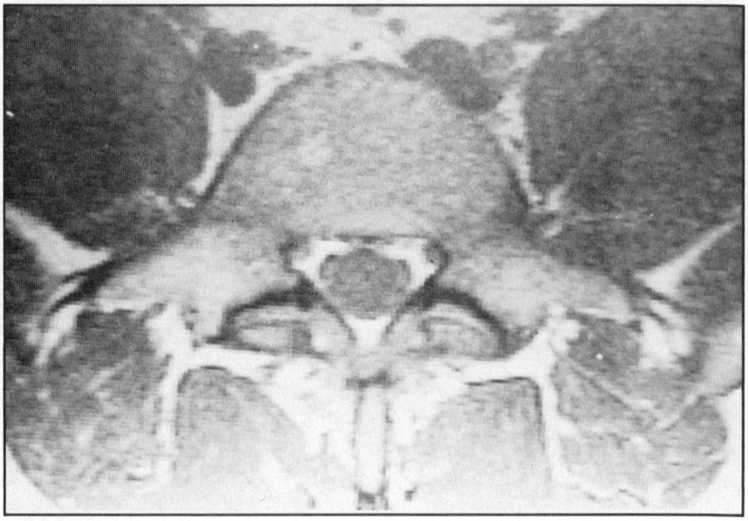

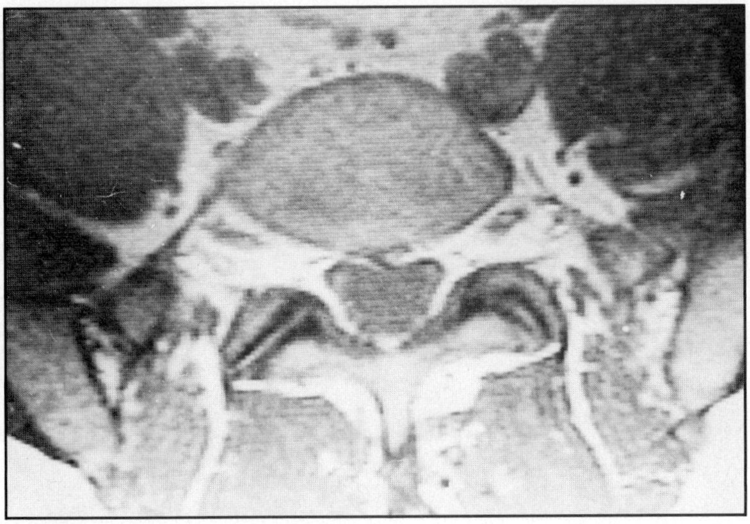

Figure 3-3C: Section through the intervertebral canals. Note asymmetry of the facet joints (facet joint tropism).

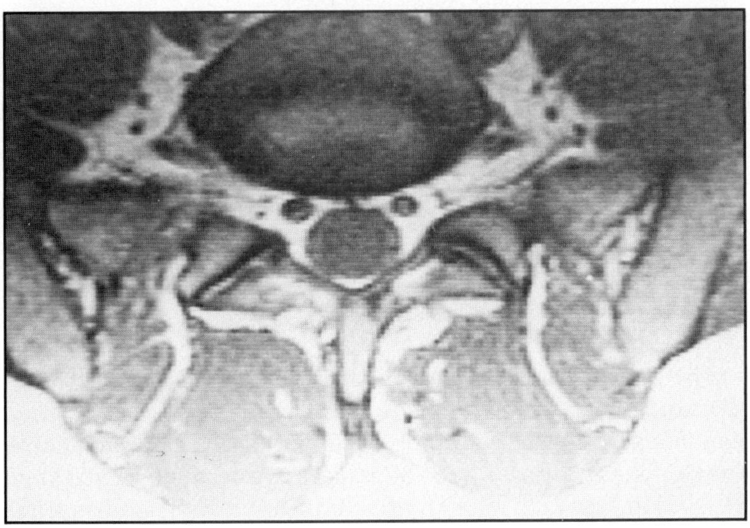

Figure 3-3D: Section through the disc plane. With this sequence the disc signal is less intense than the marrow signal (compare 3-3B & C).

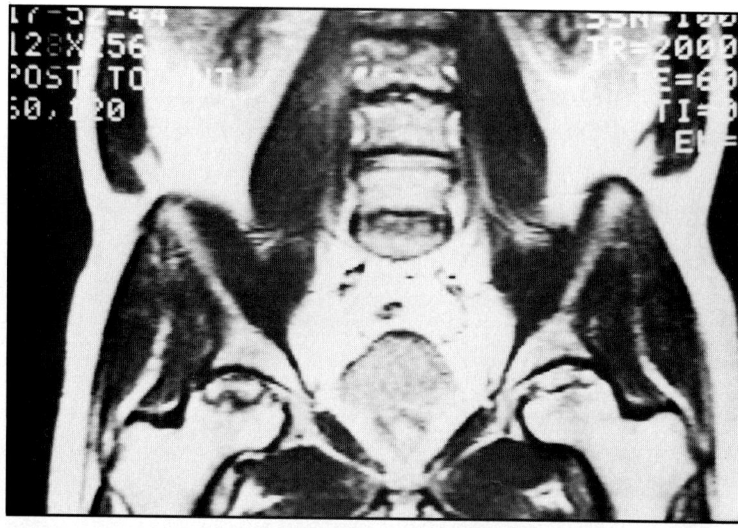

Figure 3-4: Coronal plane. Excellent depiction of topographic relationships and paraspinal region including psoas muscles.

Images in the *coronal* plane (Figure 3-4) are obtained only occasionally. These may provide helpful information in cases of paraspinal tumor or other mass, scoliosis, or congenital anomaly (Figure 6-2).

Oblique or *compound angulated* planes are occasionally utilized, to obtain sections parallel to an intervertebral disc in a patient with scoliosis.

Image Weighting

The appearance of the MR images depends upon the proton density, T1 relaxation time and T2 relaxation time of the tissue examined. In images with short TR and short TE, T1 relaxation is the dominant process and the images are termed T1-weighted (T1W) images. With long TR and TE the signal obtained depends primarily on T2 yielding T2-weighted (T2W) images. Long TR and short TE suppresses both T1 dependence and T2 dependence yielding proton density weighted (PDW) images. T1W, T2W, and PDW images are *not* maps of T1, T2, or proton density; these terms indicate the major, but not the only, factor influencing the image.

(Continued on page 47)

Figure 3-5: Effects of varying slice thickness.

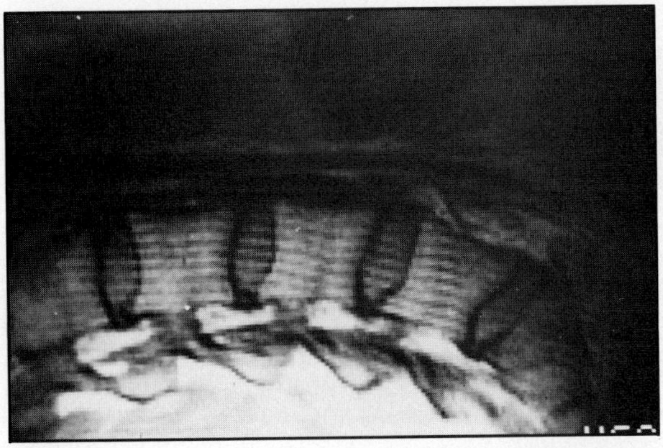

Figure 3-5A: 1cm slice/1mm gap.

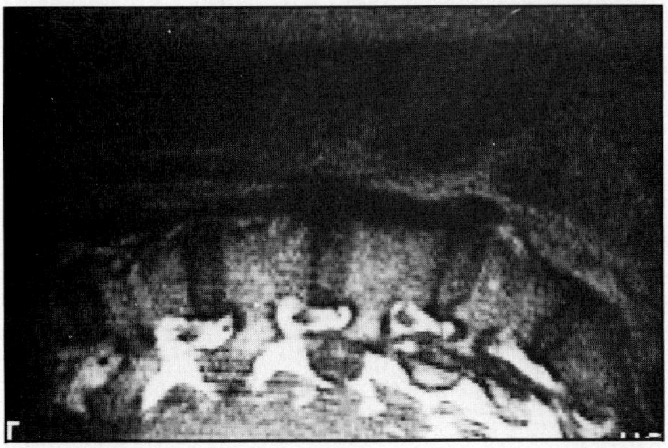

Figure 3-5B: 4mm slice/1mm gap.

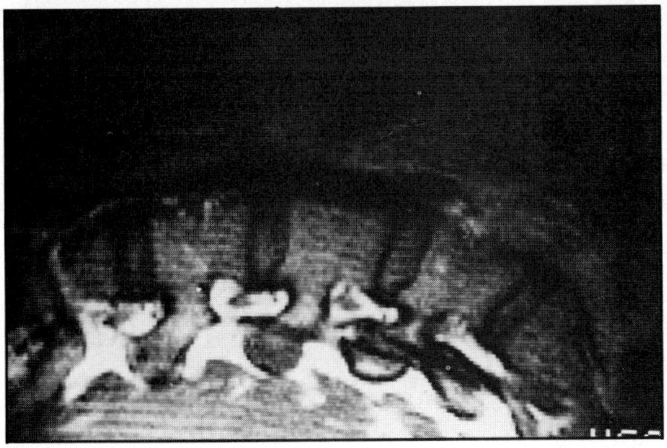

Figure 3-5C: 5mm slice/no gap.

Figure 3-6: Effect of varying TR.

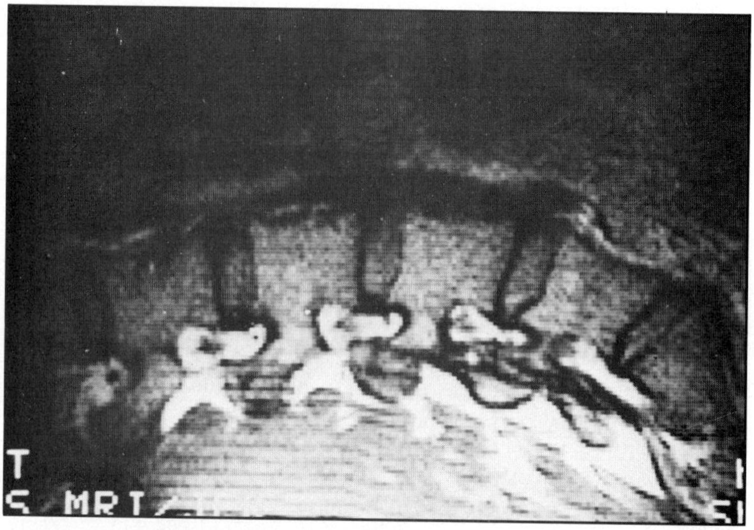

Figure 3-6A: TR300/TE40

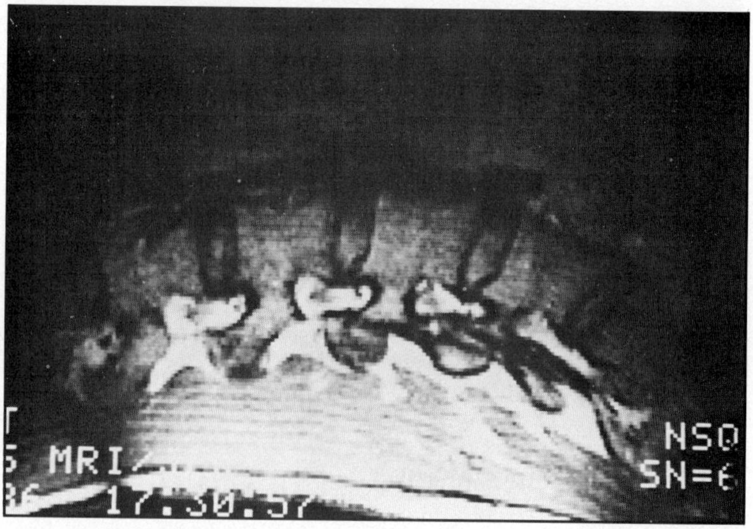

Figure 3-6B: TR900/TE40. Note differences in relative signal intensities, with the shorter TR providing a more T1 weighted image. Overall signal to noise is improved by prolonging the TR.

Figure 3-7: Effect of signal averaging.

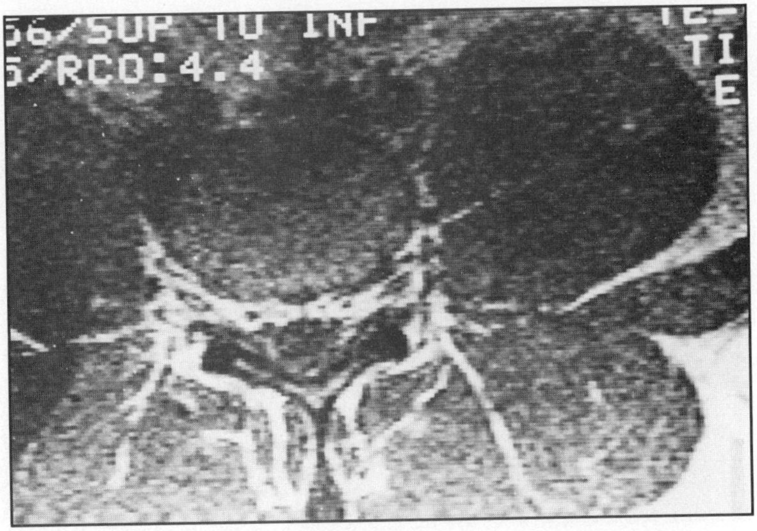

Figure 3-7A: 2 excitations

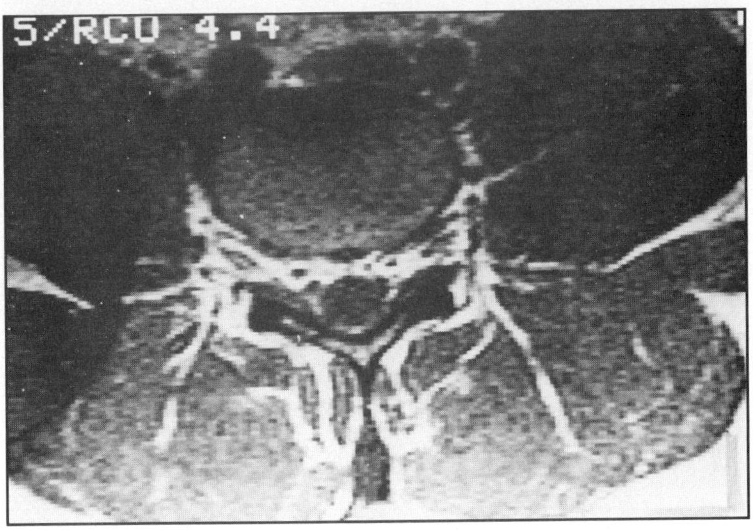

Figure 3-7B: 6 excitations

Figure 3-8: Effects of matrix size

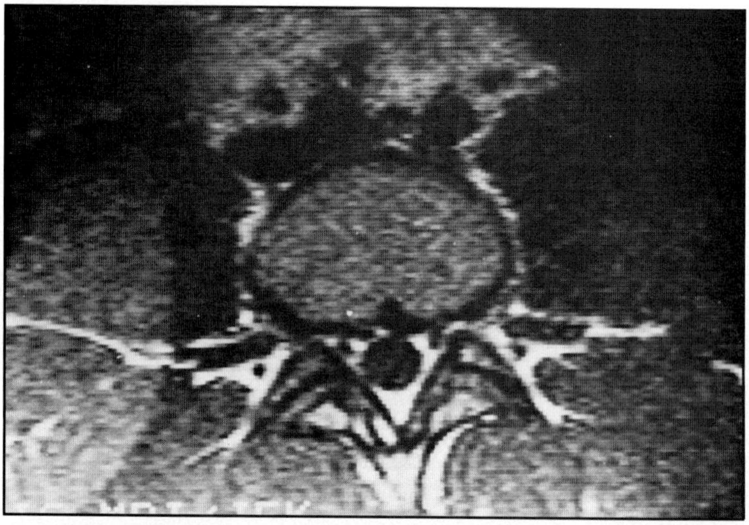

Figure 3-8A: 128 × 256

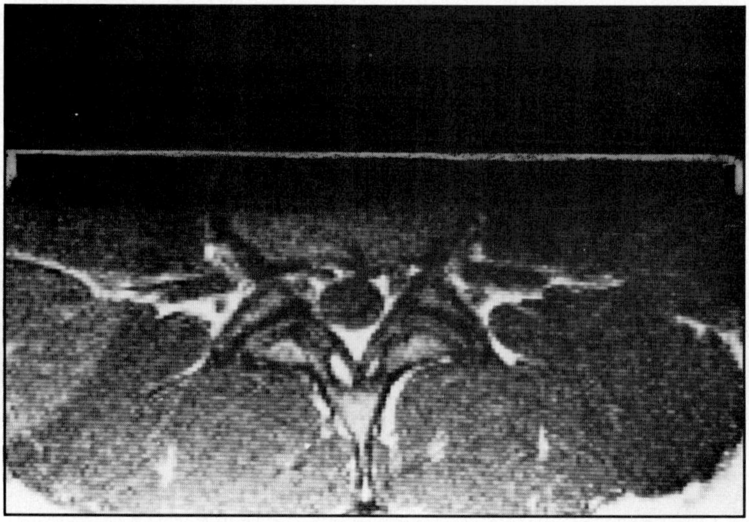

Figure 3-8B: 256 × 256

Figure 3-9: Effect of choice of receiver coil.

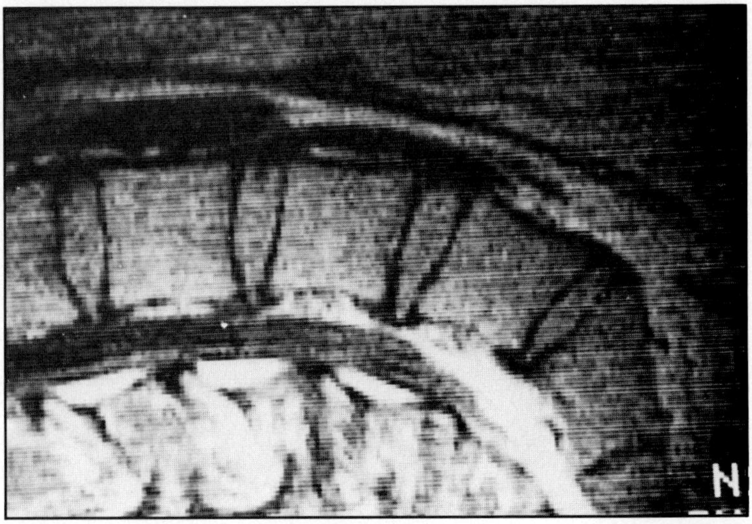

Figure 3-9A: Acquisition with surface coil

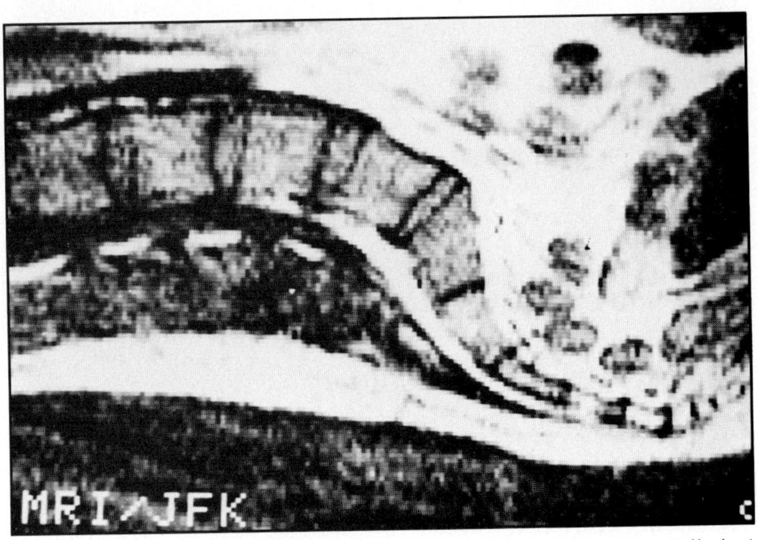

Figure 3-9B: Acquisition with body coil. Note the lesser detail, but greater field of view, of the body coil.

Figure 3-10: Transverse image of the cervical spine. Motion artifact propagates in the phase encoding direction.

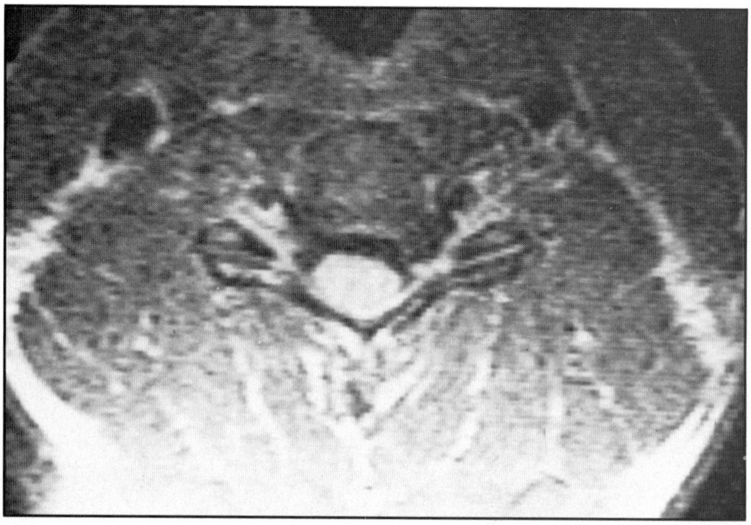

Figure 3-10A: Phase encoding in the horizontal direction.

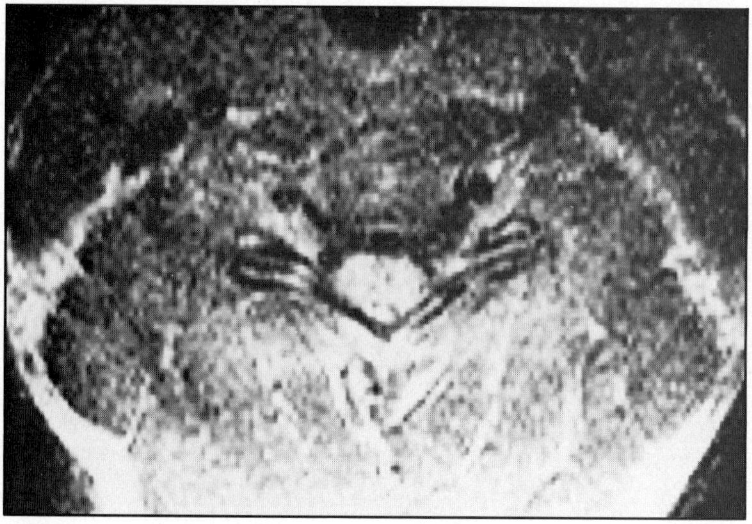

Figure 3-10B: Phase encoding in the vertical (AP) direction. Breathing and swallowing artifact degrades the image of the spinal canal. This effect is also present, although less marked, on lumbar images.

A simple key to the weighting of spinal MR images is the appearance of CSF (water). On T1-weighted images (Figure 3-1) CSF appears dark. Proton density weighted images (Figure 3-2a) show CSF as intermediate gray, and T2-weighted images (Figure 3-2c,d) show CSF as white.

Effects of Varying Image Parameters on Image Quality

The lumbar spine protocol we use (Appendix B) has evolved as a result of clinical experience and experimentation with varying acquisition parameters. Figures 3-5 through 3-10 show examples of variation in slice thickness, interslice gap, TR and TE, number of excitations, matrix size (N_y), and receiver coil. The parameters chosen for our routine study provide for an examination which may be conducted by a technologist in under one hour without physician monitoring. It is definitive in most cases and is accepted by referring physicians.

CHAPTER 4

Approach To Image Interpretation

Approach to Image Interpretation

Interpretation of lumbar spine MRI is based on the same principles as other imaging modalities. High quality images tailored to the patient's problem must be obtained. Knowledge of the relevent anatomy and pathophysiology is essential. At least a minimal knowledge of the underlying physical basis of the technique is helpful. Images must be analyzed carefully and systematically. The certainty, severity, and probable clinical significance of abnormalities present need to be assessed. Correlation to other more familiar imaging studies is helpful as well as educational.

Use a Systematic Approach

A typical lumbar MRI examination (Figure 4-1) consists of three or more acquisitions and a total of thirty or more individual images covering several spinal levels. Structures to be evaluated at each level include vertebral bodies, intervertebral discs, facet joints, nerve roots, intervertebral canals, thecal sac, etc. (Table 4-1). Adequate evaluation of these structures requires an organized approach. This may take the form of either an actual written checklist (Appendix C) or a carefully followed mental checklist.

It is helpful to review images in a fixed order. My own preference is to first review the multislice sagittal T1-weighted sequence, then the transverse images, and finally the midline sagittal T2-weighted sequence. Axial images (Figure 4-3a) are viewed as if looking up at the patient, sagittal images (Figure 4-3b) as if looking from the patient's right side with the patient supine, and coronal images (Figure 4-3c) as if facing the patient.

An important part of a systematic approach to interpretation involves the correlation of the various acquisitions so as to form a

Figure 4-1: A complete lumbar MR study.

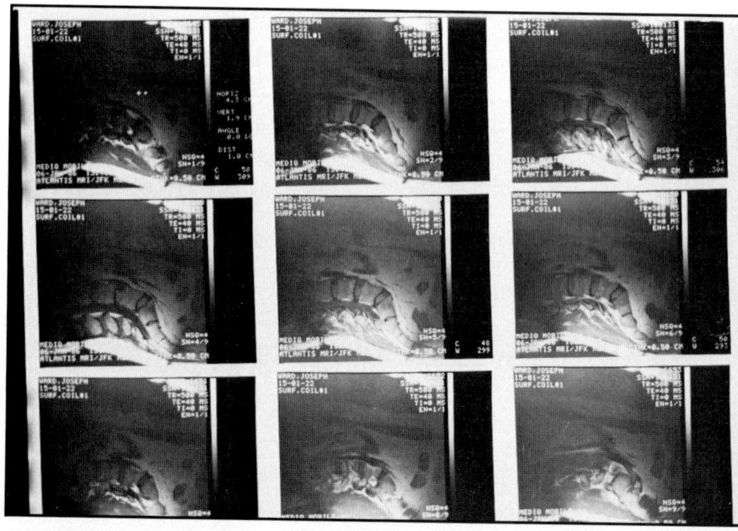

Figure 4-1A: Multislice T1 weighted sagittal.

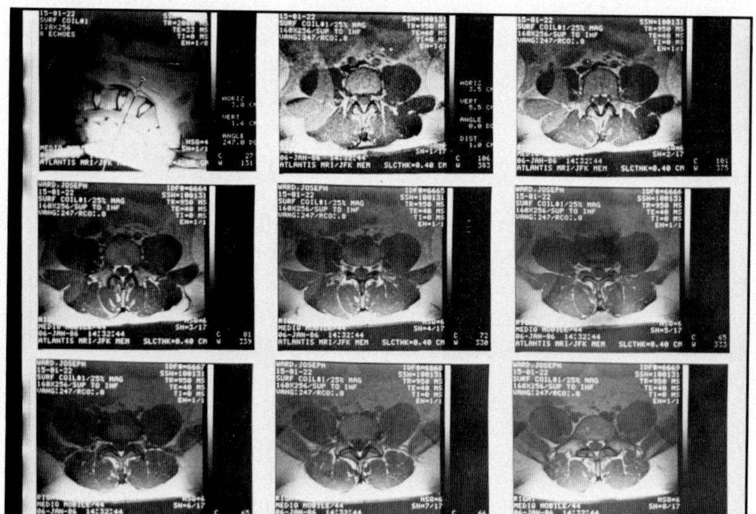

Figure 4-1B: Multislice axial including localizer view. Medium T1 weighting.

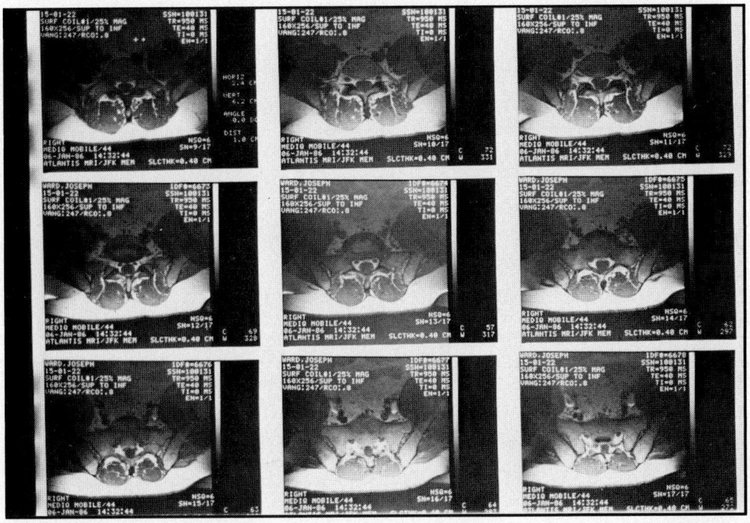

Figure 4-1C: Axial acquisition continued.

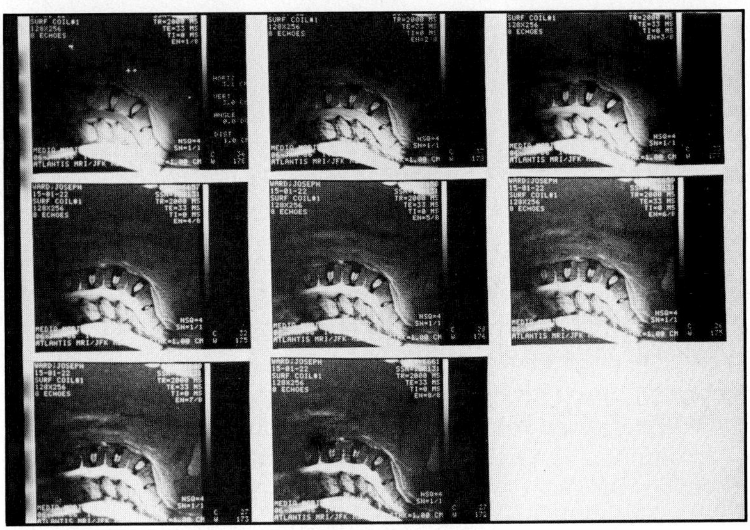

Figure 4-1D: Midline sagittal single slice with 8 echoes.

Table 4-1
Structures to be Evaluated at Each Level

Prevertebral Structures
Parvertebral Muscles
Vertebral Body
End Plates
Nucleus Pulposus
Annulus Fibrosis
Central Spinal Canal
Thecal Sac
Epidural Fat
Ligamenta Flava
Lateral Recesses
Intervertebral Canals
Exiting Nerve Roots
Superior Articular Facets
Inferior Articular Facets
Facet Joints and Capsules
Nerve Roots

mental 3-dimensional image of the structures visualized. For example, a left lateral L5-S1 disc herniation seen in sagittal view (Figure 4-4a) should also be identified in axial view (Figure 4-4b), and is also reflected by the decreased brightness of the L5-S1 disc on a T2-weighted image (Figure 4-4c).

Isolate Familiar Features

A magnetic resonance imaging study of the lumbar spine contains features familiar from other imaging studies including plain film radiography, myelography, discography, and computed tomography (Tables 4-2, 4-3, 4-4, and 4-5). The MR signal intensity (image brightness) can be regarded as analogous to radiographic density for purposes of image interpretation despite the different physical basis of the signal. Transaxial images provide the equivalent of a magnetic CT scan, with spatial resolution approaching and contrast resolution surpassing x-ray CT. Sagittal images surpass reformatted sagittal x-ray CT images in terms of both contrast and spatial resolution. The "MR discogram" yields information about the hydration (health) of the intervertebral discs not

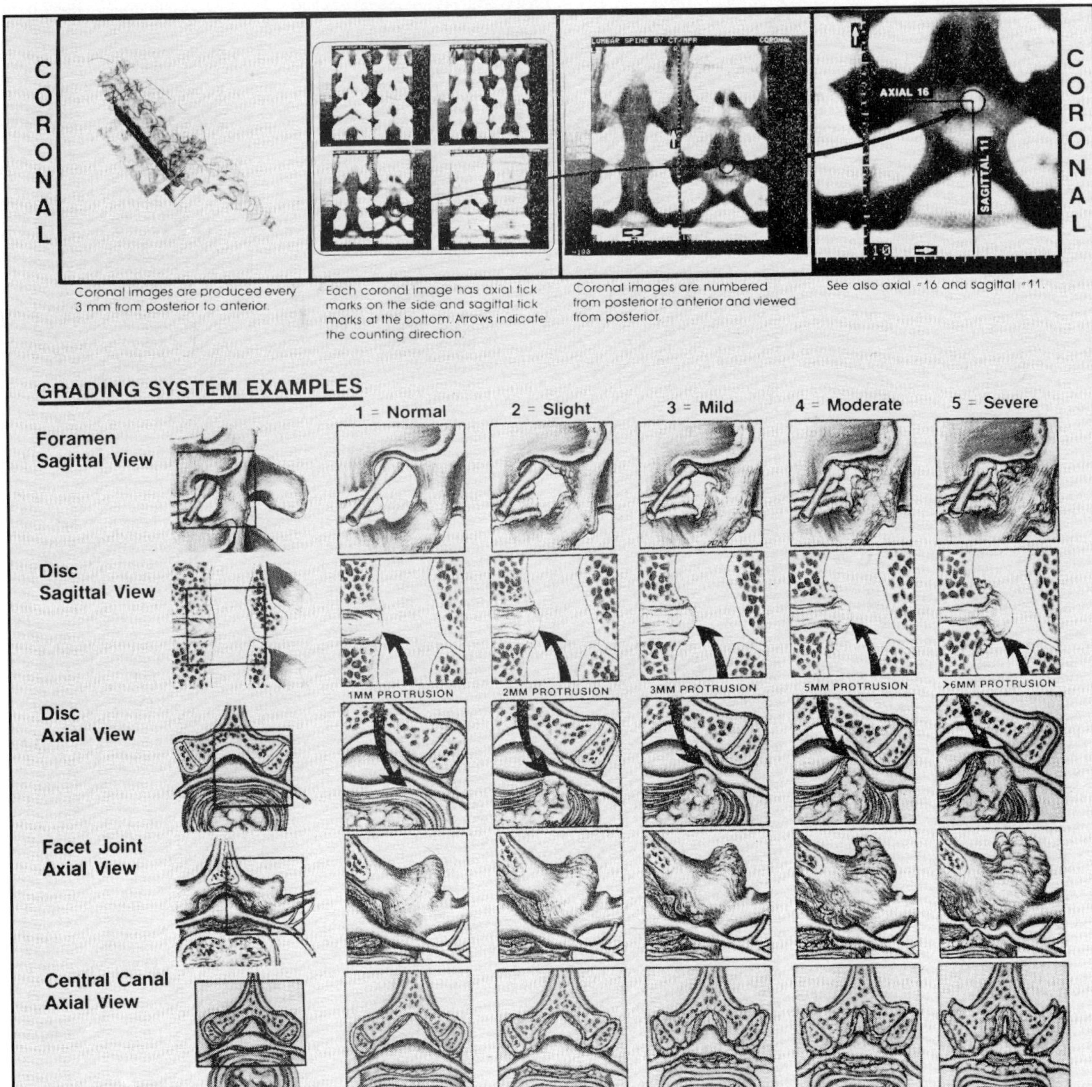

Figure 4-2: Objective grading system for lumbar spine abnormalities. This system, developed originally for CT scanning, is equally applicable to MR examinations. (Courtesy of Multiplanar Diagnostic Imaging Inc.)

Figure 4-3: Orientation of images

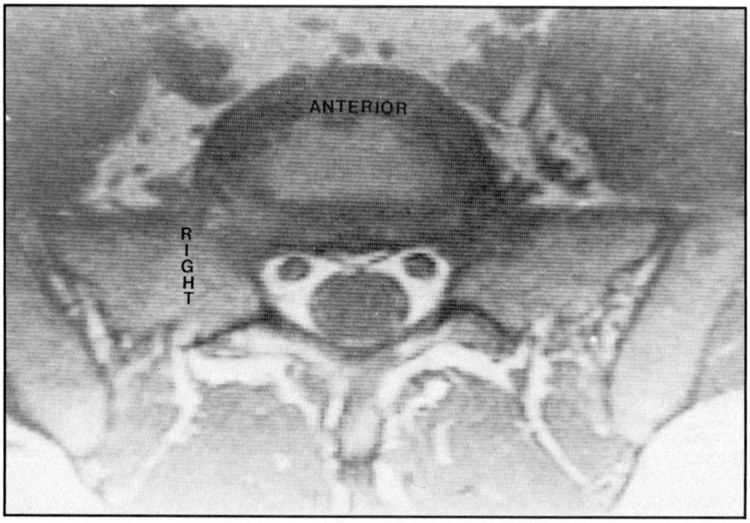

Figure 4-3A: Axial images are viewed as if looking up at the supine patient from below.

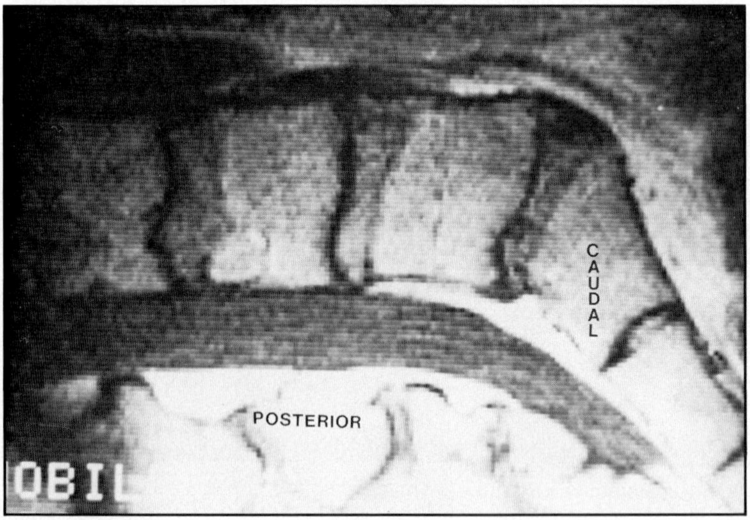

Figure 4-3B: Sagittal images are displayed as if viewing the supine patient from the right side.

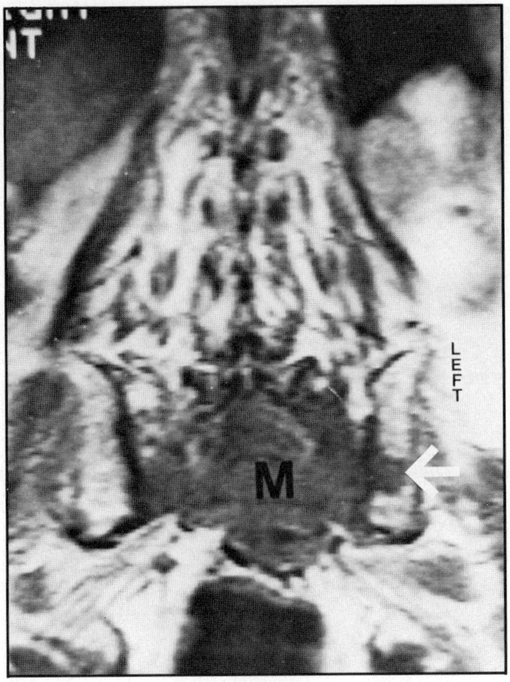

Figure 4-3C: Coronal images are displayed as if looking at the patient head on.

available from x-ray contrast discography. T2-weighted sequences produce images analagous to myelography with water-soluble contrast (Figure 4-4c).

Grading of Abnormalities

Abnormalities of the intervertebral discs and facet joints, and stenoses of the central spinal canal and intervertebral canals vary from slight to severe. Each of these structures must be assessed systematically with abnormalities graded according to a consistent scheme. Specific criteria such as those proposed by Glenn (Figure 4-2) for CT evaluation may also be used for MR interpretation and help to assure consistency among interpreters.

Correlation to Other Studies

Although the MR study may be interpreted in isolation, correlation to other available studies provides for the most accurate

Figure 4-4: Correlation of acquisitions.

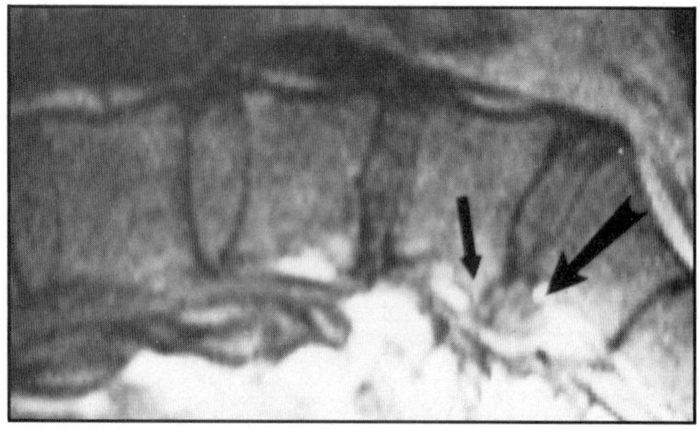

Figure 4-4A: Left parasagittal views. There is a large disc extrusion (large arrow). Osteophyte formation (small arrow) indicates chronicity.

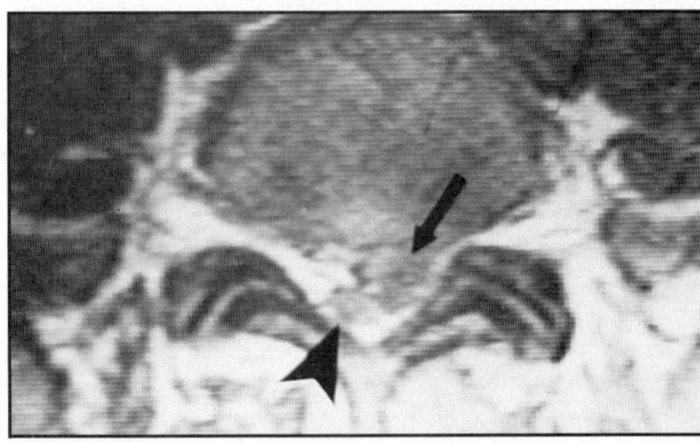

Figure 4-4B: Axial view through L5-S1 confirms the large left sided disc herniation (arrow) compressing the theca (arrowhead).

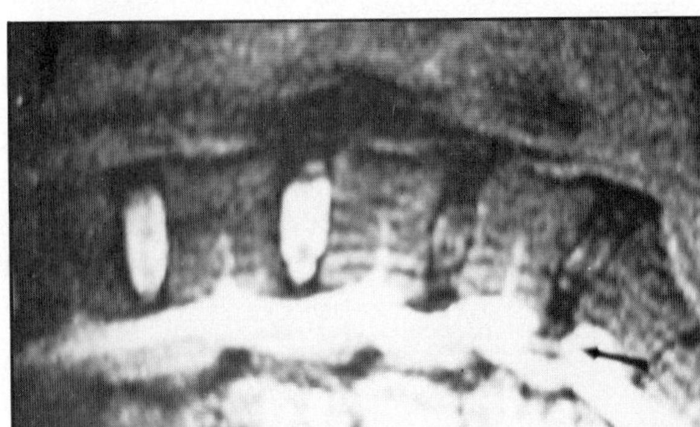

Figure 4-4C: T2 weighted midline sagittal section. The L4-5 and L5-S1 discs show diminished signal. The L5-S1 disc herniation causes an extradural defect on the myelogram-like picture (arrow).

Table 4-2
"Radiographic" Features

Alignment
Vertebral Heights
Disc Heights
Vertebral Intensity
Transitional Vertebrae

Table 4-3
"Myelographic" Features

Intradural Defects
Extradural Defects
Pseudodefects

Table 4-4
"Discographic" Features

Disc Height
Disc Intensity
"Cleft"
Extrusion
End Plates

Table 4-5
"CT" Features

Paravertebral Structures
Vertebral Bodies
Spinous Processes, Pedicles, and Laminae
Intervertebral Discs
Facet Joints and Ligamentum Flavum
Central Canal
Lateral Recesses
Nerve Exit Canals
Far Lateral Region

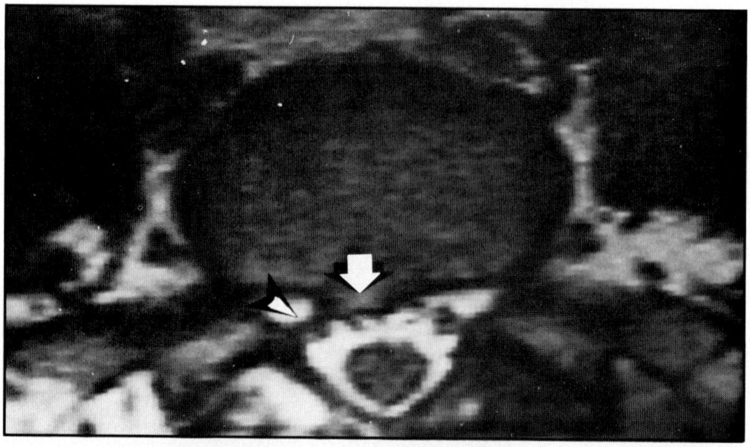

Figure 4-5: Right sided L5-S1 disc protrusion (arrow) displacing right S1 root (arrowhead). Clinical correlation indicated that this finding was not significant—the patient complained of *left sided* sciatica!

interpretation. Radiographs of the lumbar spine are particularly helpful for numbering the lumbar segments and identifying transitional vertebrae when present. In most instances CT scans and myelograms are not required, but if these have been obtained prior to referral for MR scan they should be reviewed. Any discrepancies need to be explained.

Indicate Degree of Certainty of Findings

The overall image quality of the study must be assessed realistically; findings on a high quality study are likely to be more significant than those on a blurred or limited study on an uncooperative patient. Taking the quality of the examination into account, the *existence* of suspected abnormalities should be classified as equivocal or unequivocal. Similarly the *etiology* of an area of abnormal signal intensity may be unknown or may be known with varying degrees of certainty.

Assessment of Clinical Significance

Assessment of clinical significance is the most important, and often most difficult, aspect of the evaluation of low back pain and sciatica by magnetic resonance imaging.

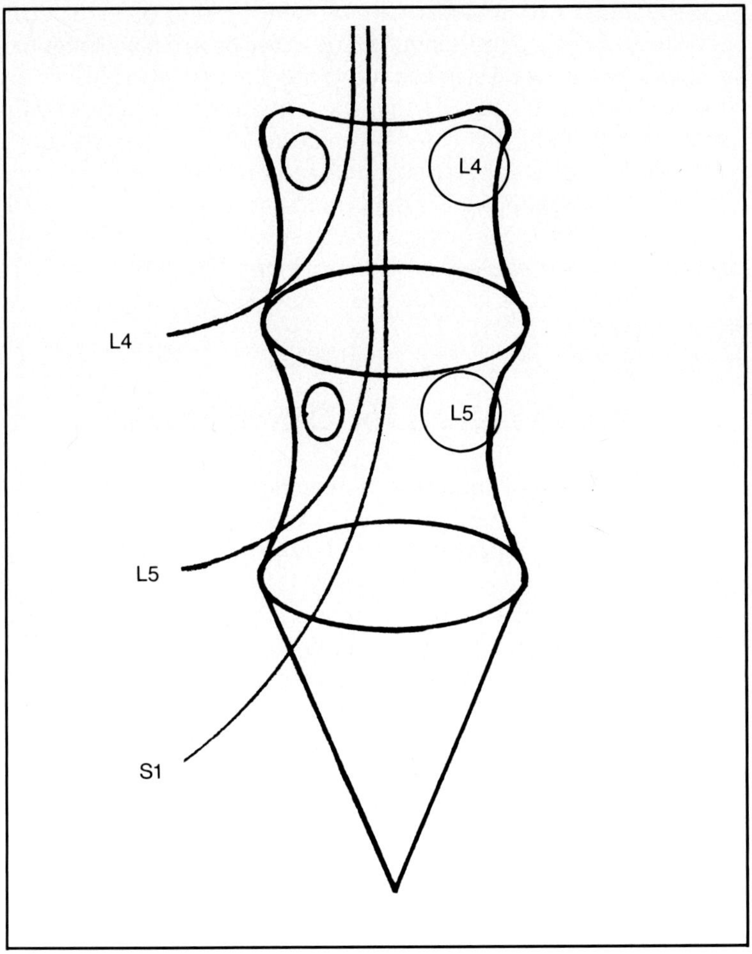

Figure 4-6: In the lumbar region the nerve roots exit beneath the corresponding pedicle. For example, the L4 root exits beneath the L4 pedicle, cephalad to the level of the L4-5 disc.

MR imaging is an extremely sensitive technique for the detection of spine abnormalities including minor degrees of disc pathology; this sensitivity creates a very real danger that the report of a herniated disc from an MR scan may lead to unnecessary surgery if careful clinical correlation is not carried out (Figure 4-5).

Correlation of the images with the clinical presentation may be carried out by the physician interpreting the images or by the referring clinician, but is ideally done by both physicians together.

In patients with sciatica, careful identification of the specific nerve root or nerve roots involved by a disc protrusion or stenosis is helpful in assessing significance of the abnormality (Figure 4-6). It is also helpful to note whether the nerve root is touched by the abnormality or still protected by epidural fat, whether the root is displaced, and whether the root is compressed. A theoretical limitation of this approach is that a nerve root appearing to be only slightly touched or compressed in the supine scanning view might be more severely involved in other positions. This has shown to be only rarely the case utilizing positional CT scanning (Heitoff & Ray, 1983).

Assess Need for Other Studies

In most cases high quality MR imaging is adequate as a stand-alone study of the lumbar spine to confirm normality, identify minor degrees of abnormality, or identify and characterize surgical lesions.

When the results of MR examination fail to correlate with clinical findings, or a patient continues to have significant unexplained symptoms following MR study, additional examinations may be required. Electrodiagnostic studies are helpful in confirming and localizing the level of nerve root irritation, particularly in patients with multilevel disease.

CT scanning remains superior to MR examination for evaluation of the integrity of spinal fusion. Patients with suspected arachnoiditis may still require myelography.

The most difficult group of patients are those with prior surgery, in whom the evaluation of a suspected recurrent disc herniation is often difficult. Definitive studies of this subgroup have not been carried out, but in our limited experience, MR scanning appears to be at least as good as contrast enhanced CT scanning in distinguishing recurrent disc herniation from postsurgical scarring. In an individual patient, however, either study may turn out to be superior so that frequently both are required.

When further information is needed following MR study with routine protocols, additional MR acquisitions may provide it.

Report Preparation

The value and acceptance of lumbar spine MRI depends upon

the quality of the reports generated. We divide our reports into 4 sections (Appendix D):

Indications: By stating the indications for the study, the interpreter indicates his knowledge (or lack of knowledge!) of the patient's symptoms to the referring clinician. This information is also helpful in expediting insurance reimbursement for these studies.

Technique: A statement of techniques utilized including pulse sequences and image planes helps the recipient of the report understand the study performed. For example, a screening sagittal survey study which may be used for evaluation of metastatic disease would have limited value for the evaluation of central spinal stenosis.

Findings: This section of the report relates the pattern of MR signal intensities to the pulse sequences utilized and to the normal and pathologic anatomy present. We use the reporting form as a worksheet for this section, but do not generally include this worksheet with the official report.

Impression: The final impression should be stated in anatomic and pathophysiologic terms; MR jargon is avoided in this portion of the report.

We routinely include a set of sample images with the report; referring physicians, particularly from other institutions, appreciate this courtesy.

Obtain Follow-Up

Obtaining follow-up may be regarded as the final step in image interpretation. Information about clinical outcome and surgical findings should improve our ability to understand the significance of abnormalities present on the MR study.

Despite the importance of follow-up information, we must be extremely careful before accepting the results of comparative studies using surgical findings as a *gold standard.* In many respects modern imaging studies provide a more accurate depiction of spinal anatomy and pathology than does the limited field of view available at surgery. Figure 4-7 presents a vivid example of this phenomenon, demonstrating a large bullet fragment not

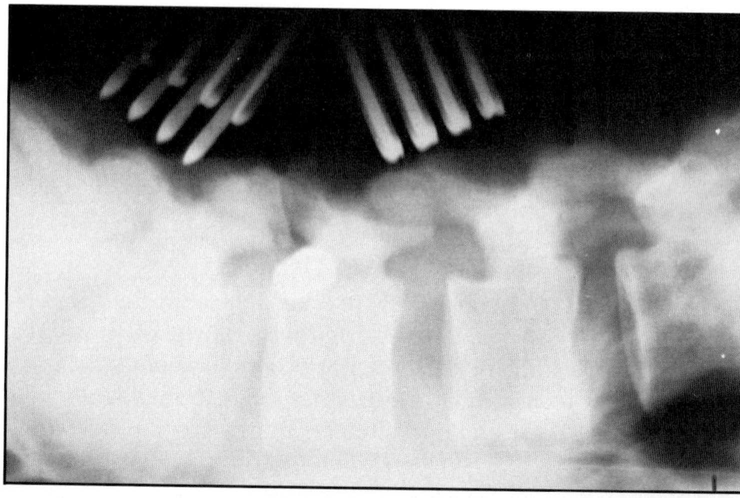

Figure 4-7A: Intra-operative lateral radiograph demonstrating bullet fragment just inferior to the level of the L4 pedicle.

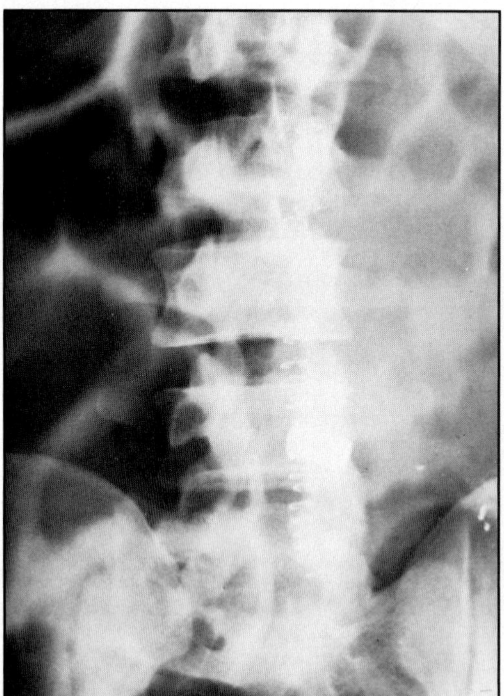

Figure 4-7B: Post-operative AP radiograph demonstrates the bullet inferior to the left pedicle of L4. At initial operation, the bullet was not located by an experienced neurosurgeon.

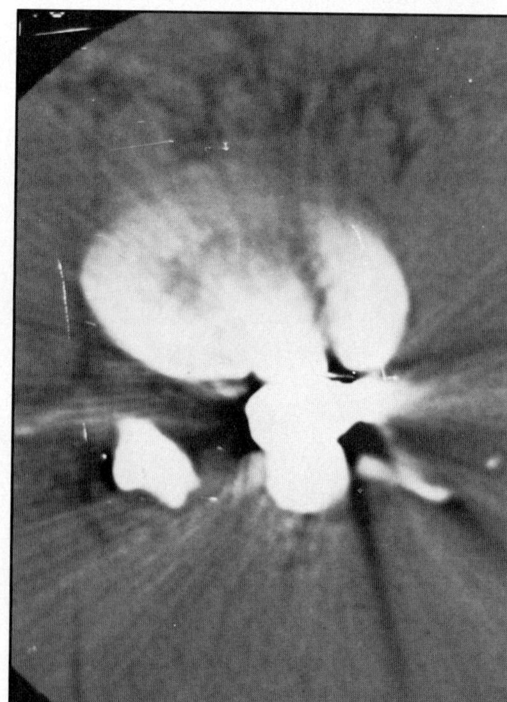

Figure 4-7C: Post-operative CT scan. Despite extensive artifact, the bullet can be seen in the left L4-5 intervertebral canal. Presumably a disc herniation could also "hide" in this location.

found by an experienced neurosurgeon during initial exploration. At the other extreme, a recent survey of 100 radiologists (attendees at Palm Beach MRI Update, West Palm Beach, Florida, February 1986) from around the United States yielded only a single case of a negative surgical exploration of the lumbar spine; this attests to either an extremely high standard of preoperative diagnostic accuracy nationwide or to the legal climate in which we function.

CHAPTER 5

Normal Anatomy

Normal Anatomy

Introduction

The anatomic relationships of the lumbar spine are complex; the multiple osseous, articular, and ligamentous structures of the central spinal canal and intervertebral canals are closely related to the critical neural elements. The existing spinal nerves and facet joints are oriented obliquely, further complicating understanding of the anatomic relationships.

Interpreting the sectional images provided by magnetic resonance requires close correlation to underlying sectional anatomy. Availability of an atlas of sectional anatomy in multiple planes is most helpful for image interpretation. I have found the work of Rauschning (1985) on detailed sectional anatomy of the spine particularly helpful in this regard. A three dimensional model of the lumbar spine also aids understanding of these complex relationships, and is useful in explaining findings to referring physicians and patients.

Sagittal Plane

Sagittal plane images survey multiple spinal levels. Structures imaged include pre-vertebral vessels and nodes, vertebrae and their articulations including associated joint capsules and ligaments, intervertebral discs, the spinal canal and its contents including the thecal sac and neural and vascular structures, and the intervertebral nerve exit canals (foramina) and their contained exiting spinal nerves.

The key sections for evaluation in the sagittal plane (Figure 5-1)

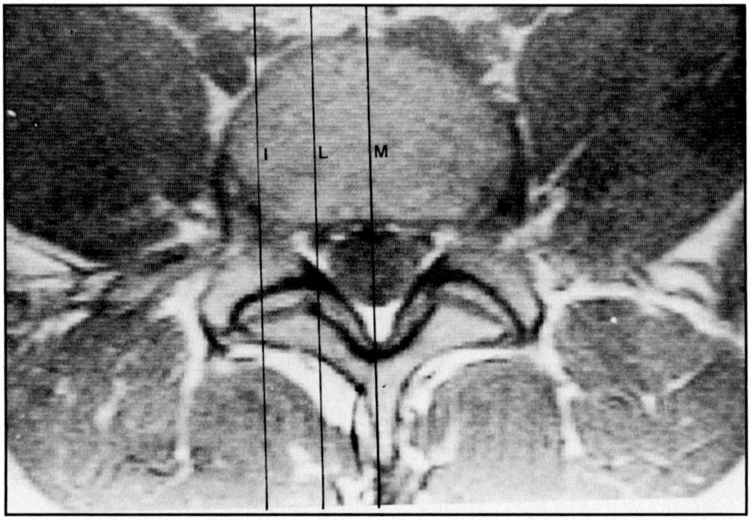

Figure 5-1: Axial reference image through the level of the L5 pedicle. Key planes include sections through the midline (M), the lateral recess (L), and the intervertebral neural canal (I). Corresponding sagittal sections are presented in Figure 5-2, 5-3, and 5-4 respectively.

include the midline sagittal plane, right and left parasagittal planes through the region of the lateral recess, and parasagittal planes through the intervertebral canals.

Midline Sagittal Plane

Midline sagittal images (Figure 5-2) permit evaluation of vertebral body size, shape, alignment, and signal intensity; of vertebral end plates and intervertebral discs; anterior and posterior longitudinal ligaments; spinal canal and its contents including thecal sac; and spinous processes with intervening ligaments.

Normal vertebral bodies are approximately rectangular in sagittal section, with mild degrees of concavity of the superior and inferior end plates as well as the anterior and posterior surfaces. The lumbar vertebral bodies are composed of coarse cancellus bone containing hematopoietic (red) marrow. On T1-weighted images, this produces an intermediate signal intensity (Figure 5-2b) and on T2-weighted images a mildly reduced intensity (Figure 5-2c). The basivertebral vein with its surrounding fat pierces the posterior surface of the vertebral body in a funnel-shaped configuration and is most prominently seen on the T2-weighted images (Figure 5-2c).

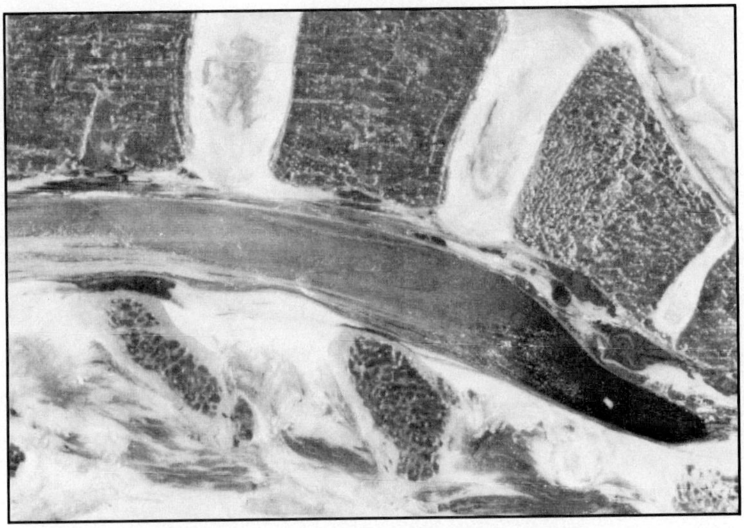

Figure 5-2A: Anatomic section. Features to note include slight normal bulging of the annulus fibrosis, the eccentric position of the nucleus pulposus within the annulus, and the indistinct margin of nucleus pulposus and annulus fibrosis (Courtesy of Wolfgang Rauschning).

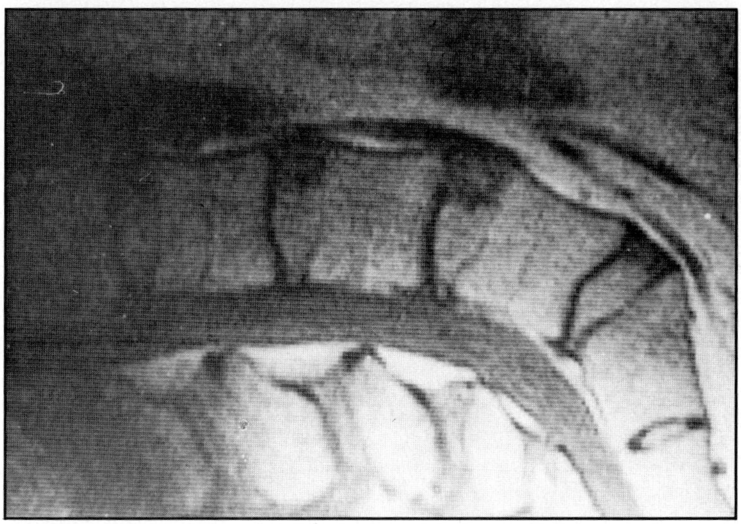

Figure 5-2B: Corresponding T1 weighted MR image. The nucleus pulposus is of similar or slightly less intensity than the vertebral marrow and the annulus fibrosis of low intensity. Apparent thickening of the inferior end plates as compared to the corresponding superior end plates represents chemical shift artifact.

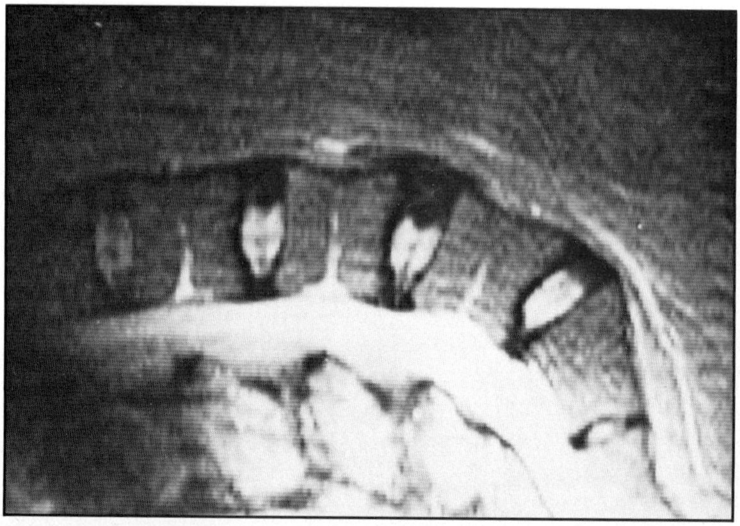

Figure 5-2C: T2 weighted image. The nucleus pulposus has a bright signal with an "intranuclear cleft". Fat surrounding the basivertebral venous plexus entering the vertebral body has high intensity.

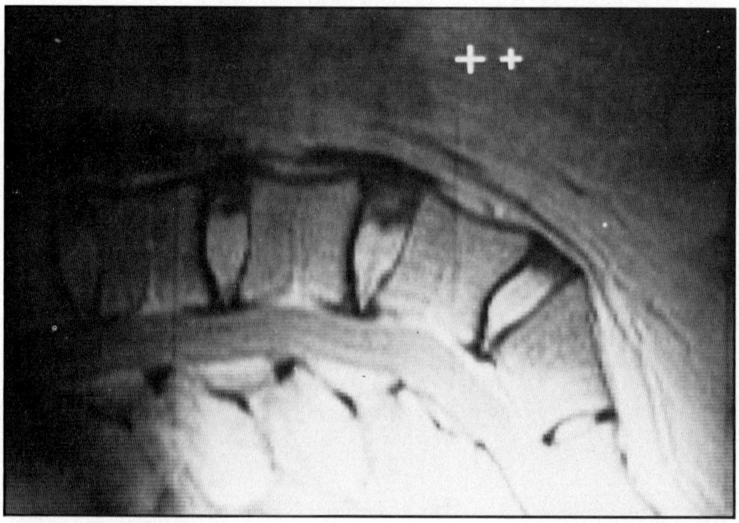

Figure 5-2D: Proton density weighted image. Extension of the bright disc signal towards the posterior margin is normal.

The low signal intensity anterior longitudinal ligament blends imperceptibly with the low signal of the thin cortical bone of the anterior vertebral body so that the anterior longitudinal ligament is only identified as a separate structure when it is elevated by a pathologic process (Figure 5-6). Similarly the posterior longitudinal ligament is not routinely distinguished from the subjacent low signal intensity of the posterior vertebral cortex or posterior margin of annulus fibrosis.

Low signal intensity of the hyaline cartilage of the vertebral end plates blends with the low signal intensity of the outer fibers of the annulus fibrosis. An apparent thickening of the inferior end plates as compared to superior (Figure 5-2b) is artifactual related to chemical shift artifact.

Lumbar intervertebral disc heights show a gradual increase progressing caudad, reaching a maximum at the L4-5 level. The discs are taller anteriorly producing the characteristic lumbar lordosis. The outer fibers of the annulus fibrosis have low signal intensity with all pulse sequences, characteristic of dense fibrous tissue and indicating lack of mobile protons. The nucleus pulposus is located eccentrically within the intervertebral disc closer to the posterior margin. On T1-weighted sequences the nucleus pulposus has signal intensity similar to or less than the vertebral bodies, whereas on T2-weighted sequences the normal nucleus (in young patients) has a characteristic bright signal indicating its water content. Correlative MR and anatomic study (Pech 1985) indicates that the central bright signal of the intervertebral disc includes not only the nucleous pulposus per se, but also a transition zone. This finding is in keeping with the indistinct annular margins demonstrated in anatomic section (Figure 5-2a). A characteristic *intranuclear cleft* with histologic and MR features similar to annular tissue has been described as a constant normal feature in subjects over the age of 30 (Aguila et al., 1985).

The normal circumference of the intervertebral disc is slightly greater than that of the subjacent vertebral end plates so that a slight (1-2mm) bulging of the intervertebral disc beyond the end plate margin may be normal.

Allowing for the mild concavity of the vertebral body margins and bulging at the disc levels normal alignment is indicated by a relatively smooth line connecting one vertebra to the next without any obvious "step-off."

The epidural space within the spinal canal contains varying degrees of fat (Figure 5-7) accounting for the variability of the

Figure 5-3: Sagittal section through the lateral recess.

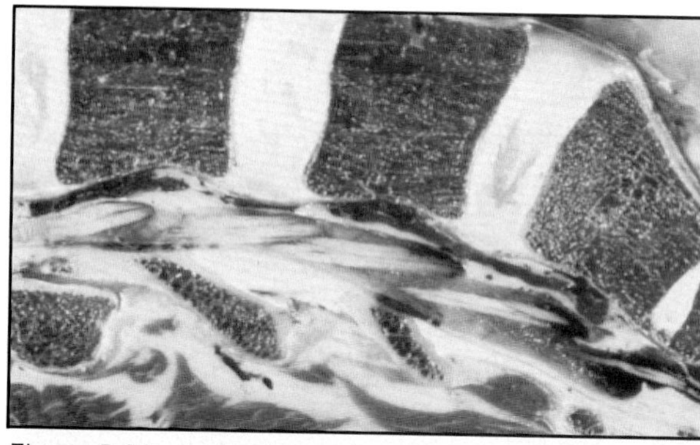

Figure 5-3A: Anatomic section. Nerve roots passing just medial to the pedicles, preparing to exit the spinal canal (Courtesy of Wolfgang Rauschning).

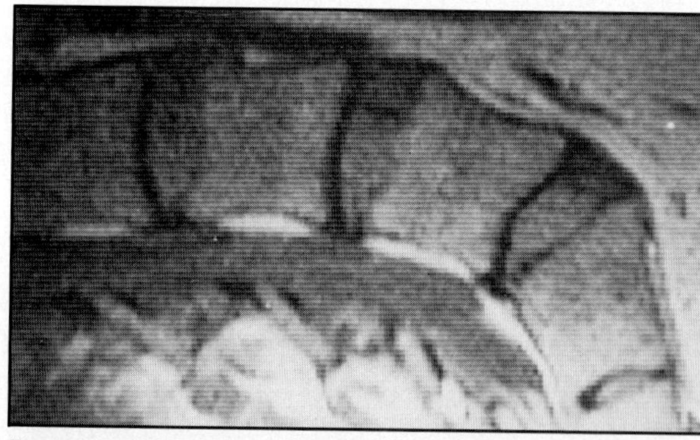

Figure 5-3B: Parasagittal MR section through the lateral margin of the theca. The axillary sleeve is just beginning to form at the L5-S1 level.

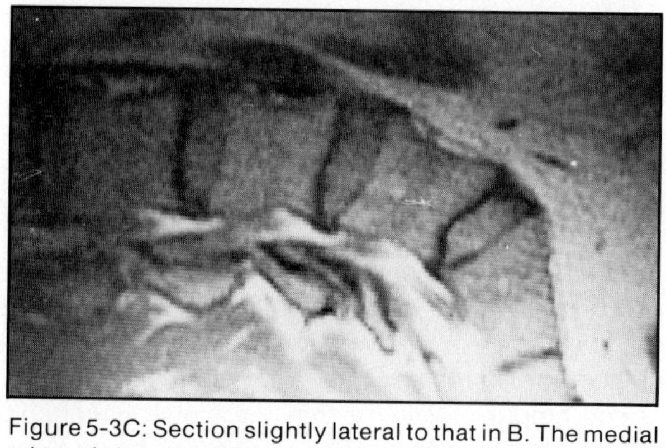

Figure 5-3C: Section slightly lateral to that in B. The medial edge of the L4 and L5 pedicles is now included in the section.

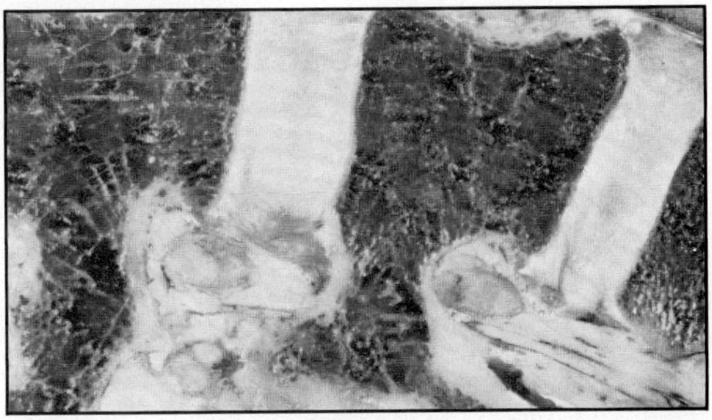

Figure 5-4A: Anatomic section through the intervertebral canal. Note the nerve roots exiting in the superior half of the canal, beneath the corresponding pedicle. The disc margin at this level may normally be either flat or outwardly convex (Courtesy of Wolfgang Rauschning).

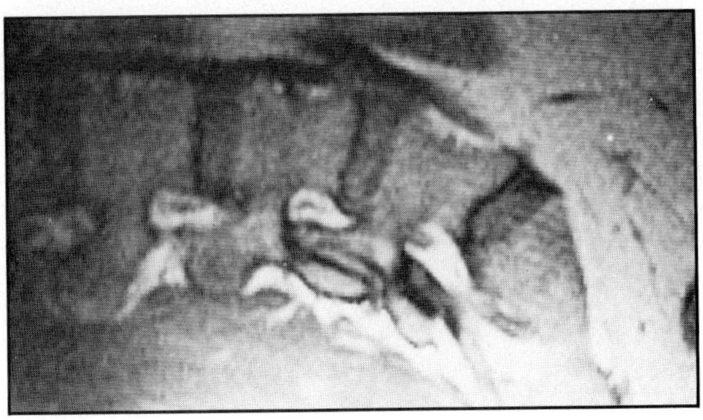

Figure 5-4B: Corresponding MR section.

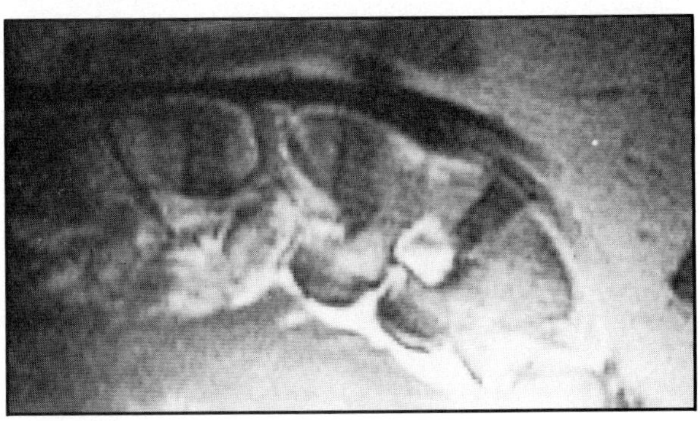

Figure 5-4C: Section 5mm lateral to B. This still includes the L5 pedicle, but passes lateral to the pedicle at L4.

Figure 5-5: MR in the midline sagittal plane—diagrammatic representation. Features to note include: 1. Slight waist-like narrowing of mid-vertebral bodies. 2. Diameter of the intervertebral disc is slightly greater than that of the subjacent vertebral end plates. 3. Blending of the nucleus pulposus with the annulus fibrosis, and the characteristic "intranuclear cleft". 4. Attachment of the annulus fibrosis at the ring apophysis of the vertebral body. 5. The eccentric position of the nucleus pulposus, located closer to the posterior disc margin. 6. Epidural veins running within the fat posterior to the concavity of the vertebral bodies. This epidural fat extends into the vertebral body surrounding the basivertebral venous plexus. 7. Apparent slight thickening of inferior end plates related to chemical shift artifact.

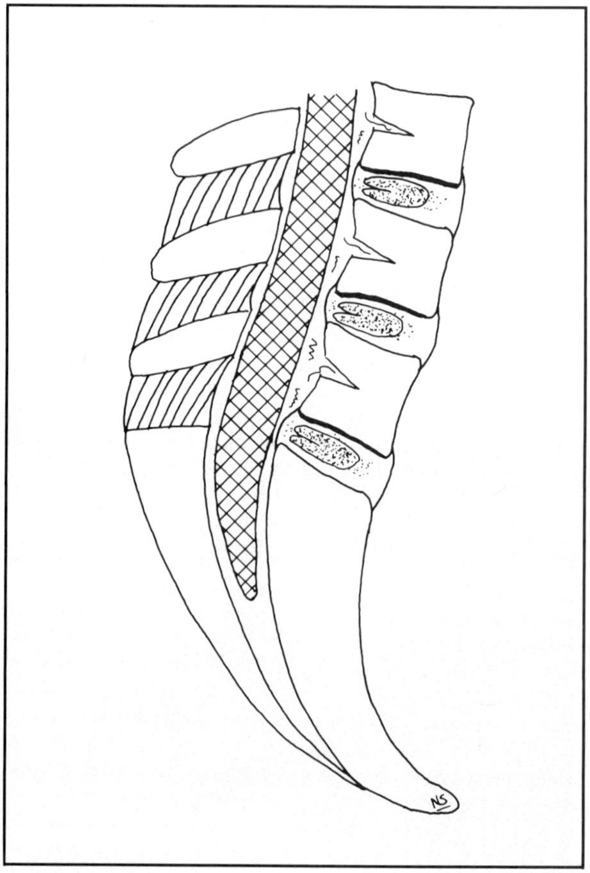

Figure 5-6: The anterior longitudinal ligament (arrow) is not normally seen. In this case, it has been elevated by an osteophyte and is thus visible.

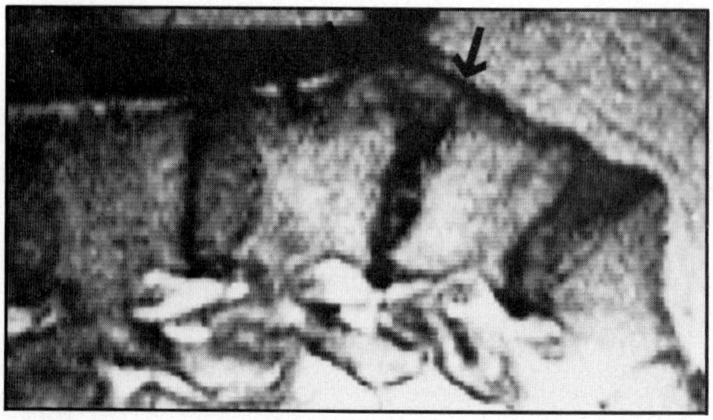

insensitive space at myelography. Typically the greatest amount of fat anterior to the theca is present at the lumbosacral level. Occasionally epidural veins may be seen within the epidural fat (Figure 5-8).

The thecal sac is a tapered conical structure with its maximum diameter at the lumbosacral level; it terminates at about the level of S2. Signal intensity varies markedly with pulse sequence (Figure 5-2); on T1-weighted sequences the spinal fluid produces relatively little signal yielding a dark structure, proton density weighted sequences yield intermediate signal, and T2-weighted sequences show a bright white signal from the water-like CSF. The individual nerve roots are not usually resolved within the theca.

Spinous processes have a bright signal due to the contained marrow with the brightness further accentuated by the near field response of the surface coil. The base of the spinous processes defines the spinal-laminar line.

Parasagittal Plane Through the Lateral Recess

The lateral recess is the region bordered laterally by the pedicle, anteriorly by the posterolateral aspect of the vertebral body, and posteriorly by the superior articular facet. The medial margin is not well defined but extends approximately through the medial margin of the thecal sac. The exiting spinal nerves pass through the lateral recess before turning laterally beneath the corresponding pedicle.

Sections through the medial portion of the lateral recess (Figure 5-3b) include the lateral margin of thecal sac and the axillary sleeves of the exiting nerve roots, with sections through the more lateral portion of the recess (Figure 5-3c) including a partial volume of the pedicles as well as the superior articular facets at the entrance to the intervertebral nerve exit canal.

Parasagittal Plane of the Intervertebral Canals

The spinal intervertebral canals are continuous with the lateral recess of the central spinal canal medially. The superior border is formed by the inferior surface of the pedicle above with the inferior margin formed by a notch in the superior margin of the pedicle below. The anterior margin is formed by the inferolateral portion of the vertebral body as well as the slightly bulging intervertebral disc, with the posterior margin formed by the superior articular process of the vertebra below and its associated joint

Figure 5-7: Variation in epidural fat (myelographically insensitive space).

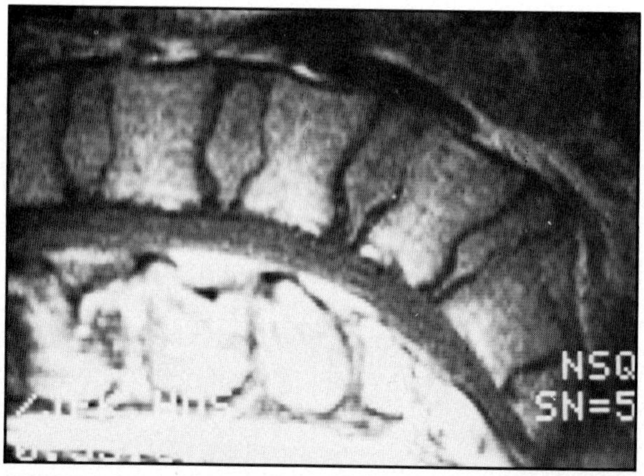

Figure 5-7A: Scant epidural fat. Myelography would be sensitive to L5-S1 disc herniation.

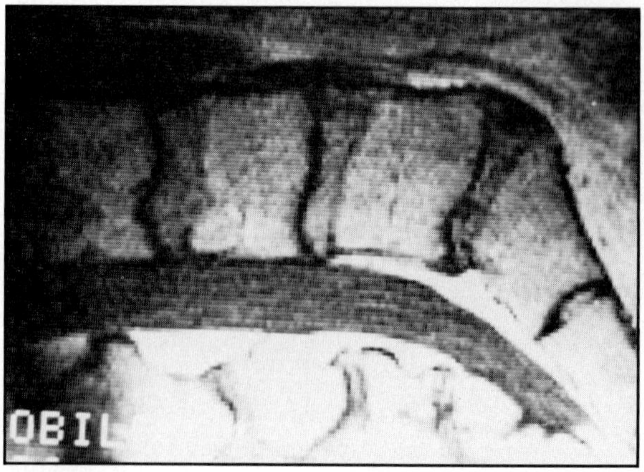

Figure 5-7B: Abundant epidural fat with a wide insensitive space at L5-S1.

capsule and ligamentum flavum. The intervertebral canal may be regarded as a *tunnel* through which the segmental vessels and nerves emerge from the spinal canal. It is a three dimensional structure with the entrance continuous with the lateral recess and the exit at the lateral margin of the vertebral body and superior articular process. Because of this three dimensional nature, the term intervertebral canal is preferable to the often used expression *neural foramen*.

In the lumbar region the intervertebral canal is directed laterally

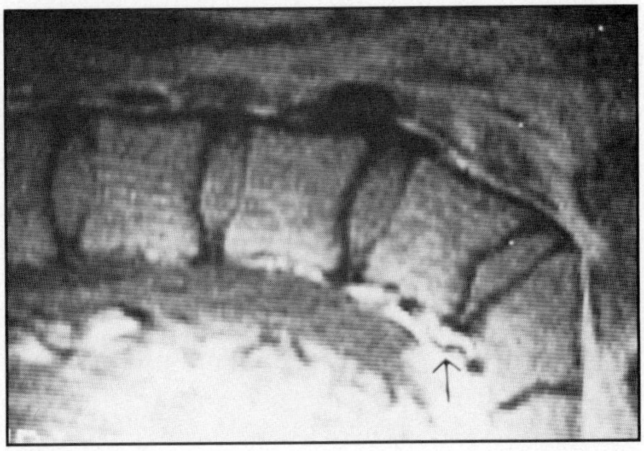

Figure 5-8A: Epidural veins (arrow) seen as serpiginous structures coursing through the epidural fat in the sagittal view near the midline.

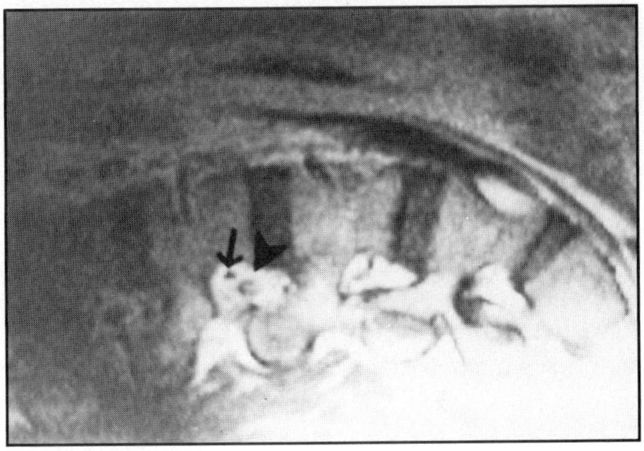

Figure 5-8B: Parasagittal section through intervertebral canal. Small low density structure (arrow) adjacent to the L3 nerve root (arrowhead) probably represents an epidural vein.

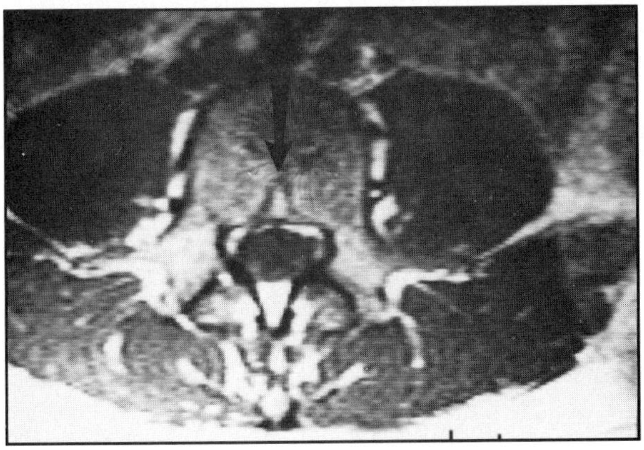

Figure 5-8C: Cross section through the level of the pedicles showing the funnel-shaped basivertebral venous plexus and surrounding fat (arrow) piercing the posterior vertebral body.

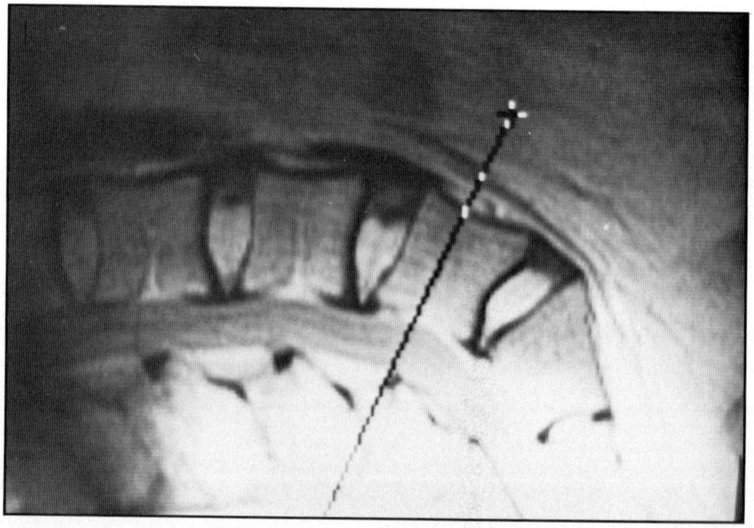

Figure 5-9: Sagittal scout view. The cursor line through the level of the L5 pedicles indicates the obliquity of the axial sections in Figure 5-10 through 5-13.

and slightly anteriorly and inferiorly. Although the shape changes with position, it is basically an inverted tear drop configuration widest superiorly. In the lumbar region (in contradistinction to the cervical) the exiting spinal nerves occupy the superior one-half of the foramen.

Sagittal MR sections through the intervertebral canals (Figure 5-4) show the exiting spinal nerves surrounded by epidural fat. The nerves, visualized in slightly oblique or true cross section as they course through the intervertebral canals, appear round or eliptical on sagittal images. Note that the structure identified as the *nerve* on the MR images represents a combination of the ventral spinal root and dorsal root ganglion within their dural sheath. Also traversing the intervertebral canals are the spinal branches of the segmental arteries, radicular veins, and the recurrent sinuvertebral nerves which arise from the dorsal divisions of the spinal nerves and reenter the spinal canal to innervate the annulus fibrosis and posterior longitudinal ligament. These other exiting structures are not routinely identified, but may be suggested as dots of low signal intensity surrounded by fat within the intervertebral canals (Figure 5-8b).

The L5 vertebra commonly has the widest interpedicular

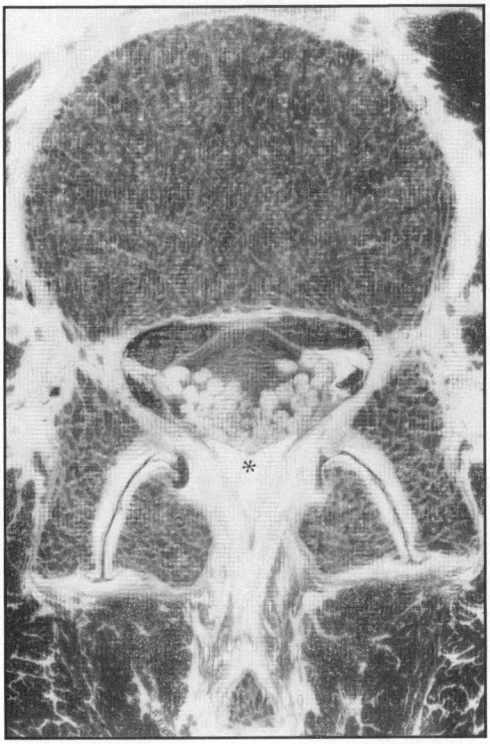

Figure 5-10A: Anatomic section through the level of the pedicles. Nerve root seen to the pedicles (Courtesy of Wolfgang Rauschning).

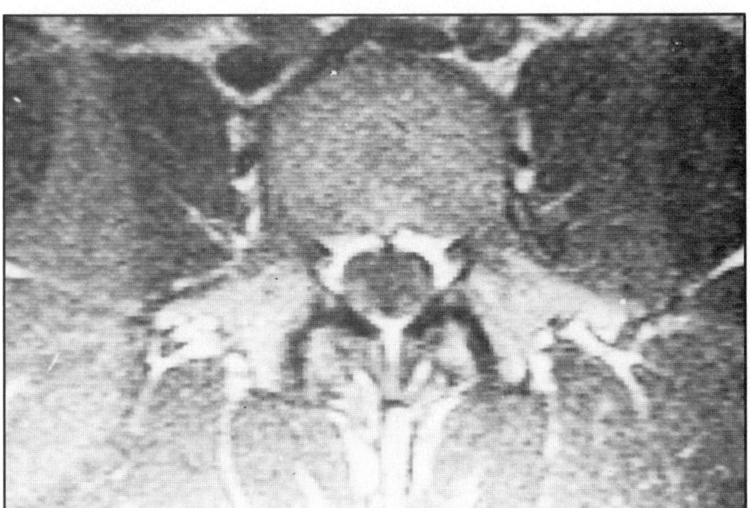

Figure 5-10B: Corresponding MR section.

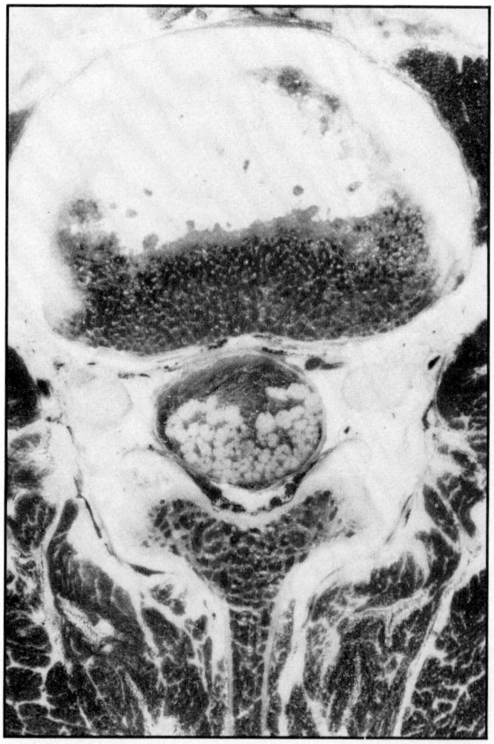

Figure 5-11A: Anatomic section through the exiting nerve roots (Courtesy of Wolfgang Rauschning).

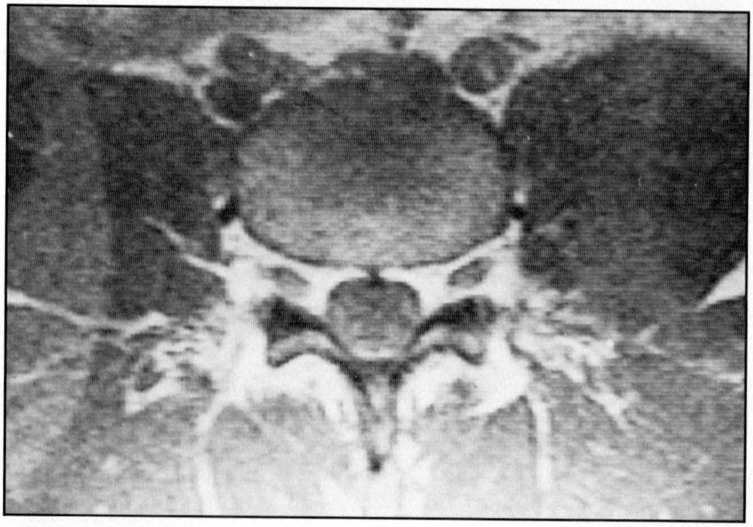

Figure 5-11B: Corresponding MR sections. The nerve root ganglia are seen within the intervertebral canal.

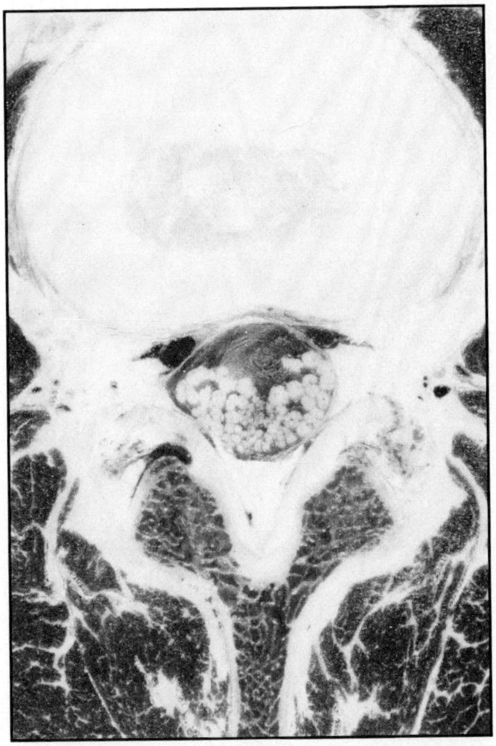

Figure 5-12A: Anatomic cross section through the level of the intervertebral disc (Courtesy of Wolfgang Rauschning).

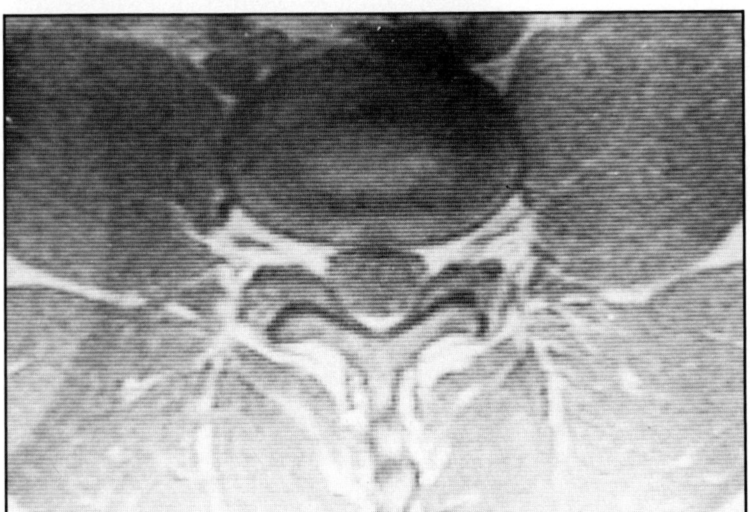

Figure 5-12B: Corresponding MR sections. The nucleus is seen as having slightly greater intensity than the surrounding annulus. The inferior nerve root margins are cut tangentially.

Figure 5-13A: Anatomic section through the level of superior end plate. The facet joints and ligaments are well displayed (Courtesy of Wolfgang Rauschning).

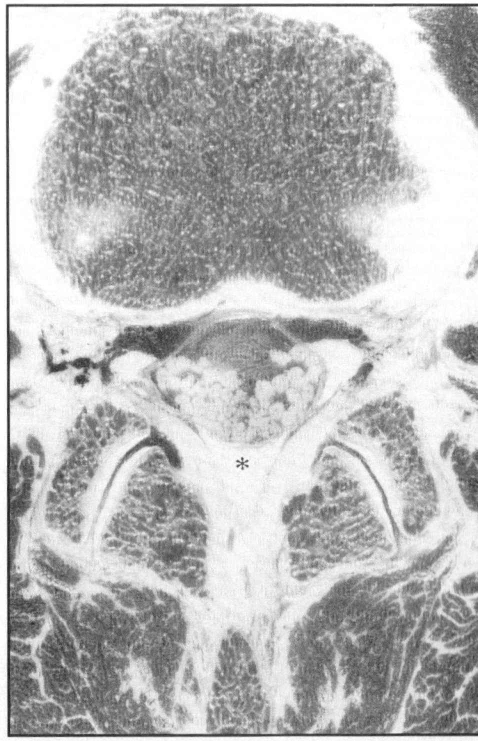

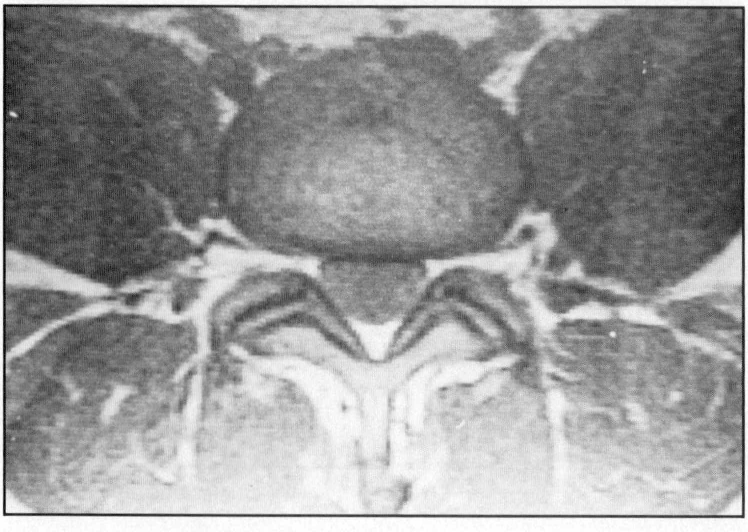

Figure 5-13B: Corresponding MR section.

diameter in the lumbar spine, so that sagittal sections through the exit of the L5-S1 intervertebral canal pass lateral to the vertebral bodies at higher levels (Figure 5-4c).

Axial Plane Anatomy

Axial images are obtained in an oblique plane angled so as to approximate the plane of the lower lumbar discs (Figure 5-9).

The key anatomic levels studied include sections through the pedicle or osseous ring level (Figure 5-10), sections through the superior half of the intervertebral canal including the exiting nerve roots (Figure 5-11), sections through the plane of the interverte-bral discs (Figure 5-12), and sections through the level of the superior end plate (Figure 5-13).

A section throughout the inferior portion of the pedicles of L4 (Figure 5-10b) demonstrates the L4 nerve roots cut in cross section just medial to the pedicles. Spinal nerves within the thecal sac are not individually resolved but are suggested as an area of slightly greater signal intensity than the CSF. Epidural fat sur-rounds the theca and nerve roots. The vertebral body marrow shows a uniform signal intensity pattern. The inferior portion of the L3-4 facet joints are included within the section.

A section through the inferior end plate of L4 (Figure 5-11b) shows a blending of marrow and end plate signal due to partial volume effect. The exiting nerve root ganglia are clearly seen surrounded by fat within the intervertebral canals. The spinous process and lamina of L4 are seen posteriorly.

A T1-weighted section through the L4-5 intervertebral disc (Figure 5-12b) shows a slightly higher signal centrally than periph-erally. The reduced peripheral signal probably represents a combination of annulus fibrosis and vertebral end plates averaged together, producing a lower signal than the central disc space. The inferior margins of the exiting L4 spinal nerves are just cut tangentially in the lateral halves of the intervertebral canals. The L4-5 facet joints are included but better demonstrated in the next section inferiorly.

A section through the level of the superior end plate of L5 (Figure 5-13b) includes the most inferior portion of the interverte-bral canals. The central spinal canal is approximately triangular in cross section at this level, with the anterior margin formed by the vertebral end plate and the posterolateral margins by the facet

Figure 5-14: Following the nerve roots.

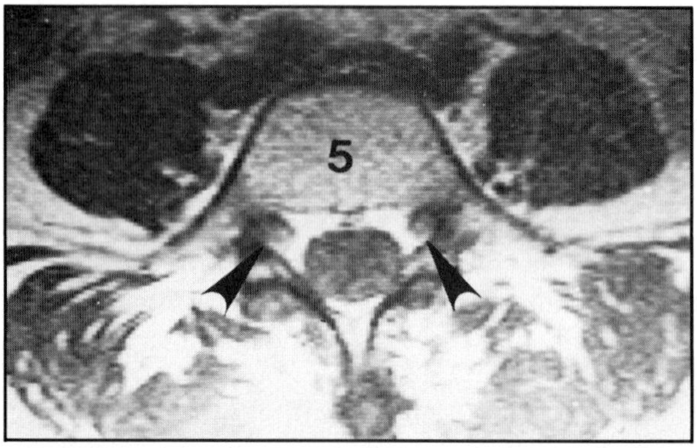

Figure 5-14A: L5 nerve roots (arrowheads) medial to the pedicles of L5.

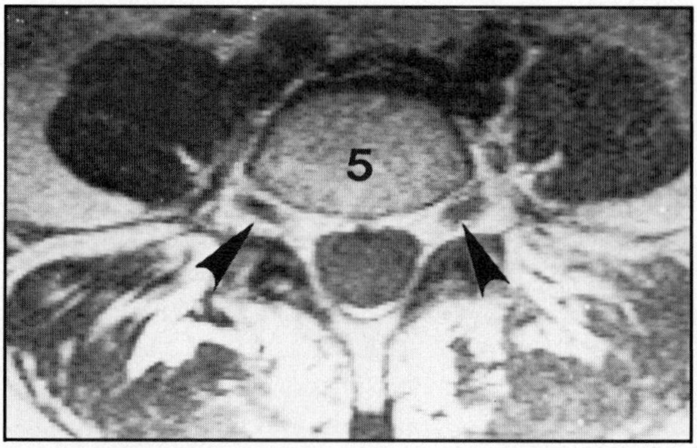

Figure 5-14B: The L5 nerve roots (arrowheads) are exiting the L5-S1 intervertebral canals.

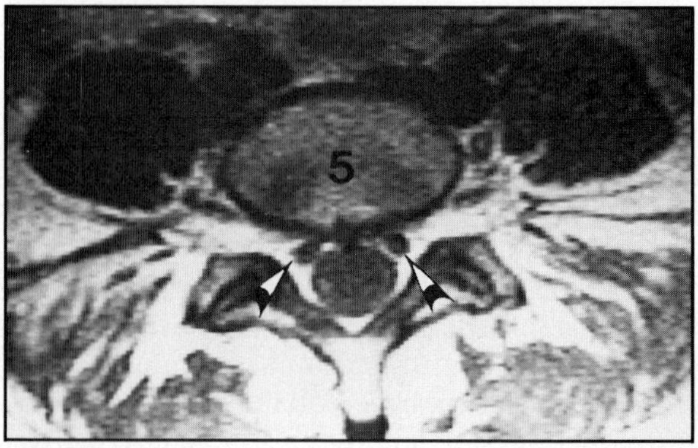

Figure 5-14C: Section through the L5-S1 disc. The S1 nerve roots (arrowheads) have now separated from the thecal sac.

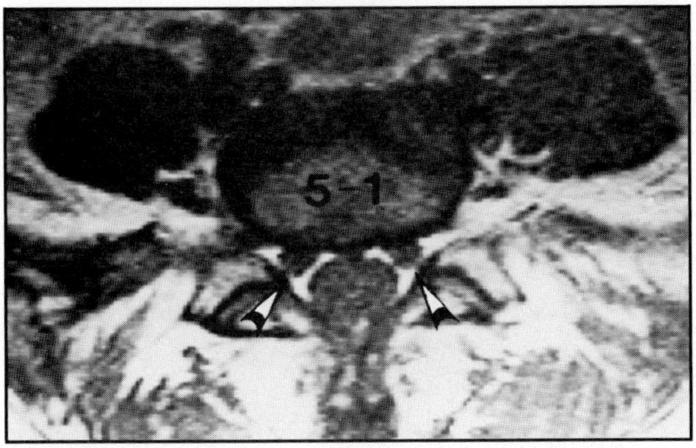

Figure 5-14D: Slightly inferior section through the L5-S1 disc. S1 nerve roots again depicted (arrowheads).

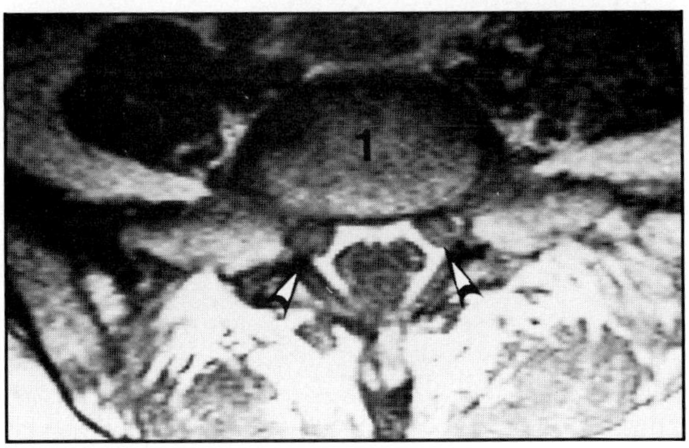

Figure 5-14E: Section through S1. The S1 nerve roots (arrowheads) are seen. The S2 roots are about to separate from the thecal sac.

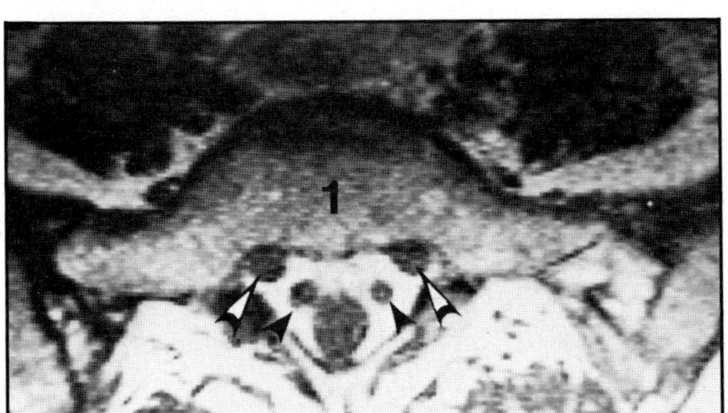

Figure 5-14F: More inferiorly through S1. The S1 roots (large arrowheads) are still seen, and S2 roots (small arrowheads) are now well separated from the theca.

Figure 5-15: Coronal image depicting the relationships of the vertebral bodies, discs, and psoas muscles (P).

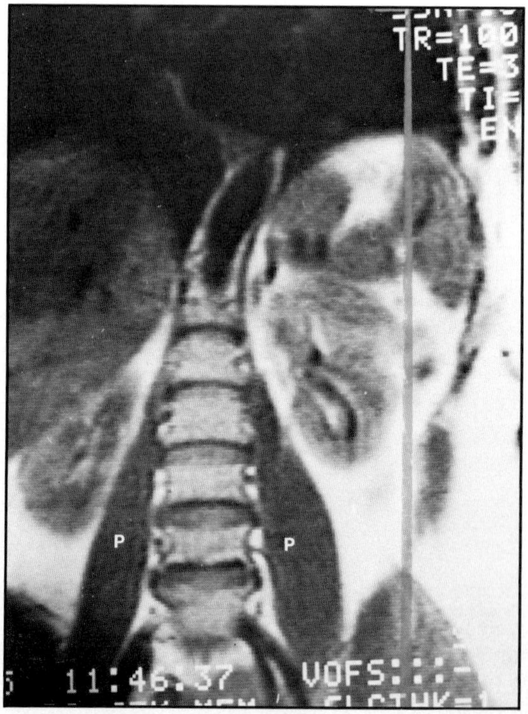

joints, joint capsules, and ligamenta flava. A triangular fat pad posterior to the theca, bounded laterally by the ligamenta flava, is characteristic.

Note that the inferior articular facets of L4 are located posteromedial to the superior articular facets of L5. The superior articular facets are seen forming the posterior margin of the intervertebral canals and lateral recesses. The ligamenta flava are normally 2-4mm in thickness.

Utilizing 4mm thick sections with 1mm intervals between the sections, the intervertebral canals are normally visualized on either 2 or 3 adjacent transverse sections. Failure to visualize the intervertebral canals in at least two adjacent sections has been described as an indirect sign of superior to inferior narrowing of the intervertebral canals by CT scanning. This sign is less important when direct sagittal images are available.

Transaxial images through the lumbar spine offer the advantage of being able to *follow the nerve roots* (Thoen et al., 1982). By

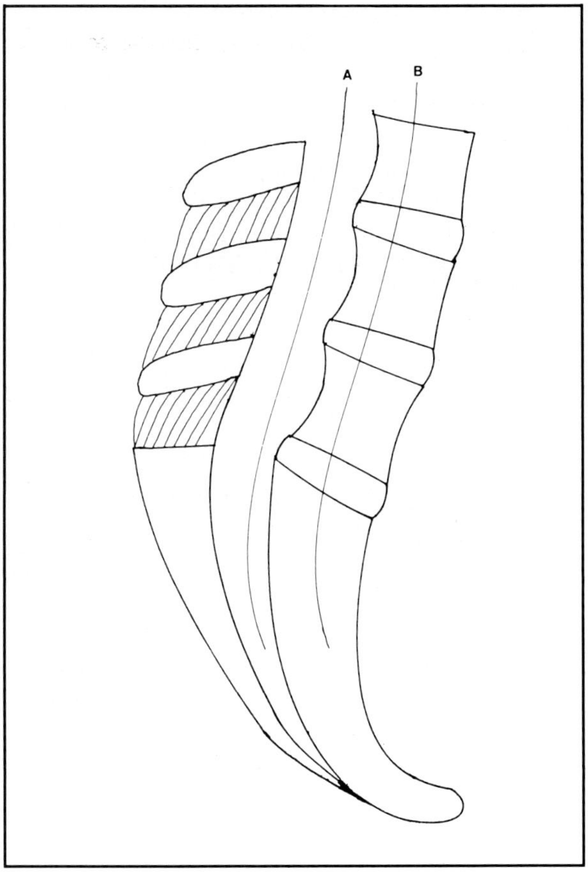

Figure 5-16: Projection of the "curved coronal" plane on a sagittal section. Surface A passes through the spinal canal, and surface B through the vertebral bodies.

following the nerve roots one can accurately determine whether they are significantly compromised by a disc protrusion or other abnormality and thus estimate the likelihood that a particular lesion is clinically significant. The sequence of images in Figure 5-14 illustrates this principle.

Coronal Plane

Images in the coronal plane are not obtained routinely but are helpful in sorting out complex anatomy. Sections through the vertebral bodies (Figure 5-15) show an excellent depiction of the paraspinal region and psoas muscles, as well as delineation of the vertebral bodies and discs. These are particularly helpful in cases of scoliosis (Figure 10-2), trauma, or congenital hemivertebra (Figure 6-2).

Because of the lumbar lordosis true coronal sections through the lower lumbar region cut the spinal canal obliquely. When *curved coronal* MR images (Figure 5-16) analagous to the reformatted curved coronal images now available with CT (Rothman & Glenn, 1985) become available, these may be helpful in evaluating the nerve roots passing out the intervertebral canals.

CHAPTER 6

Congenital Variations and Abnormalities

Congenital Variations and Abnormalities

Transitional Vertebrae

Any uncertainty as to the number of spinal segments should be clearly indicated in reports of MR examinations, particularly when radiographs are unavailable.

The diagnosis of a transitional vertebra on the MR examination is not made from a single image, but rather requires the correlation of multiple images (Figure 6-1). Clues to the possible presence of a transitional lumbosacral vertebra on sagittal images (Figure 6-1a) include a decrease in the degree of vertical orientation of the lowest well-formed disc interspace, and an apparently high termination of the thecal sac in relation to the lowest well-formed interspace.

On axial images, the identification of a "sacral" shaped vertebral body and spinal canal (Figure 6-1c) located cephalad to the level of a disc interspace (Figure 6-1b) indicates a transitional form.

Abnormalities of Vertebral Body Formation

Abnormalities of vertebral body formation range from severe to subtle. The presence of a congenital hemivertebra (Figure 6-2) presents a confusing appearance on sagittal and axial images, but is readily resolved in the coronal plane. In this situation, oblique, angled axial images provide the best view of the disc levels.

The sagittal diameters of the vertebral bodies from L4 to the sacrum demonstrate a slight, gradual, narrowing (Figure 6-3). The vertebral bodies are aligned in such a manner that the *envelope* of

Figure 6-1: Transitional lumbosacral vertebrae.

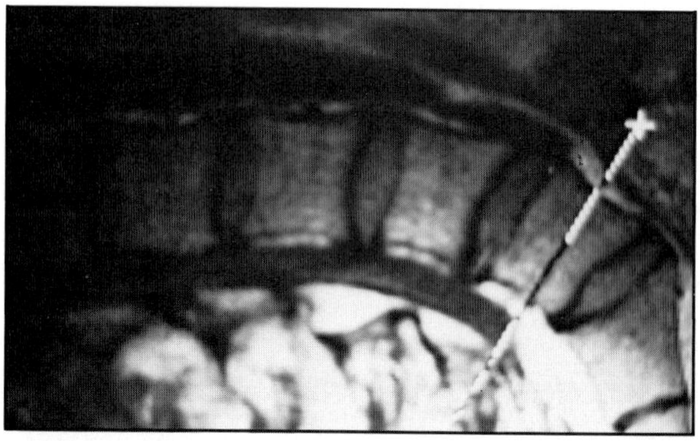

Figure 6-1A: Sagittal views. The cursor line passes through the transitional vertebra. Note that the disc space caudal to the cursor line has a relatively horizontal configuration, and that the thecal sac terminates at this level.

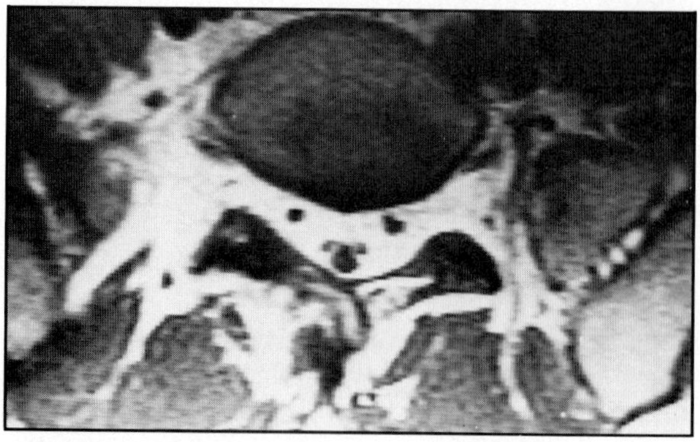

Figure 6-1B: Axial image through the well-formed disc space caudal to the cursor line in A. Note intervertebral canal.

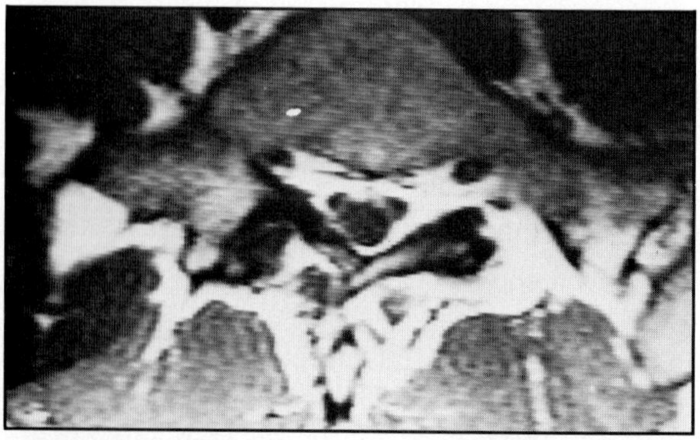

Figure 6-1C: Section through the vertebral body cephalad to the disc in B. Note the sacral type configuration.

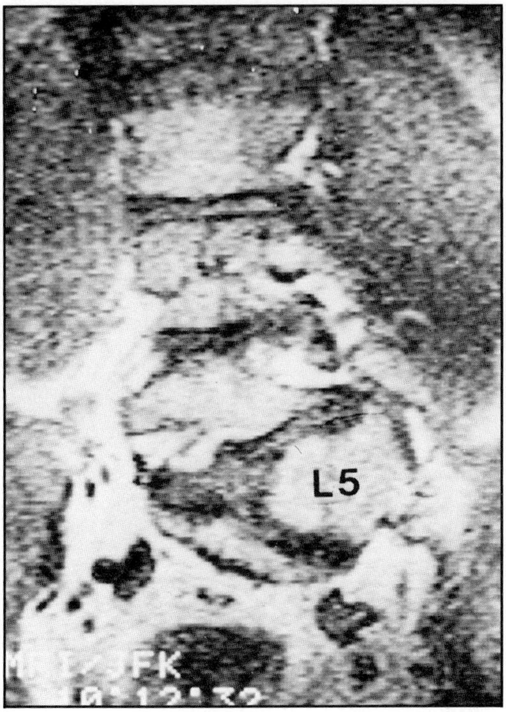

Figure 6-2: Congenital left L5 hemivertebra, coronal view. On the right there is an L4-S1 disc interspace, continuing in a Y-shaped configuration as a left L4-5 and left L5-S1 disc.

the vertebral bodies would fit within a curving, smoothly tapered funnel.

At each vertebral level, the AP diameter of the superior end plate should be only minimally greater than that of the inferior end plate, and at each disc level the AP diameter of the inferior end plate of the body above should only minimally exceed that of the superior end plate of the body below. The AP diameter of each vertebral body is slightly less at its mid-section than at the end plate levels, and the AP diameter of the intervertebral discs slightly greater than the subjacent end plates.

Spondylolisthesis indicates an abnormality of alignment of *normal sized* vertebral bodies as visualized in the sagittal plane, with the upper body displaced anteriorly with reference to the body below. This will be discussed further in Chapter 9. Retro-spondylolisthesis or retrolisthesis indicates the reverse of this situation.

Abnormalities of the sagittal diameter of vertebral bodies, with

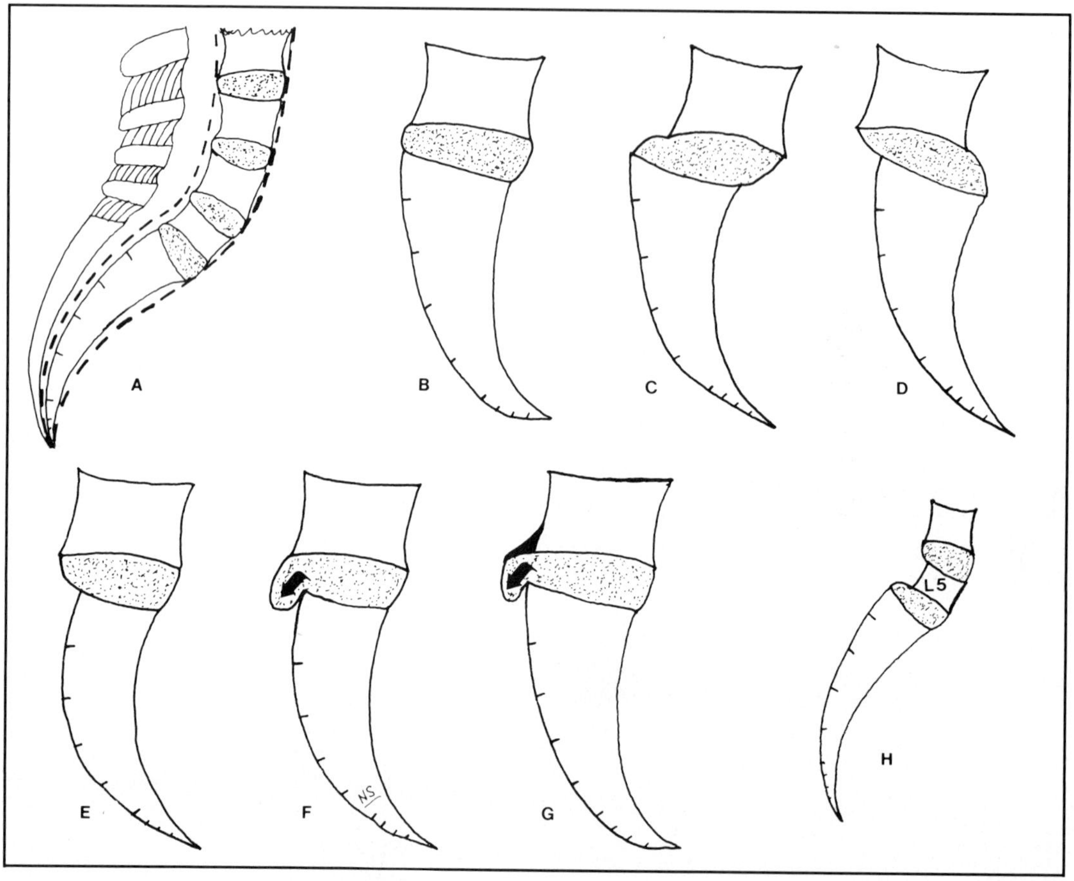

Figure 6-3: Schematic diagram of alignment abnormalities. A. Normal vertebral alignment. The vertebrae show a curving, "tapered funnel" (dotted lines) configuration. The discs are slightly taller anteriorly than posteriorly, and have a slightly greater AP diameter than the vertebral bodies. The end plates on either side of each disc are approximately of equal length, with the superior end plate of each vertebra slightly greater than the corresponding inferior end plate. B. Normal alignment at lumbosacral level. C. Spondylolisthesis. Anterior displacement of normal size L5 on normal size S1. D. Retrolisthesis. Posterior displacement of L5 on S1 with normal size relationships. E. Pseudoretrolisthesis. Congenitally short superior end plate of S1 as compred to the inferior end plate of L5. The AP diameters of the superior and inferior end plates of L5 are approximately equal. Along the *posterior* vertebral margin the appearance is similar to that in true retrolisthesis, but with pseudoretrolisthesis the *anterior* relationships remain normal. No significant disc abnormality. F. Pseudoretrolisthesis with associated disc protrusion. The overhanging inferior end plate of L5 directs the typical downward (caudad) disc protrusion. G. "Pseudopseudoretrolisthesis" with disc protrusion. Acquired degenerative reaction secondary to disc protrusion (with normal vertebral body size) creates a situation which resembles pseudoretrolisthesis. The appearance along the posterior vertebral margin is similar to that in F, except that the posterior inferior corner of L5 is involved by an osteophyte. The size discrepancy between the inferior and superior end plates of L5 distinguishes this situation from congenital pseudoretrolisthesis (E & F). H. Congenital anomally with a shortened AP diameter of L5, causing an appearance of "pseudospondylolisthesis" of L5 on S1 as well as pseudoretrolisthesis of L4 on L5.

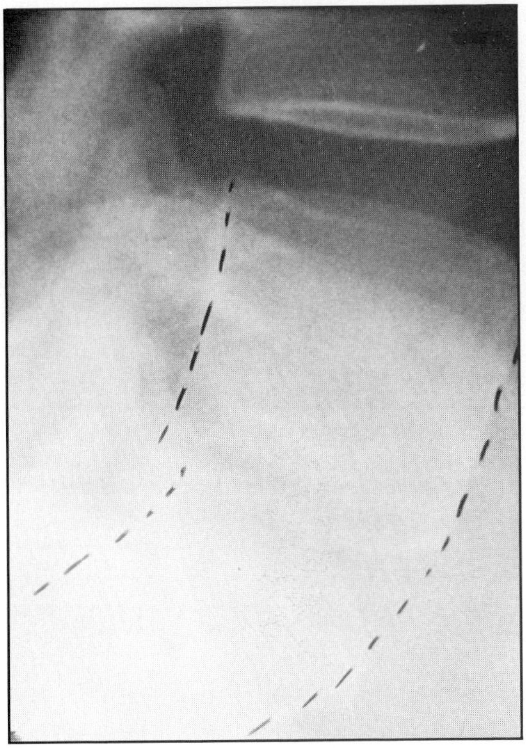

Figure 6-4: Lateral radiograph of lumbosacral junction showing pseudoretrolisthesis (emphasis added).

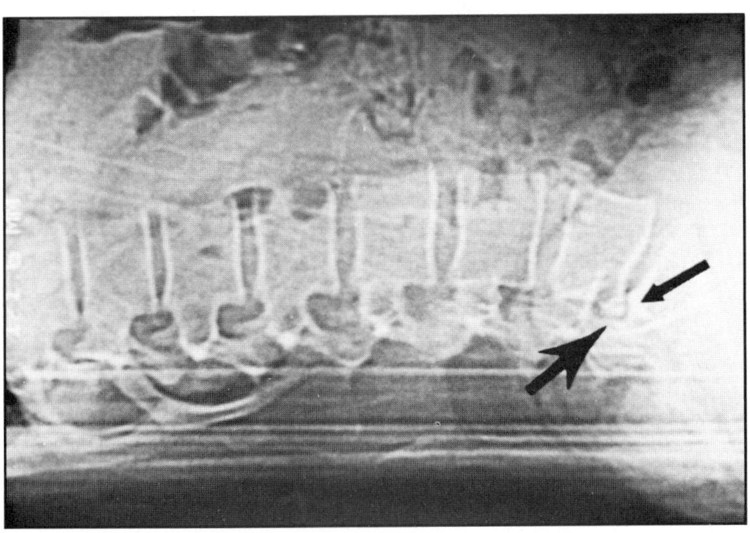

Figure 6-5: Pseudoretrolisthesis demonstrated on CT localizer view.

Figure 6-6: Examples of pseudoretrolisthesis.

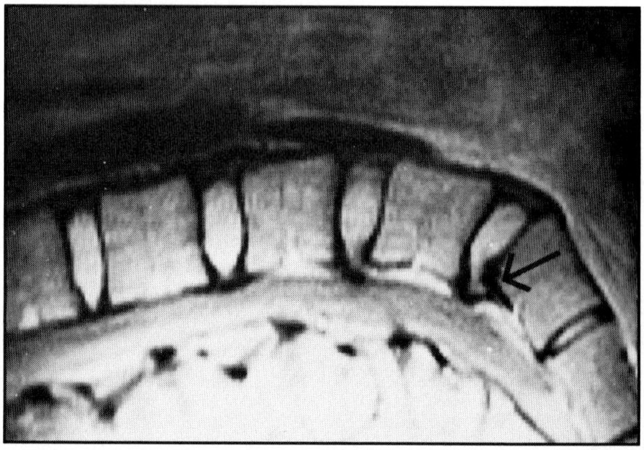

Figure 6-6A: Arrow indicates the posterior superior corner of S1 indenting the L5-S1 disc and causing abnormal stress. The AP diameter of the inferior end plate of L5 exceeds that of the superior end plate of S1.

Figure 6-6B-E: Another example of pseudoretrolisthesis.

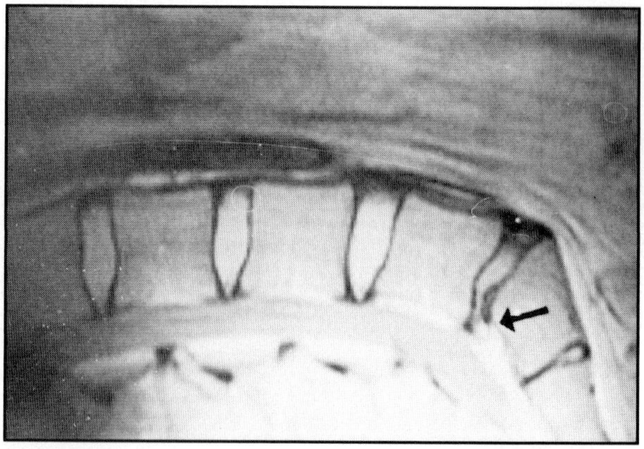

Figure 6-6B: Shows the end plate inequality and a small central disc protrusion. The T2 weighted image (C) shows loss of signal of the L5-S1 disc. A triangle of fat posterior to S1 ("fat wedge sign") is characteristic. Section D, through the disc level, shows no protrusion. Section E, through the superior end plate of S1, shows the small central disc protrusion. The theca and S1 roots remain protected by epidural fat.

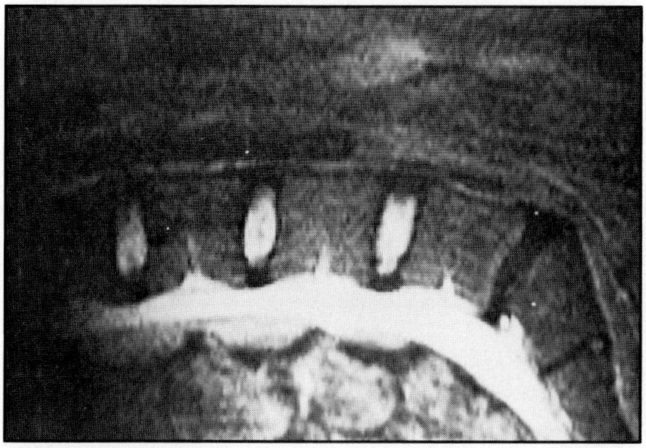

Figure 6-6C

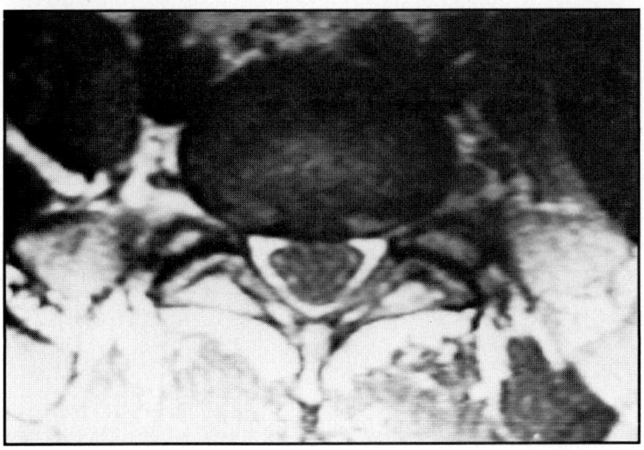

Figure 6-6D

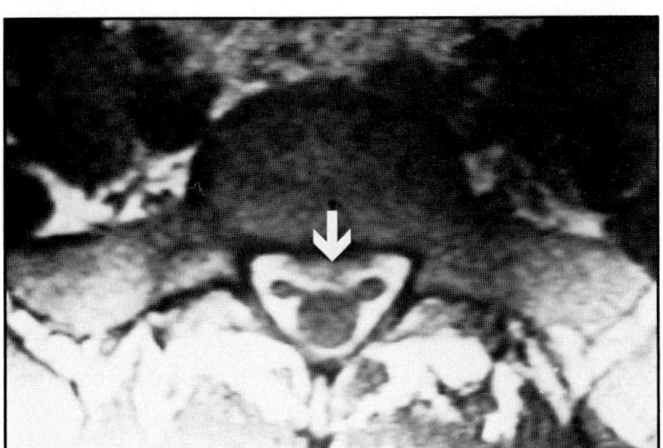

Figure 6-6E

Figure 6-6F and G: Additional examples.

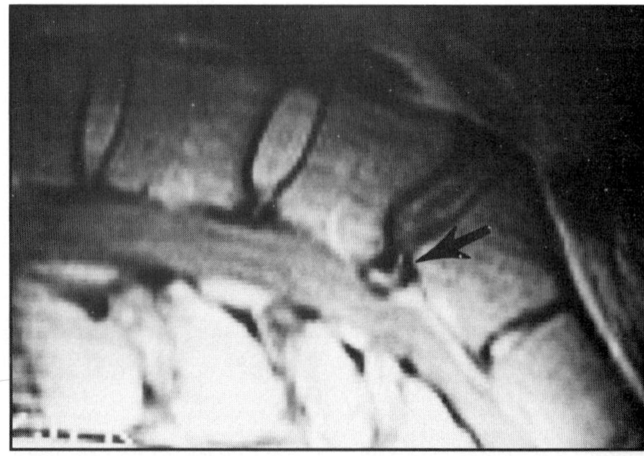

Figure 6-6F: Sagittal MR showing pseudoretrolisthesis of L5 on S1 with associated L5-S1 disc protrusion (arrow).

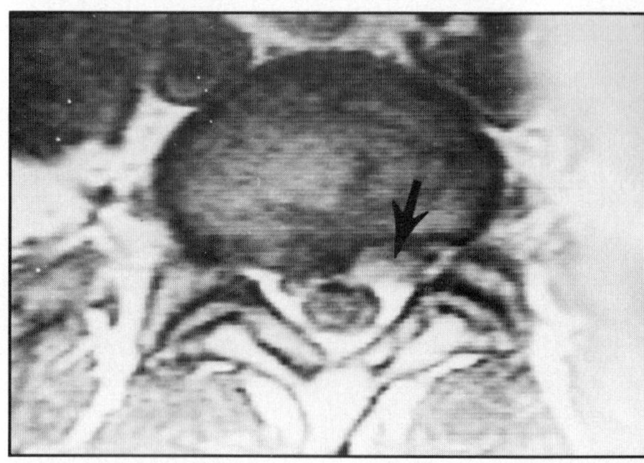

Figure 6-6G: Axial MR of the same patient as in "F" showing the left sided disc extrusion (arrow).

loss of the normal smooth tapered progression, can create a situation superficially resembling spondylolisthesis or retrolisthesis if only the posterior vertebral body and disc margins are examined (Figure 6-3e-h). Although this anomaly can be detected on lateral radiographs (Figure 6-4) or CT scan (Figure 6-5), it is much more readily identifiable on MR studies (Figure 6-6).

In our experience the most common anomaly of this type has been an increased AP diameter of the inferior end plate of L5 as

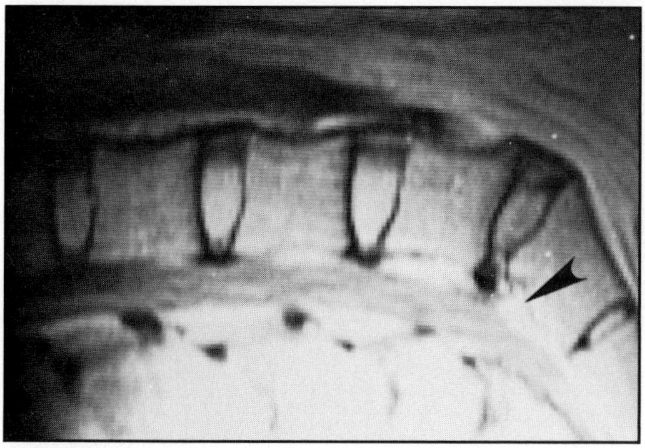

Figure 6-7: Pseudopseudoretrolisthesis. Central L5-S1 disc protrusion with accompanying degenerative reaction indicated by the dark area at the posterior inferior corner of the L5 vertebral body. Although this appearance is similar to the congenital type of pseudoretrolisthesis, the mechanism is different (see Figure 6-3). Again the "fat wedge sign" is present (arrowhead).

compared to the superior end plate of S1, often but not always associated with an increased lumbosacral angle. This situation creates an abnormal force on the posterior aspect of the L5-S1 disc and has frequently, although not always, been associated with loss of signal of the disc. Only when the intervertebral disc margin extends significantly posterior to the posterior margin of the vertebral body above (Figure 6-3f) is a disc herniation diagnosed in this situation. Under these circumstances disc herniation is generally downward, posterior to the superior end plate of the vertebral body below, with the overriding vertebral body preventing upward herniation.

Note that with true retrolisthesis there is an abnormality of *position* of normal sized vertebral bodies, whereas with the *pseudoretrolisthesis* (Dihlmann, 1966) described above a discrepancy of vertebral *size* is the basic abnormality. The appearance of the posterior vertebral margins is indistinguishable, but with pseudoretrolisthesis the anterior vertebral margins remain in alignment.

With chronic disc herniation a buttressing osteophyte may form at the posterior - inferior corner of the vertebral body above (Figure 6-3g) producing a situation superficially resembling pseudoretrolisthesis. However, close analysis will reveal a discrepancy between the AP diameter of the superior and inferior end plates of the vertebral body above, yielding a correct understanding of the etiology of the appearance of the posterior vertebral margins. This situation might be termed "pseudo-pseudoretrolisthesis" (Figure 6-7). Of course, degenerative reaction may also be superimposed on true pseudoretrolisthesis.

Figure 6-8: Congenitally short AP diameter of the L5 vertebral body.

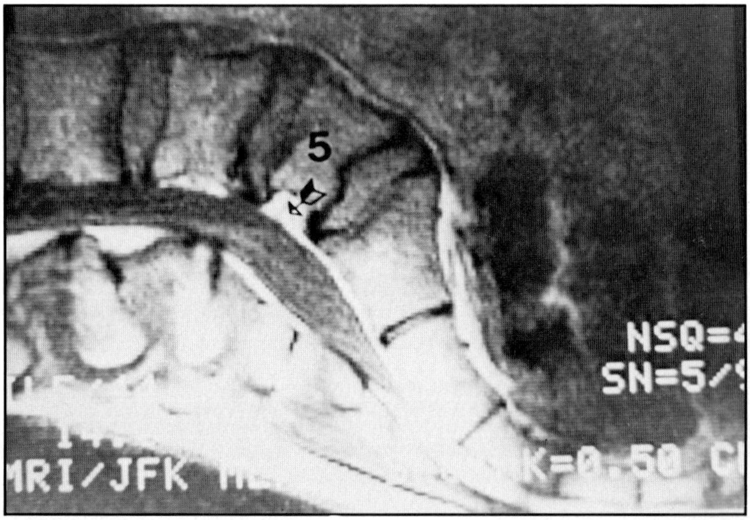

Figure 6-8A: T1 weighted sagittal view. Epidural fat (arrow) seen filling in the space between the theca and the shortened L5 body.

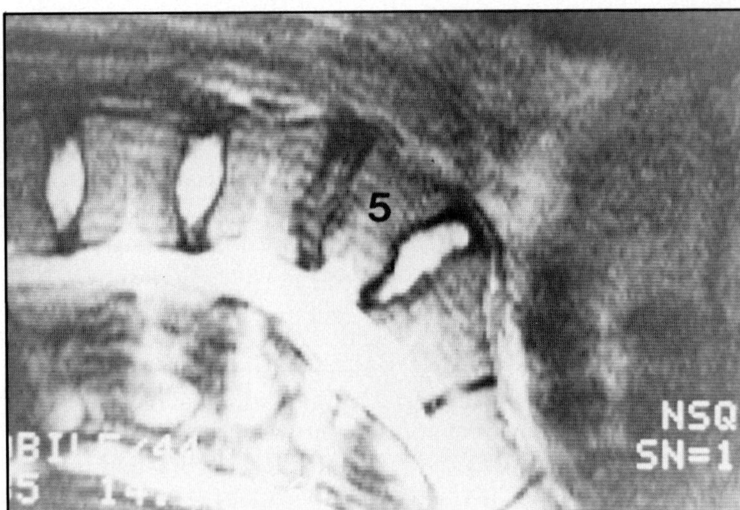

Figure 6-8B: T2 weighted image shows equal signal of the CSF and epidural fat. The L4-5 disc has lost hydration.

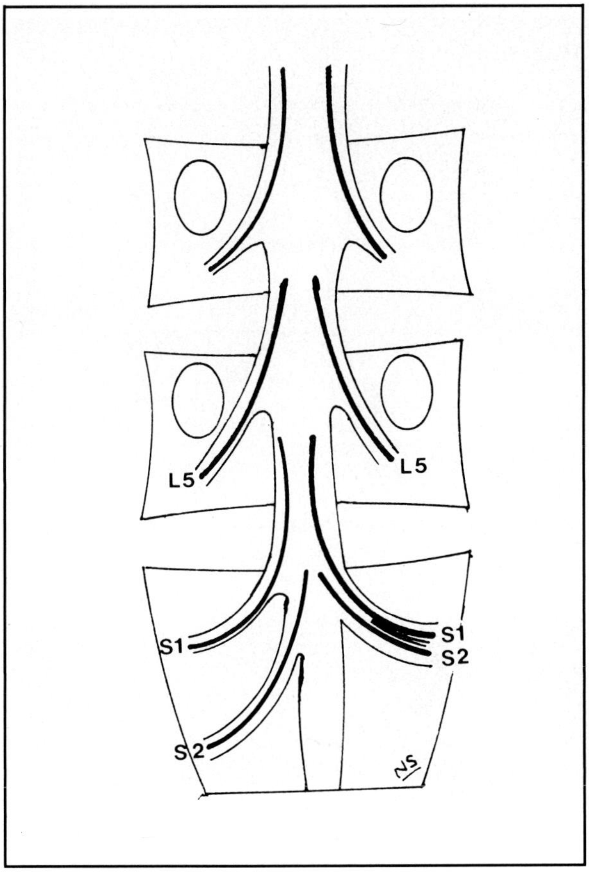

Figure 6-9: Conjoined nerve roots. The left S1 and S2 roots exit together.

When the AP diameter of the L5 vertebral body is short in relation to both S1 and L4 (Figure 6-8), the posterior vertebral margin shows an appearance of "pseudospondylolisthesis" at L5-S1 and pseudoretrolisthesis at L4-5 (Figures 6-3h and 6-8).

Abnormalities of Nerve Roots

Conjoined Roots

Occasionally two nerve roots take origin at a common level or within a common sheath (Figure 6-9). This situation may be identified by analysis of sequential MR sections (Figure 6-10), and must not be confused with disc herniation.

Figure 6-10: Conjoined nerve roots—axial MR images.

Figure 6-10A-D: Progressively more caudal sections from the L5-S1 disc into the sacrum. The right S1 root (small arrow) exits normally. The left S1 root (medium arrowhead) and left S2 (large arrowhead) have a common origin.

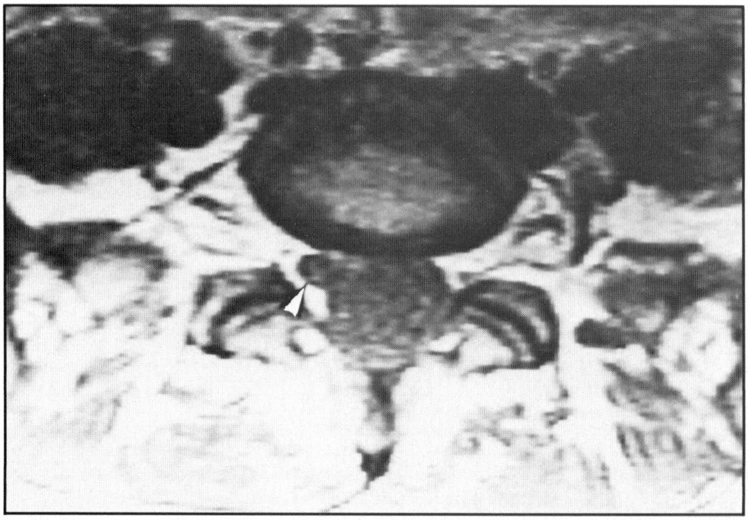

Figure 6-10A

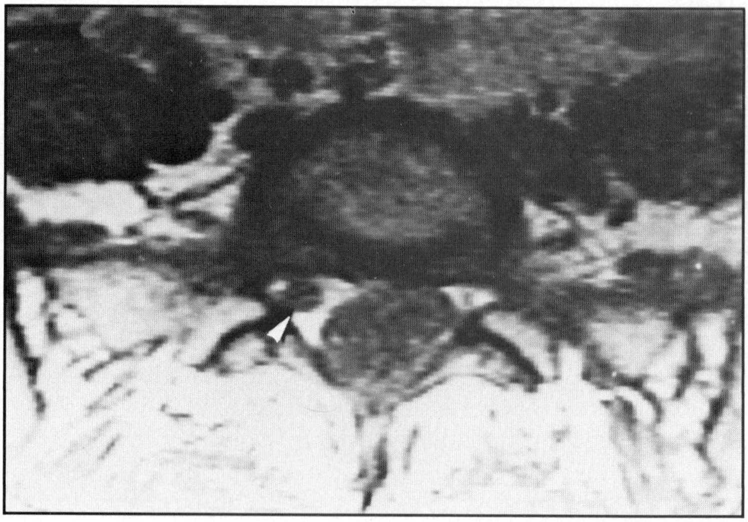

Figure 6-10B

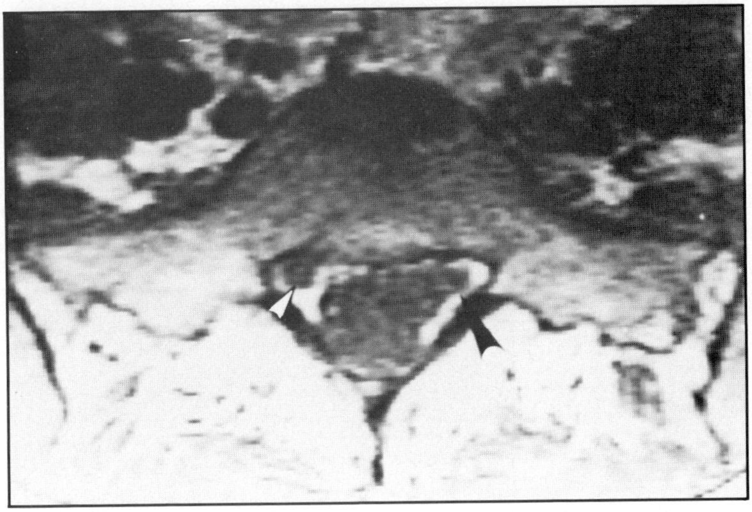

Figure 6-10C

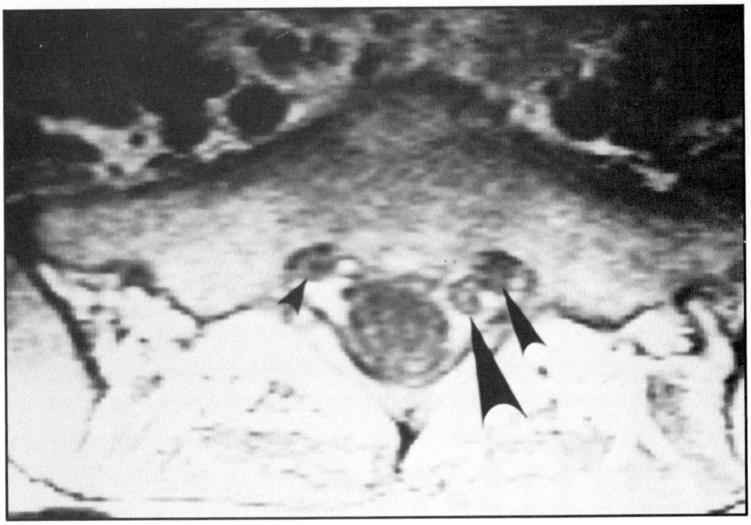

Figure 6-10D

Figure 6-10E: Myelography with water soluble contrast demonstrating the S1 nerve root (small arrowhead) and S2 nerve root (medium arrowhead).

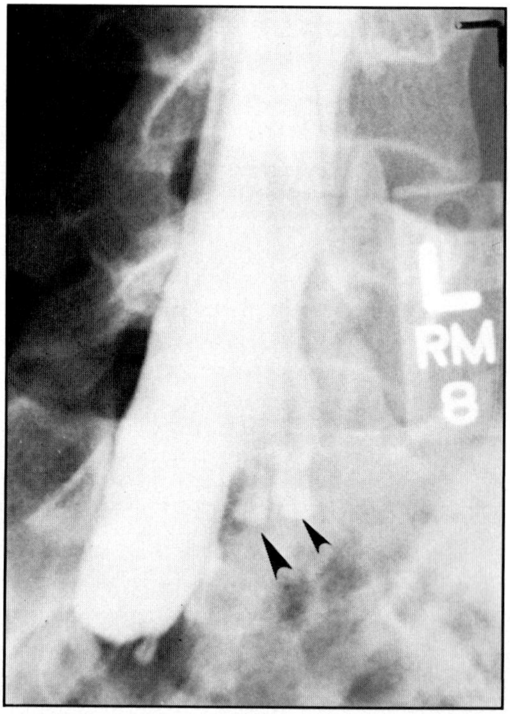

Nerve Root Cysts

Nerve root cysts (Tarlov cysts) can be identified as characteristic rounded structures iso-intense with CSF on all pulse sequences (Figure 6-11). These are not clinically significant and must not be confused with solid masses. Although no individual image is completely diagnostic, the presence of signal intensity iso-tense with CSF on multiple different sequences is characteristic.

Spinal Dysraphism

Magnetic Resonance Imaging provides an excellent screening examination for children with dysraphic myelodysplasia (Barnes et al., 1986). Utilizing appropriate pulse sequences and imaging planes the soft tissue elements of a myelodysplastic abnormality can be localized and characterized, with identification of associated findings of tethered spinal cord, spinal lipoma, or dural

(Continued on page 113)

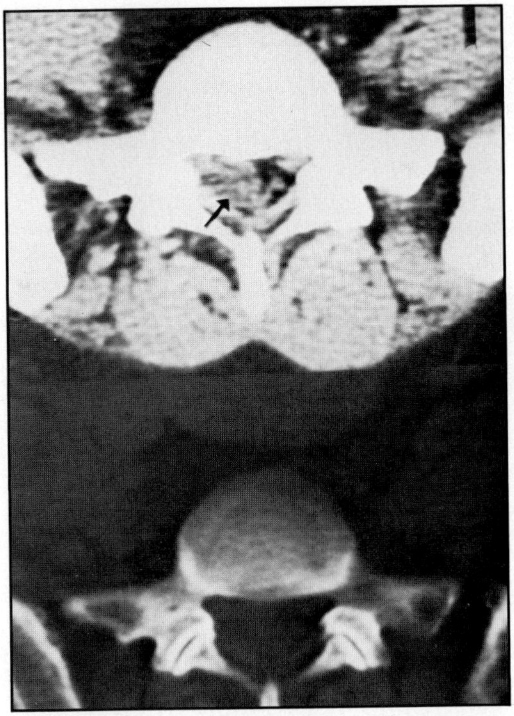

Figure 6-11A

Figure 6-11: Congenital nerve root cysts (Tarlov cysts). A. CT scan demonstrating soft tissue density (arrow) filling the right side of the spinal canal.

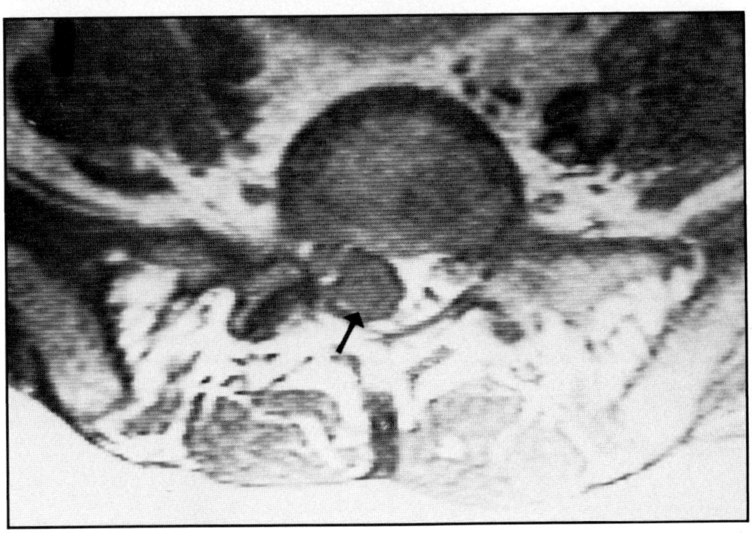

Figure 6-11B: Transaxial MR through the same level again showing the same structure (arrow).

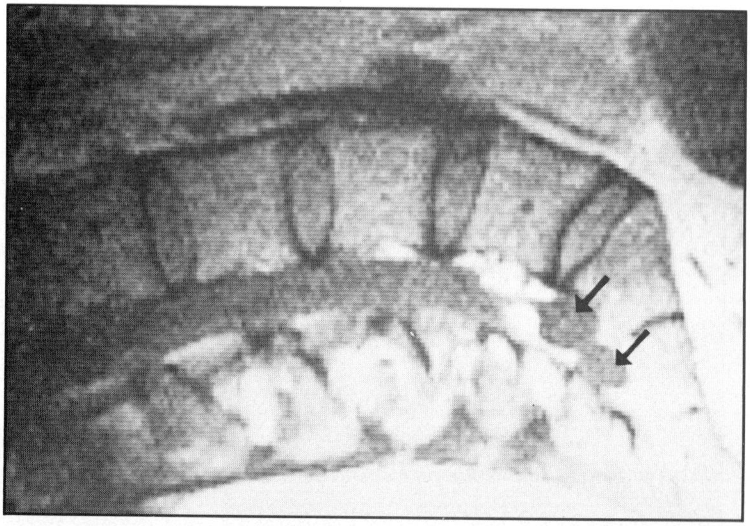

Figure 6-11C: T1 weighted MR showing two rounded structures (arrows) iso-intense with CSF.

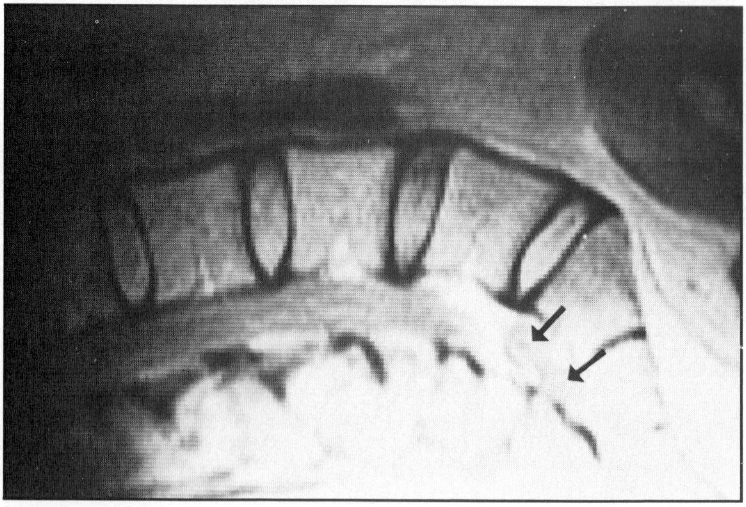

Figure 6-11D: These structures remain iso-intense with CSF on proton weighted image.

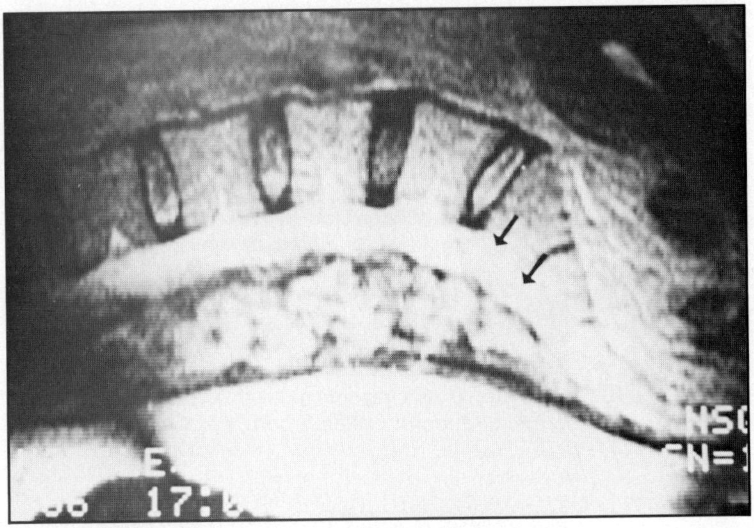

Figure 6-11E: They are again iso-intense with CSF on T2 weighted image.

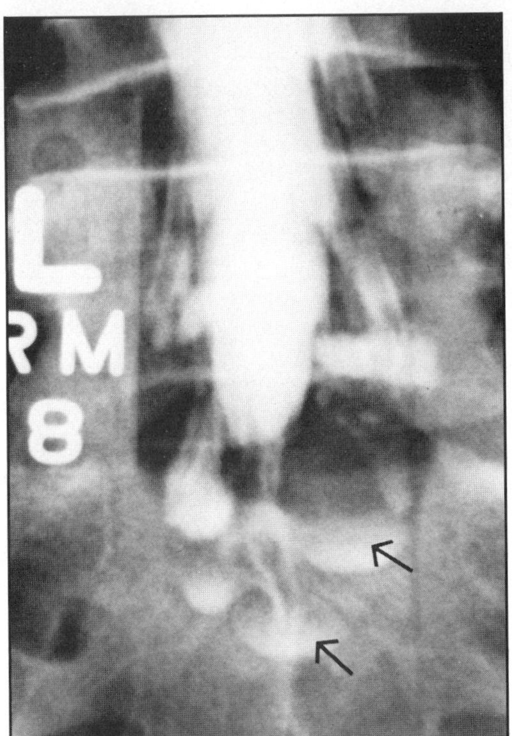

Figure 6-11F: Myelography with water soluble contrast demonstrating multiple nerve root cysts (arrows).

Figure 6-12: Myelodysplasia.

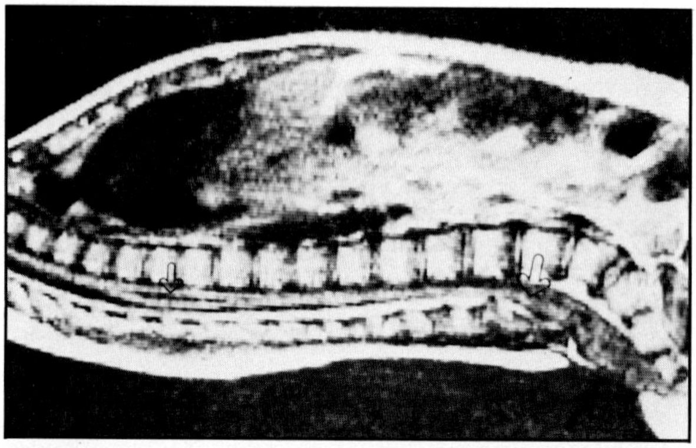

Figure 6-12A: Six year old girl with myelomeningocele. MR demonstration of tethered cord (large arrow) as well as previously unsuspected thoracic syrinx (small arrow).

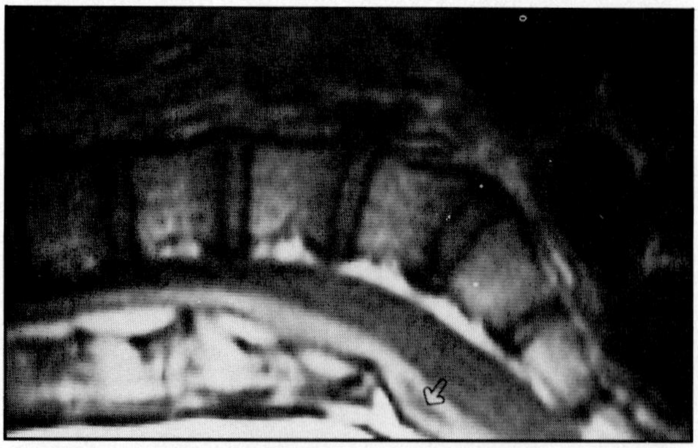

Figure 6-12B: Surface coil image demonstrating a small syrinx or cystic collection within the tethered cord.

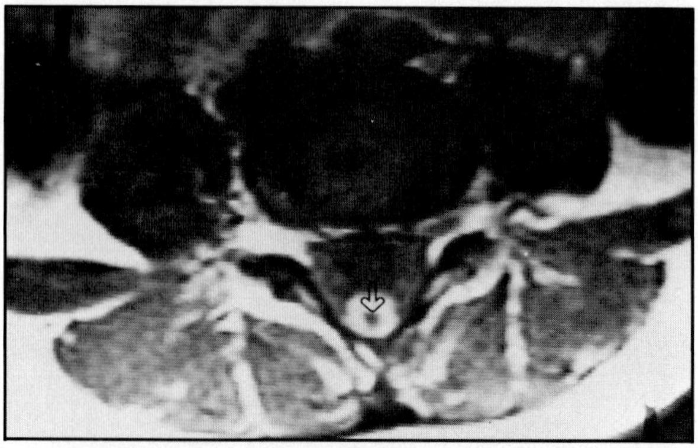

Figure 6-12C: Cross section through the lumbosacral level again demonstrates the tethered cord with the small cystic collection (arrow).

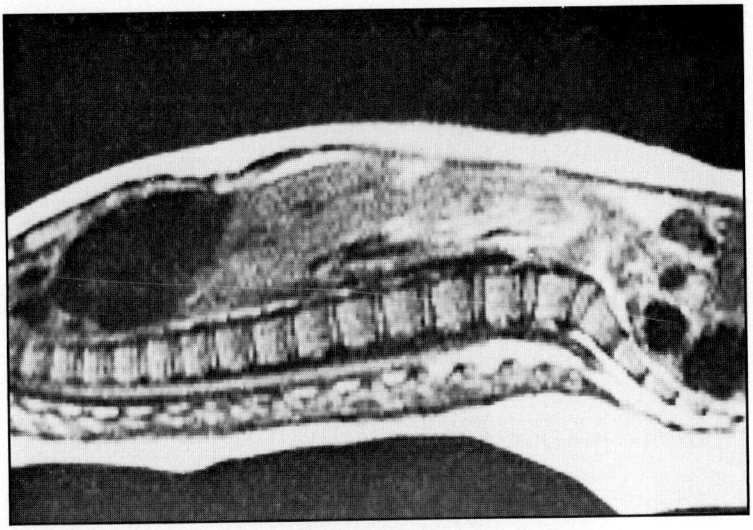

Figure 6-13A: Another example of tethered cord, associated with lipoma at the lumbar level.

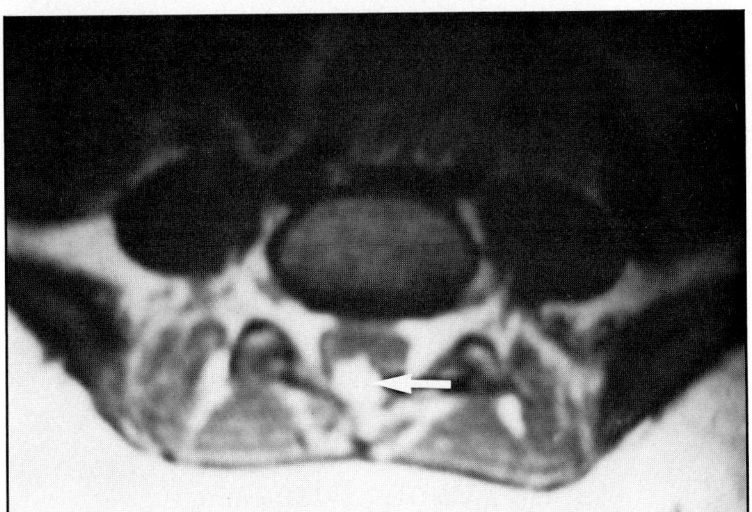

Figure 6-13B: Transverse image through the lipomatous tethered cord at L4 (arrow).

Figure 6-14: Myelomeningocele and scoliosis successfully imaged by MR despite presence of Harrington rod. A. Radiograph demonstrating the Harrington rod.

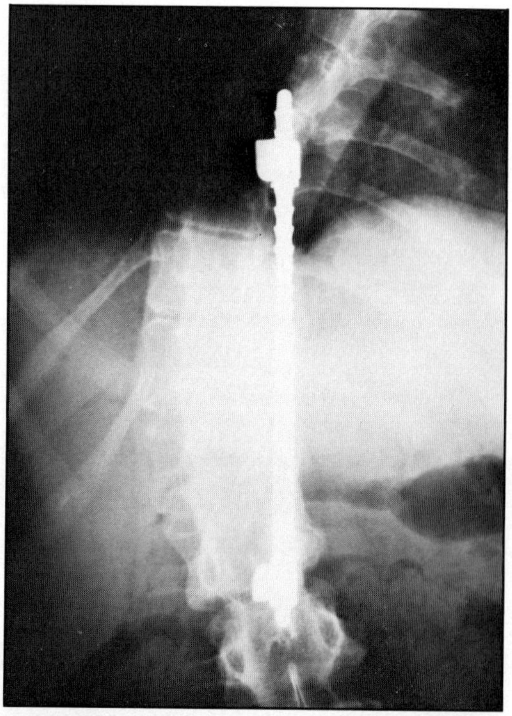

Figure 6-14A

ectasia (Figures 6-12 through 6-14). Associated diastematomyelia can be identified (Hahn, et al., 1985) and the associated hemicords visualized, although conventional radiography or plain CT study provide better detail of the osseous anatomy.

Complete or partial sacral agenesis, a form of spinal dysraphism with anterior myelomeningocele, is well evaluated by MR scanning (Figure 6-15).

Systemic Diseases Affecting Signal Intensity

Inherited diseases affecting spinal morphology to produce abnormalities on MR images analogous to those on conventional radiographs and will not be discussed here.

Some inherited systemic diseases causing diffuse biochemical abnormality of the vertebral marrow or intervertebral discs have a

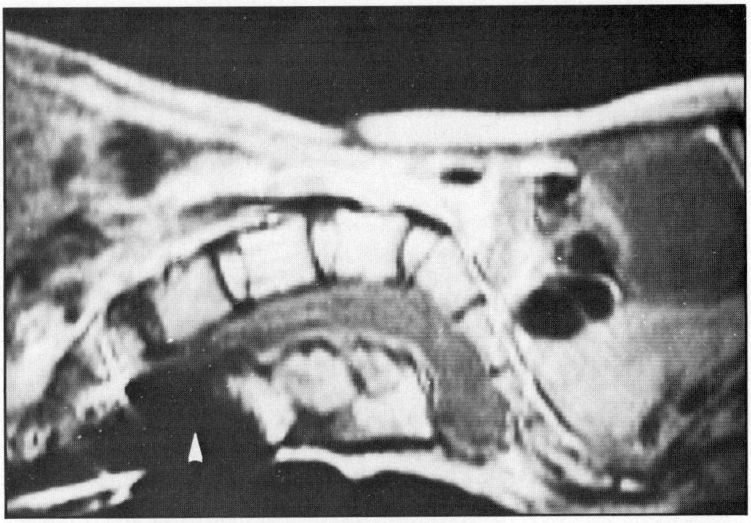

Figure 6-14B: T1 weighted MR study. The postoperative sacral myelomeningocele is well demonstrated. The Harrington rod causes local artifact on the MR study (arrowhead).

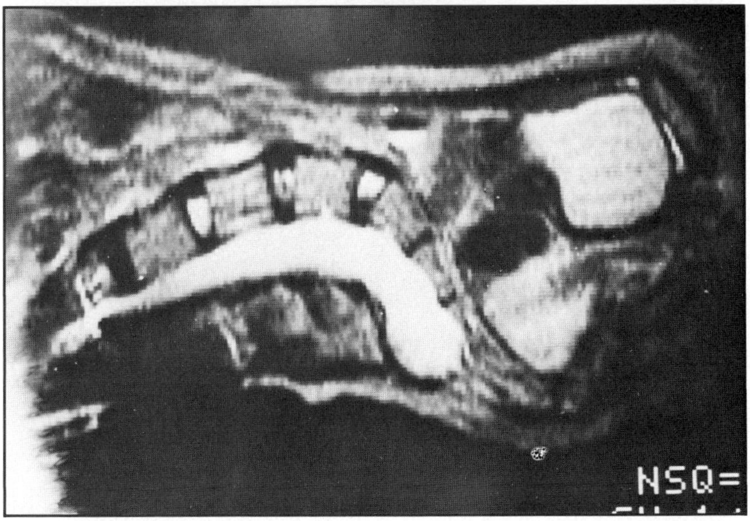

Figure 6-14C: T2 weighted MR study again demonstrating the dilated thecal sac.

Figure 6-15: Partial sacral agenesis. A. MR scan. Two and one half sacral segments are visualized.

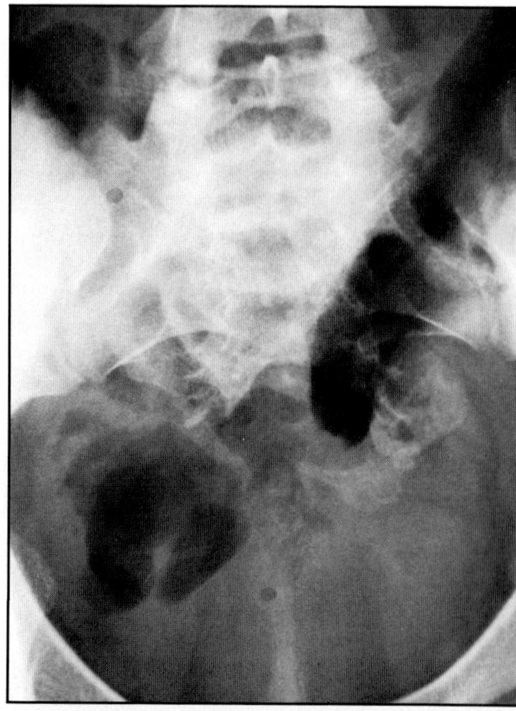

Figure 6-15A

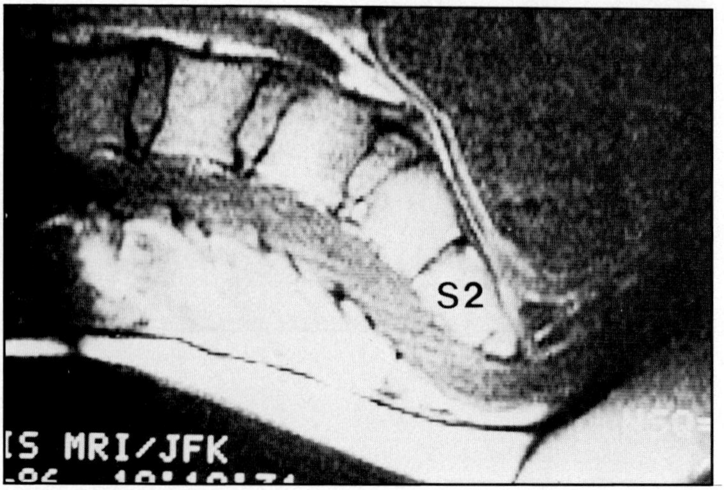

Figure 6-15B: AP radiograph.

characteristic appearance on MR studies. The increased marrow iron in thallassemia has been reported to show a diffuse decrease in the signal intensity of the vertebral marrow related to the paramagnetic effects of iron (Modic et al., 1986). Transfusional siderosis would be expected to show a similar appearance.

Extensive disc space calcification such as occurs in ochronosis would be expected to produce a marked loss of signal intensity of intervertebral discs due to the lack of mobile protons in the calcified disc.

CHAPTER 7

Intervertebral Disc Disease

Intervertebral Disc Disease

In our experience the most common clinical indication leading to referral for lumbar magnetic resonance imaging studies is "rule out HNP." This chapter will review the applied anatomy and pathophysiology of the intervertebral disc as it relates to acute and chronic disc injury and degeneration.

Applied Anatomy and Pathophysiology of the Intervertebral Disc

The human intervertebral disc has evolved as a well organized structure composed of specialized fibrocartilaginous connective tissue. Organization at both the macroscopic and microscopic levels allows the disc to firmly join the adjacent vertebrae, simultaneously absorbing shock and yet able to transmit forces from all directions.

The normal lumbar intervertebral disc is a biconcave wedge-shaped structure tallest anteriorly (Figure 7-1, Table 7-1). In total the lumbar discs account for approximately one third the length of the lumbar spine.

Inferiorly and superiorly the hyaline cartilage end plates are surrounded by a boney epiphyseal ring. These perforated cartilaginous end plates are located eccentrically, closer to the posterior vertebral margins, and can be seen separating the nucleus pulposus from the vertebral body.

The annulus fibrosis is a circular ligament composed of concentric layers of collagen fibers at right angles to one another running in oblique fashion between the vertebral bodies (Brown, 1971). The outermost fibers (Sharpey's fibers) attach the annulus to the vertebral bodies, inserting to the vertebral bodies at their

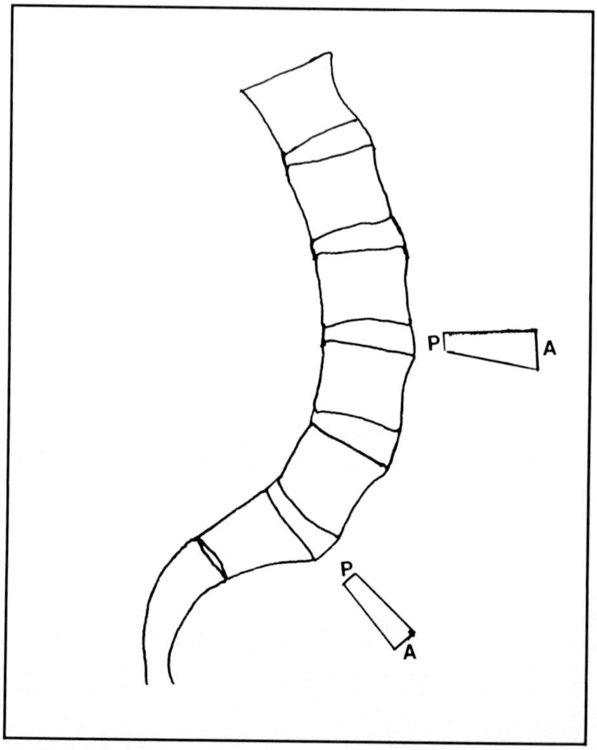

Figure 7-1: The disc is a biconcave wedge shaped structure tallest anteriorly.

junction with the epiphyseal ring. The middle group of fibers connect the epiphyseal ring of one vertebral body to the next, and the inner fibers connect the cartilaginous end plates. Since the nucleus pulposus is located relatively posteriorly within the annulus fibrosis, the posterior lamellae of the annulus are thinner and more closely packed between the nucleus and the dorsal aspect of the disc (Park & Schiff, 1971).

The nucleus pulposus is the definitive remnant of the embryonic notocord. It is composed of loose delicate fibrous strands imbedded in a gelatinous matrix (Park & Schiff, 1971). These show no geometric preference centrally, forming a felted mesh, but do display a more definite geometric organization as they attach to the cartilaginous end plates. The presence of a considerable number of cells within the nucleus pulposus attests to its vital nature despite the lack of vascular elements.

There is no definite structural interface between the nucleus pulposus and the annulus fibrosis. Rather, the composition of the

Table 7-1
Dimensions of the Normal Intervertebral Disc in the Upright Position

	Anterior Disc Height	Posterior Disc Height	Disc Depth
Level	**Mean**	**Mean**	**Mean**
L1-L2	8	4	34
L2-L3	11	4.5	34
L3-L4	12.5	4.5	33
L4-L5	14	5.5	33
L5-S1	13	4.5	31

Modified from Tibrewal and Pearcy

two tissues blends imperceptibly, frustrating any attempt to cleanly extirpate the entire nucleus with blunt dissection (Park & Schiff, 1971). This transition zone is narrower in young subjects and becomes broader to non-existent in older subjects, as demonstrated by dissection studies (Brown, 1971) as well as MR images.

From a functional standpoint the annulus fibrosis serves to resist tensile forces, whereas the nucleus pulposus, contained within the annulus, acts as a "shock absorber" to resist compressive forces. This elastic or shock absorbing capability of the nucleus pulposus is dependent upon its water content. The acid mucopolysaccharides of the nucleus are able to imbibe many times their own weight in water. Hydration of the nucleus pulposus is highest at birth, measured at 88%, decreasing to 80% at 18 years and 65% at 77 years (Naylor, 1971). Corresponding values for annulus fibrosis are 78% water at birth decreasing to 70% at 30 years.

This ability to imbibe water, with associated increase in intradiscal pressure, accounts for the ability of the nucleus pulposus to resist compressive forces. The dynamic living nature of the nucleus pulposus, and the chemical properties of the acid mucopolysaccharides, provide for the maintenance of intradiscal pressure. This osmotic effect, with the disc losing water with loading and gaining water when unloaded (Kramer et al., 1984) accounts for the diurnal variation in human height. This pumping action also accounts for the nutrition of the intervertebral disc, with nutrients passing from the vertebral spongiosa through the cribriform end plates into the disc.

The anterior longitudinal ligament is a strong band of fibers connecting the vertebral bodies anteriorly. Its deepest fibers blend with the vertebral body periosteum, with the tightest attachment at the end plate level. It is only loosely adherent to the underlying intervertebral disc.

The posterior longitudinal ligament has a denticulate segmental configuration. It is most closely adherent to the midportion of the vertebral bodies and the lateral extensions overlying the disc spaces, with the fibers of the ligament *bowstrung* across the intervertebral disc in the midline.

Innervation of the articular connective tissue, periosteum, meninges, and epidural venous sinuses is provided by the recurrent sinuvertebral branch of each spinal nerve. This nerve originates just distal to the dorsal root ganglion and returns back through the intervertebral canal into the spinal canal. The sinuvertebral nerve at each level probably provides anastomosing fibers to the levels above and below analogous to arterial distribution. Numerous nerve endings are distributed in the posterior longitudinal ligament, including its lateral extensions, and in the periosteum. Some but not all investigators report nerve fibers within the outer layers of the annulus fibrosis, whereas the nucleus pulposus and inner layers of the annulus lack nerve endings. Thus discogenic pain may relate to damage or irritation of the outer fibers of the annulus fibrosis or to the overlying posterior longitudinal ligament, periosteum, venous sinuses, and/or meninges.

Disc Injury and Degeneration

Terminology

Terminology used to describe disc abnormalities has been imprecise, inconsistent, and sometimes confusing. It is in the best interest of a patient that all those involved in his care and evaluation including radiologists, referring clinicians, and attorneys utilize a common, consistent terminology. Words should be used with their generally accepted meanings. The diagnosis made should be the most exact possible from the available evidence but no more exact. When precise pathophysiologic details cannot be ascertained from imaging studies, general terms should be used (Figure 7-2, Table 7-2).

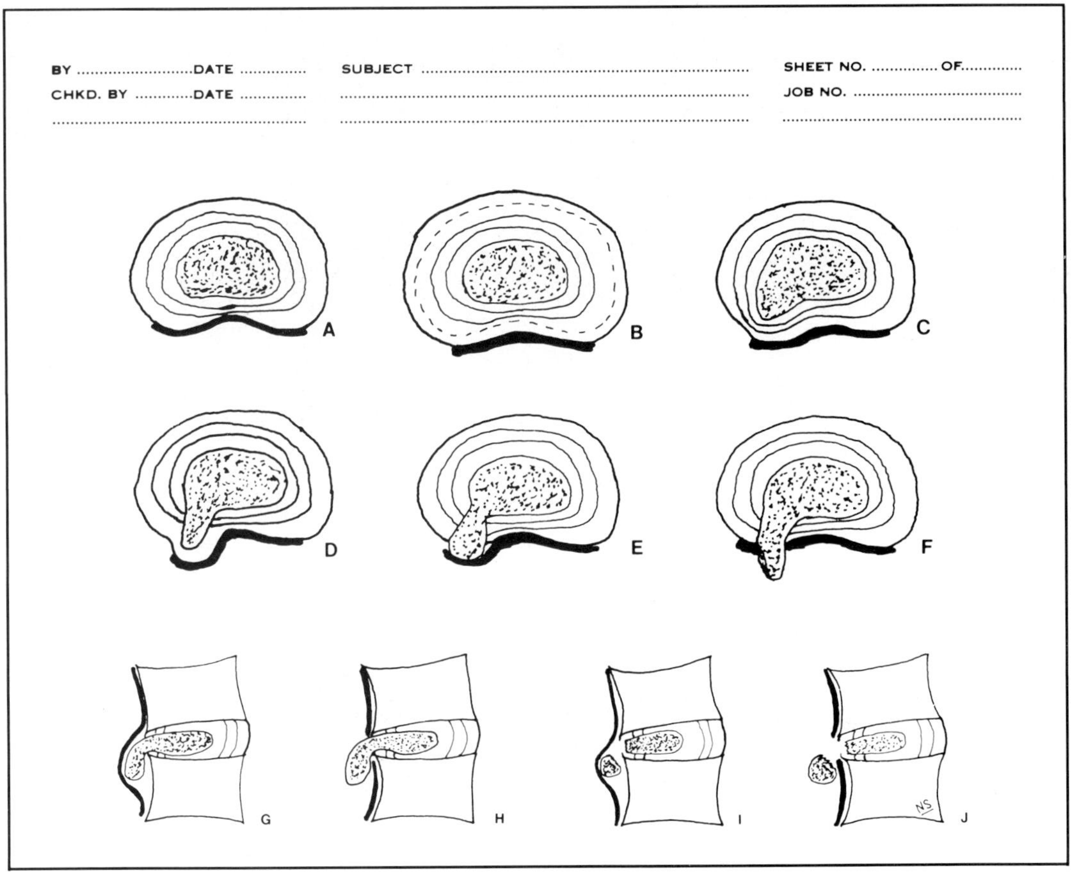

Figure 7-2: Pathology of the intervertebral disc. A. Normal disc. The nucleus pulposus (stippled) is eccentrically located closer to the posterior margin. The inner fibers of the annulus fibrosis are more closely spaced along the posterior margin. Note the posterior longitudinal ligament (heavy line). B. Diffuse annular bulging. The annulus bulges circumferentially beyond the normal expected position (dotted line). Normal central position of nucleus. C. Focal annular bulge. There is thinning and stretching of intact annular fibers, with the nucleus bulging toward the thinned area. D. Focal protrusion. The inner annular fibers are torn, with the outer fibers of the annulus intact. The nucleus protrudes through the ruptured inner fibers of the annulus. Posterior longitudinal ligament intact. In practice, this form of "intradiscal herniation" is difficult to distinguish from the situation in C. E. Ruptured annulus fibrosis with herniated (extruded) nucleus pulposus, subligamentous. All layers of the annulus are ruptured, with the herniated nuclear material contained by the posterior longitudinal ligament. F. Ruptured annulus fibrosis with herniated nucleus pulposus, sequestered. The ruptured nucleus has extruded through (or around) the posterior longitudinal ligament. Note that some authors reserve the use of the term sequestered to describe free fragments. G. Subligamentous extrusion with migration. Either extruded disc material in continuity with the nucleus pulposus or free fragments of the nucleus may migrate (move away from the site of extrusion) in either the subligamentous or the epidural space. H. Sequestered extrusion with inferior migration. Note that in this instance the posterior longitudinal ligament is ruptured. I. Migration of a subligamentous free fragment. J. Migration of a sequestered free fragment in the epidural space.

Table 7-2
Annulus Fibrosis and Nucleus Pulposus in Various Disc Abnormalities Diagnosis on MR Scans

	Nucleus Pulposus				
Annulus Fibrosis	**Normal**	**Decreased Signal**	**Protruded**	**Extruded**	**Sequestered**
Intact	Normal	Dessication			
Diffuse Thinning		Diffuse Annular Bulge			
Focal Thinning			Focal Annular Bulge*		
Partial Tear			Focal Protrusion*		
Complete Tear				Ruptured Annulus Fibrosis with Herniated Nucleus Pulposus	Ruptured Annulus Fibrosis with Herniated Nucleus Pulposus and Sequestered ("free") Fragment

*In practice Focal Annular Bulge and Focal Protrusion ("Intradiscal Herniation") are often indistinguishable.

Protrusion may be defined as the state of being thrust forward (Stedman, 1966). A *bulge* is a swelling or protruberant part. A *prolapse* is a falling forward or sinking down. A *hernia* is defined as the protrusion of an organ or part of an organ or other structure through the wall of the cavity normally containing it. *Rupture* refers to a tear or break in continuity of a structure. *Extrude* is to thrust forth or to force out, as toothpaste is extruded from the tube.

Utilizing these elementary definitions one can classify disc abnormalities precisely (Figure 7-2). The annulus fibrosis may be normal, it may show a localized area of thinning without discontinuity of its fibers but associated with focal bulging (focal annular bulge), or it may show a generalized degenerative change and extension beyond the expected margins, usually associated with a loss of disc space height and termed a *generalized annular bulge*. Note that a mild degree of annular bulging is physiologic.

Ruptures of the annulus fibrosis may be partial or complete. Partial ruptures may involve minor degrees of radial or circumfer-

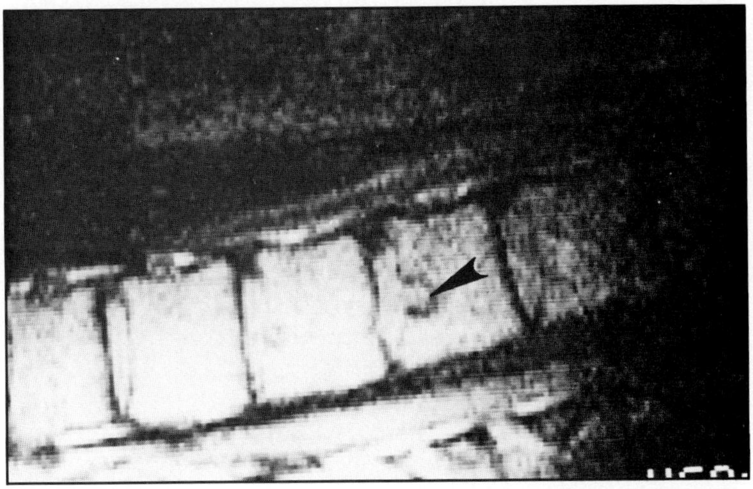

Figure 7-3: Disc herniation into vertebral end plate (Schmorl's node) associated with old vertebral compression fracture.

ential tearing (difficult to detect), or may extend so as to leave only the outer annular fibers intact. Under these circumstances nuclear material will tend to fill in the defect, and the weakened annulus will protrude locally at the site of the partial tear.

With a complete rupture of the annulus fibrosis, nuclear material may be extruded. This material may remain beneath the anterior longitudinal ligament, creating a subligamentous extrusion, or it may pass through or around the anterior longitudinal ligament creating a sequestered extrusion. Movement of the extruded portion of the nucleus pulposus, either subligamentous or sequestered, is referred to as *migration*. When an extruded portion of the nucleus pulposus separates from the main body of the nucleus it is denoted a *freu fragment*. Such free fragments may be either subligamentous or sequestered, and may migrate cephalad or caudad either in the subligamentous space or the epidural space. Rarely free fragments may become intradural.

In clinical cases the most precise anatomic diagnosis possible should be made. Identification and localization of free fragments is particularly important. On MR images annular thinning with intact annular fibers with a focal annular bulge may be indistinguishable from partial annular rupture with intact outer fibers and a focal protrusion (intradiscal herniation). Under these circumstances the terminology focal disc bulge or focal disc protrusion may be utilized.

The anatomy of the annulus fibrosis and longitudinal ligaments helps to determine the vectors of lumbar disc herniations. The most common site of herniation is in the posterior paramedian zone (85%-90%), with 5%-12% of herniations in the posterior midline and 5% posterolateral in the intervertebral canal (Williams, et al., 1982). Anterior disc herniations (Figure 9-4) are rare. Disc herniation into the vertebral end plates (Schmorl's nodules) may occur on an idiopathic basis or as a result of a discrete traumatic episode (Figure 7-3). Figures 7-4 through 7-21 present examples of disc protrusions demonstrated by MR.

Disc Degeneration

Disc herniation can occur as a result of a recognized injury. This explains the sudden onset of back pain and sciatica following bending or lifting incidents, and has been confirmed experimentally with cadaver discs (Adams & Hutton, 1985). More commonly, however, patients with back pain and sciatica have no history of discreet antecedent trauma. Their presentation is more in keeping with a gradual process of disc degeneration. Even those patients with acute herniations soon undergo secondary disc degenerative changes.

With aging there is a gradual but progressive loss of hydration of the intervertebral discs, particularly the nucleus pulposus, as previously mentioned. An intranuclear cleft develops by age thirty in most individuals. The distinction between nucleus pulposus and annulus fibrosis becomes progressively less distinct. These changes of normal aging are accelerated following disc injury. Although multiple complex biochemical changes occur within the intervertebral disc with normal aging, or following injury, progressive loss of hydration is primarily responsible for the loss of signal intensity of the nucleus pulposus on T2-weighted MR images (Aguila et al., 1985).

With aging the nucleus pulposus undergoes a gradual loss of its gel-like properties related to subtle alterations in the mucopolysaccharide matrix and associated water loss, and is gradually replaced by fibrocartilage. The annulus fibrosis, as a result of mechanical and metabolic insults, undergoes biochemical changes leading to mechanical weakening (Brown, 1971). The earliest macroscopic disruption of the annulus fibrosis generally consists of small concentric tears. These may coalesce so as to form tears oriented in the radial direction. When these radial tears extend to the end plates, with detachment of the annulus from the end plate along the direction of the tear, nuclear material is then extruded. This material, relieved of mechanical loading, is actually able to imbibe water and expand, increasing its mechanical effects and eliciting an inflammatory response.

It is likely that most herniated discs degenerate and lose water content *prior* to the episode of herniation. Following herniation of a previously normal disc, the exact time course of desiccation is not known but is probably rapid, occurring within weeks. Certainly the presence of a herniated lumbar intervertebral disc showing normal hydration signal by MR imaging is rare.

Adequate data are not yet available on the incidence of dehydration of lumbar discs at various levels at different ages, but discs displaying decreased hydration without herniation are not rare in young adults (Figure 7-22). This lack of good data about relative hydration of the discs creates difficulty in assigning a cause and effect relationship between a particular injury and the findings present on a magnetic resonance study.

The Postoperative Disc

Both CT and MR evaluation of the lumbar intervertebral discs, and their relationship to adjacent nerve roots, depends heavily on the presence of epidural fat (Figure 7-23). Following surgical disc removal, this fat is commonly replaced by epidural fibrous tissue complicating follow-up evaluation.

In patients with persistent or recurring symptoms following disc surgery the distinction between residual or recurrent disc herniation and post-surgical epidural fibrosis is important because of the potentially good surgical response of the former and poor surgical response of the latter. Myelography is rarely helpful in making this distinction. CT scanning, even with intravenous and/or intrathecal contrast, is often difficult to interpret in this situation. Magnetic resonance studies with direct visualization of the disc in multiple planes (Figure 7-24) may better differentiate epidural fibrosis from recurrent disc herniation than any other study available (Mikhael et al., 1985).

With magnetic resonance studies the level, size, and extent of bone removal can be assessed in a manner approximating that of CT (Figure 7-25). Although both epidural fibrosis and recurrent disc herniation are manifest as areas of less signal than the normal

Figure 7-4A: MR demonstration of posterolateral disc protrusion (arrow) causing nerve root (arrowhead) displacement.

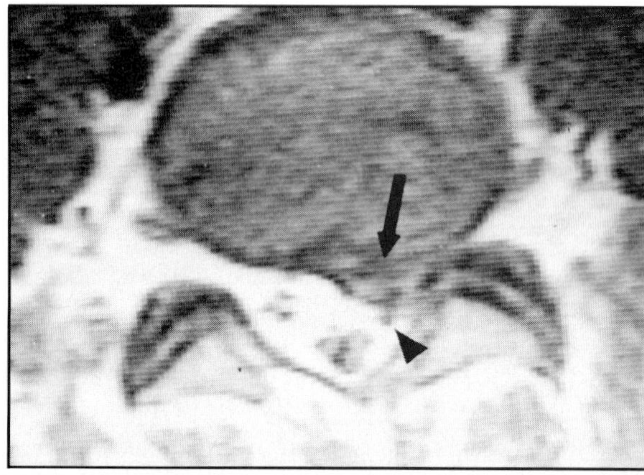

Figure 7-4B: CT scan of the same level shows similar findings.

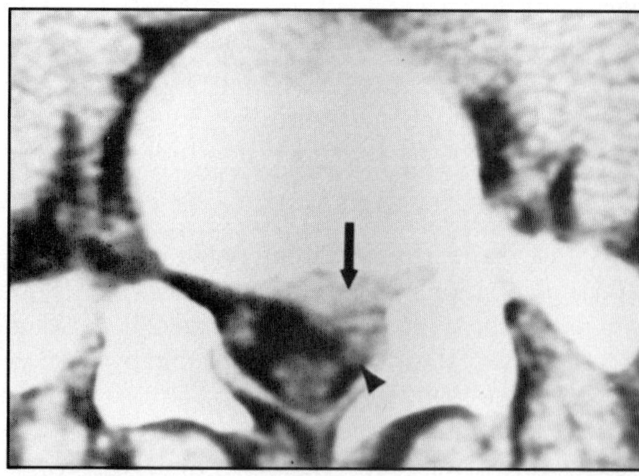

Figure 7-4C: Sagittal MR. The cross sections in A and B were obtained through the level between the transitional vertebra (T) and the sacrum. Disc extrusion (arrowhead) is confirmed. At the next highest level, there is pseudoretrolisthesis with the posterior inferior corner of the vertebra above (large arrow) displaced posteriorly with respect to the posterior superior corner of the transitional vertebra below (small arrow). Associated inferior disc extrusion at this level (blunted arrowhead).

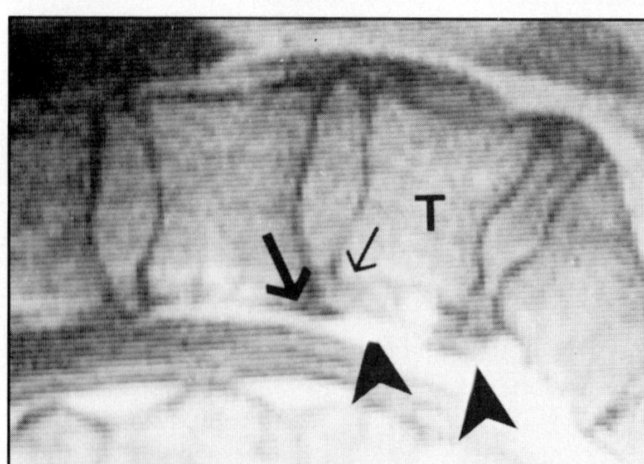

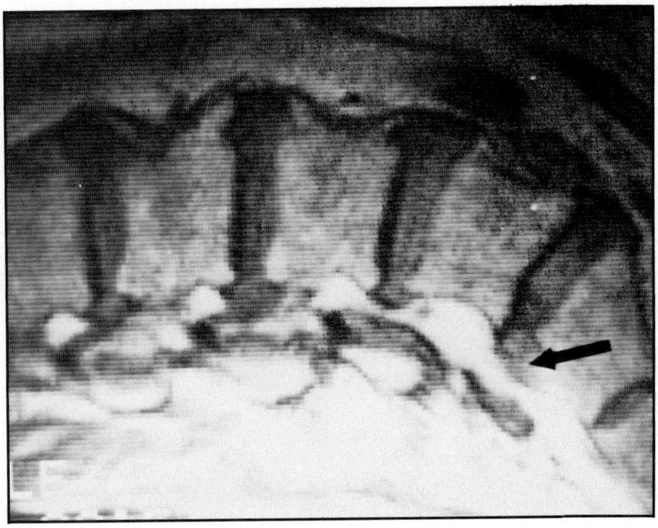

Figure 7-5A: Left parasagittal section. There is slight pseudoretrolisthesis of L5 with respect to S1. Extruded disc material (arrow) extends posterior to the superior end plate of S1.

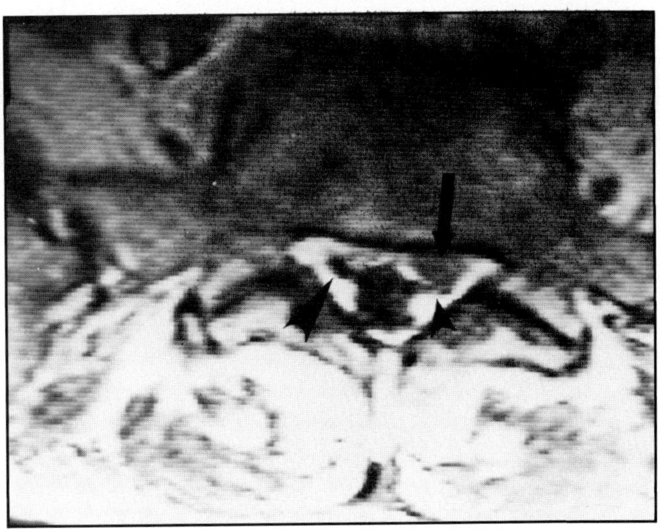

Figure 7-5B: Axial section through the superior end plate of S1. The extruded disc material (arrow) is displacing the left S1 nerve root (small arrowhead) posteriorly; the right S1 nerve root (large arrowhead) is normal.

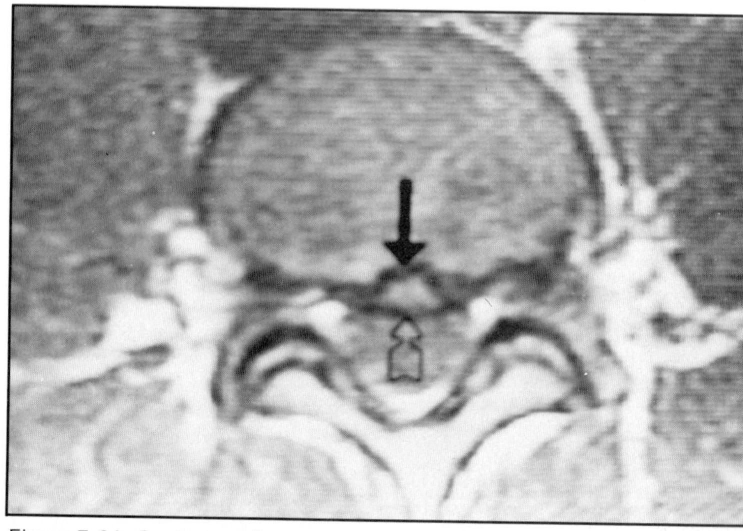

Figure 7-6A: Central subligamentous herniation (solid arrow) elevating the posterior longitudinal ligament (open arrow).

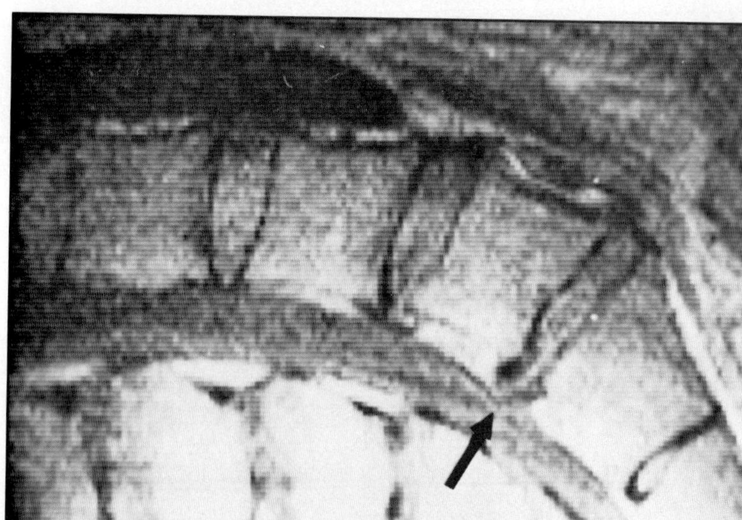

Figure 7-6B: Sagittal view. Elevation of PLL again noted.

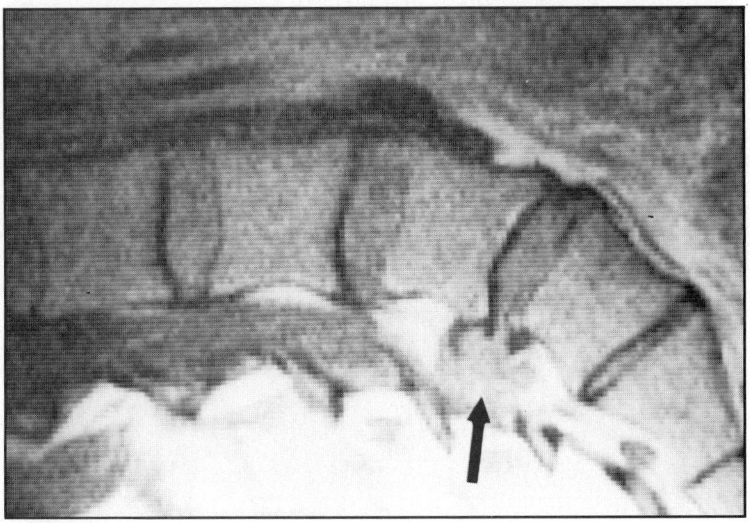

Figure 7-7A: Huge L5-S1 disc extrusion (arrow).

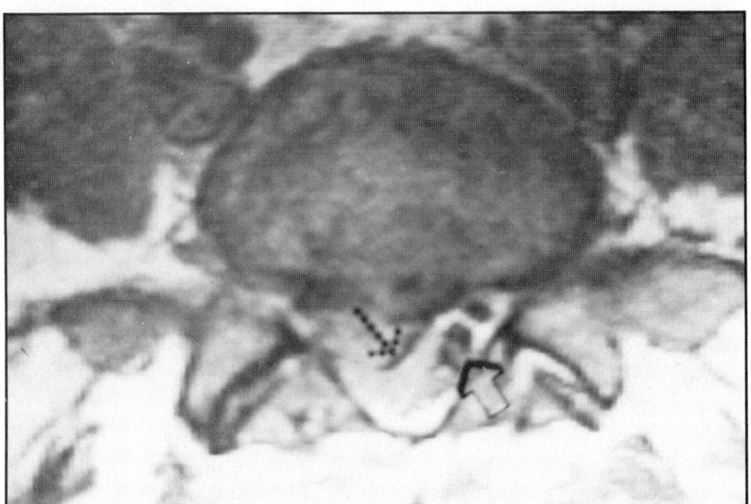

Figure 7-7B: Transverse section shows ment is associated with marked displacement and compression of the theca (open arrow) and "flap tear" of posterior longitudinal ligament (dotted arrow).

Figure 7-8: Extruded fragment.

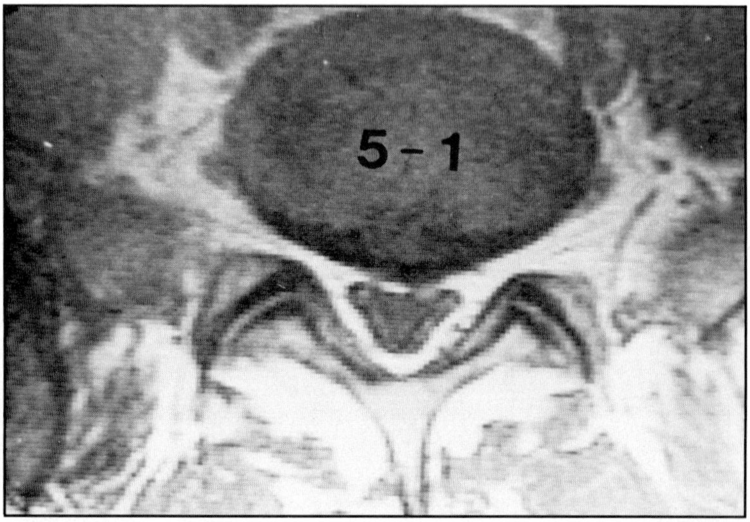

Figure 7-8A: Section through the L5-S1 interspace shows minimal abnormality.

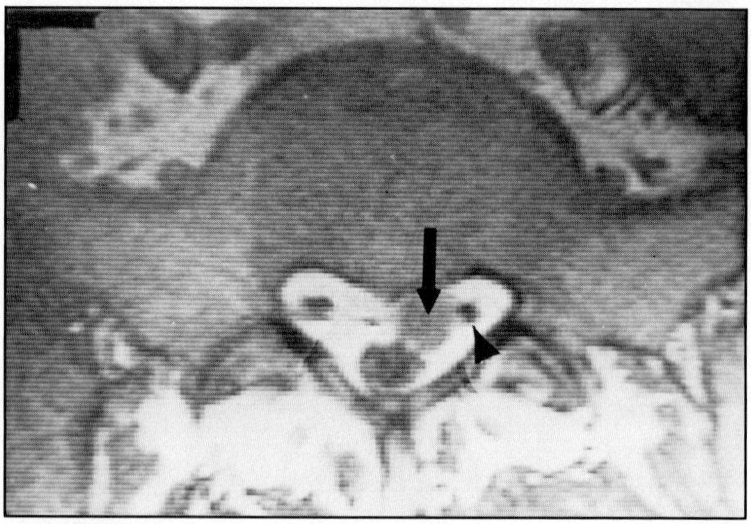

Figure 7-8B: Next section caudad through the upper portion of S1 shows free fragment (arrow) medial to the left S1 nerve root (arrowhead).

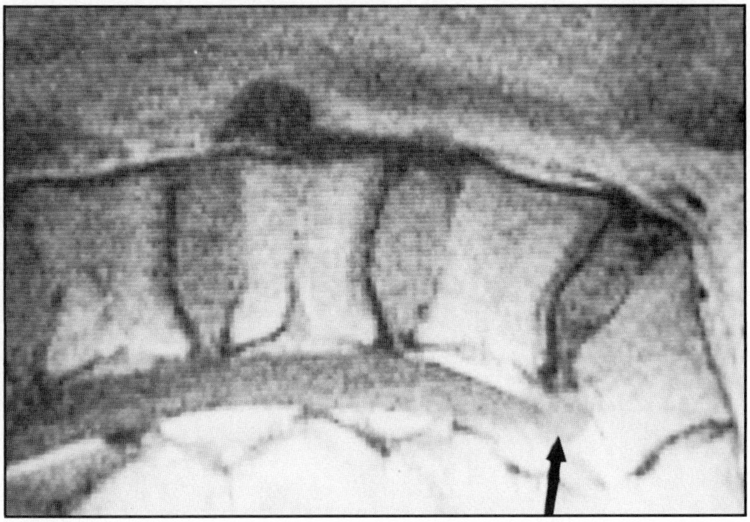

Figure 7-8C: Sagittal section showing the extruded fragment (arrow).

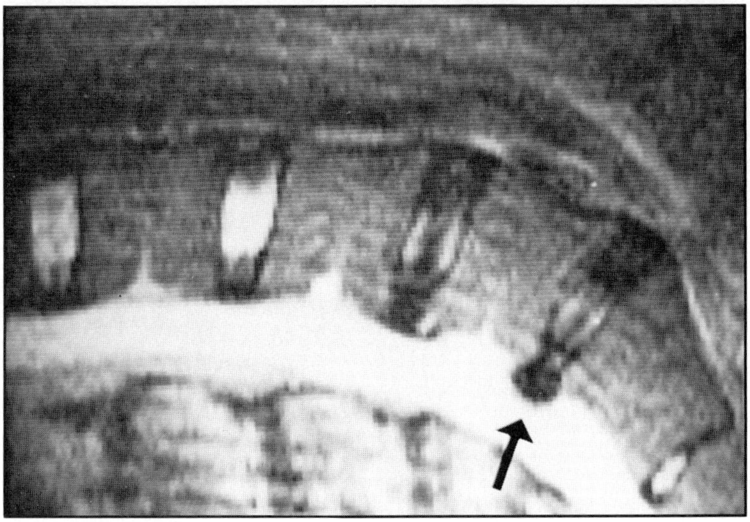

Figure 7-8D: T2 weighted image shows the loss of signal of the L4-5 and L5-S1 discs as well as the extradural defect (arrow).

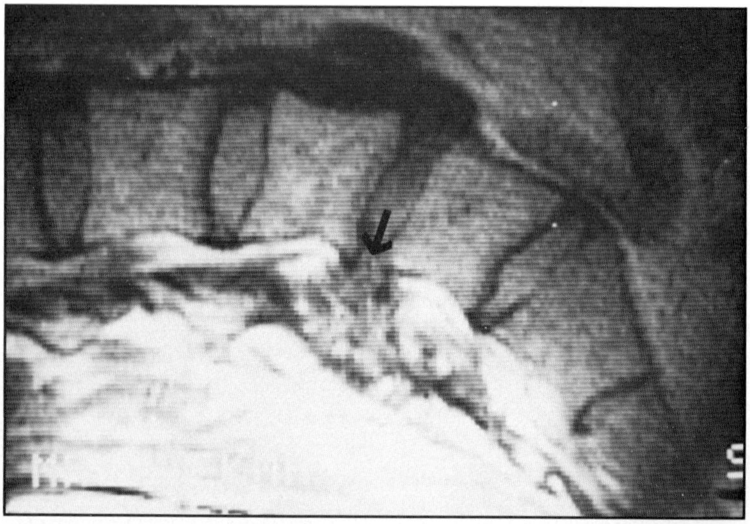

Figure 7-9A: Right parasagittal section through an extruded disc (arrow).

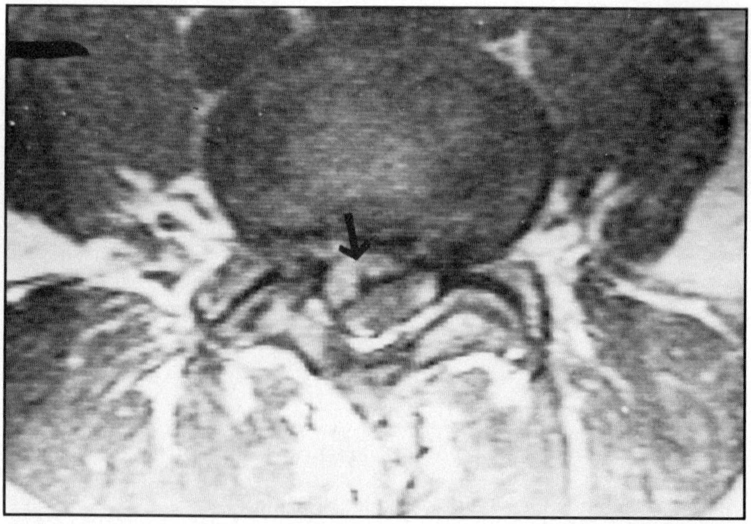

Figure 7-9B: Transverse section shows the disc fragment (arrow) with slightly increased signal. Note associated osteophyte spurs on right facet joint also impinging on the right lateral recess.

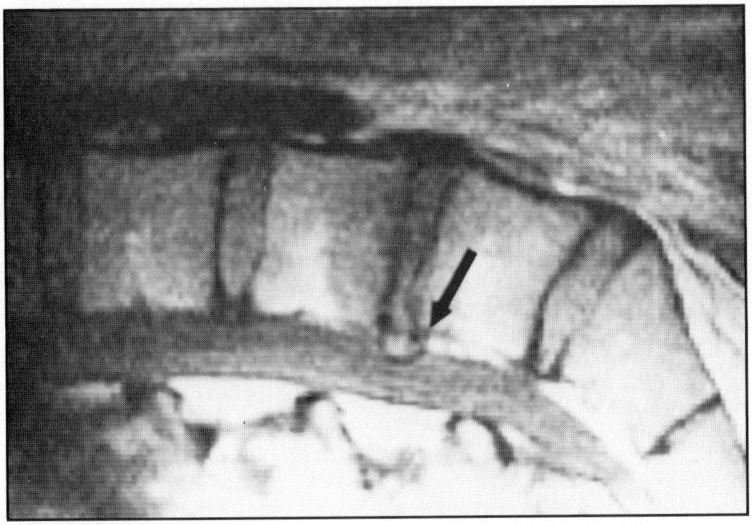

Figure 7-10: Postoperative recurrent disc (arrow) elevating posterior longitudinal ligament. A. TR2000,TE30.

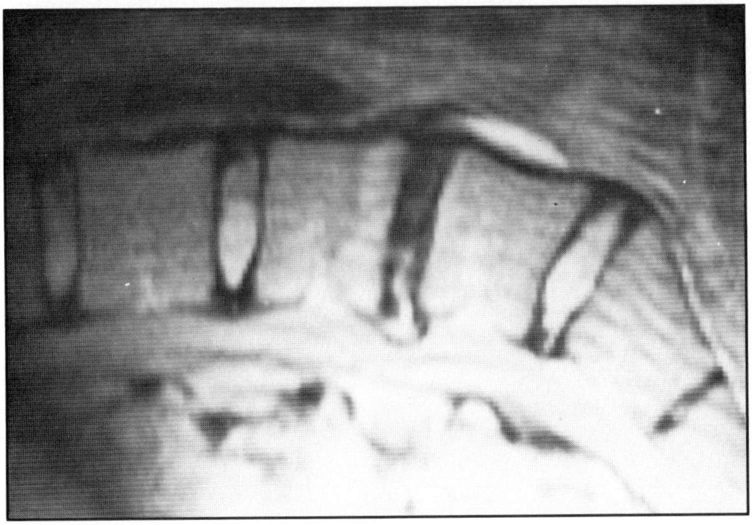

Figure 7-10B: TR2000,TE120. The recurrent disc shows bright signal as does the inferior marrow of the L4 body. No clinical evidence of infection.

Figure 7-11: Small central L4-5 disc protrusion. A. Axial MR.

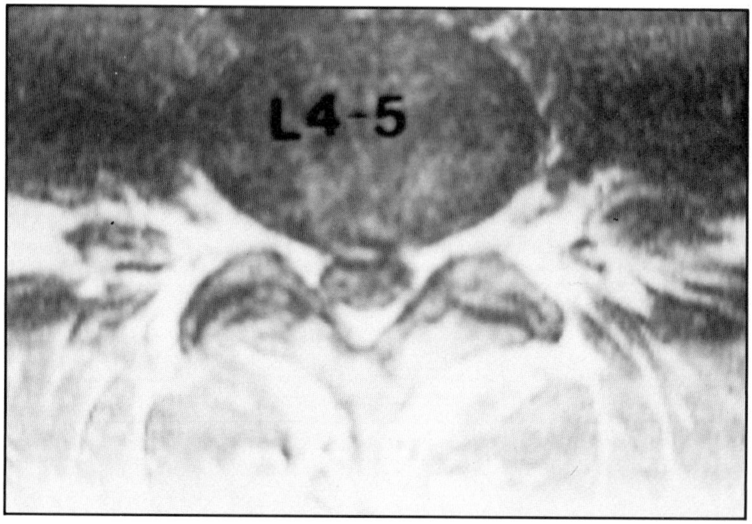

Figure 7-11A

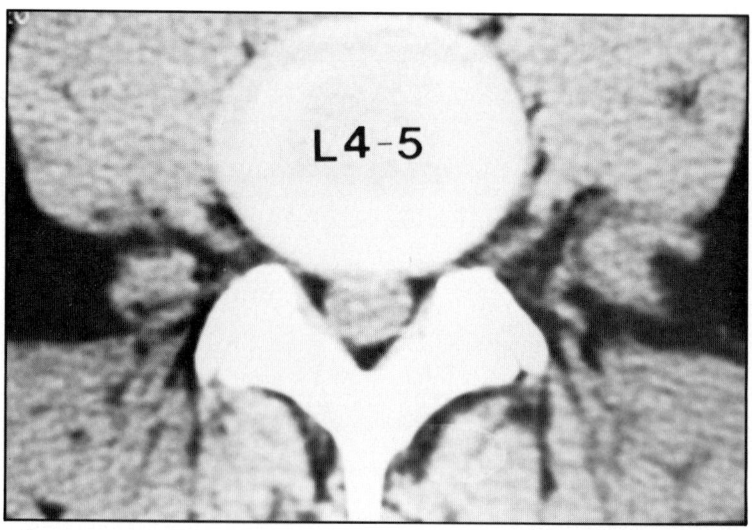

Figure 7-11B: Axial CT.

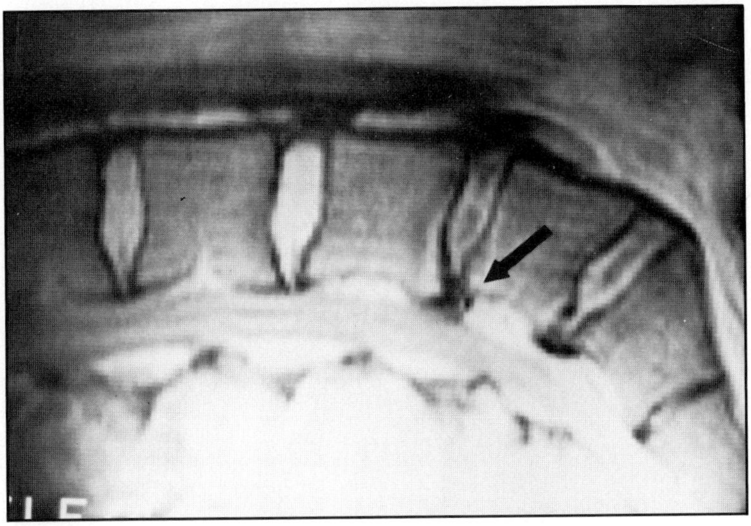

Figure 7-11C: Sagittal MR with TR2000,TE90. Note relative loss of disc signal and mild increased end plate signal as well as the disc protrusion (arrowhead).

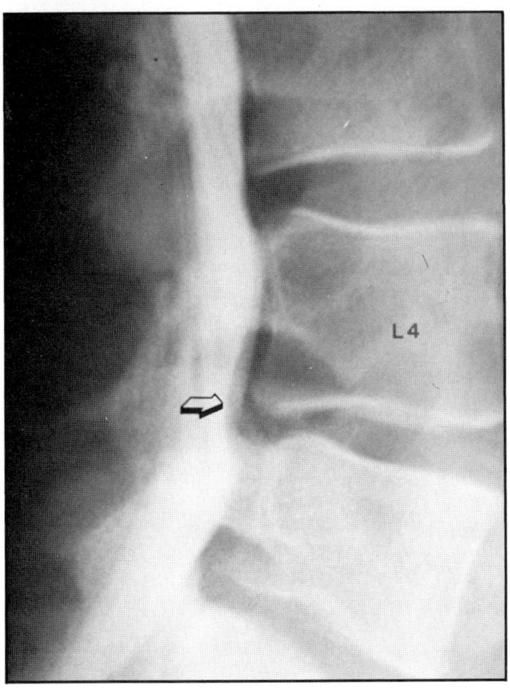

Figure 7-11D: Water soluble contrast myelogram with the anterior double density indicating extradural defect (open arrow).

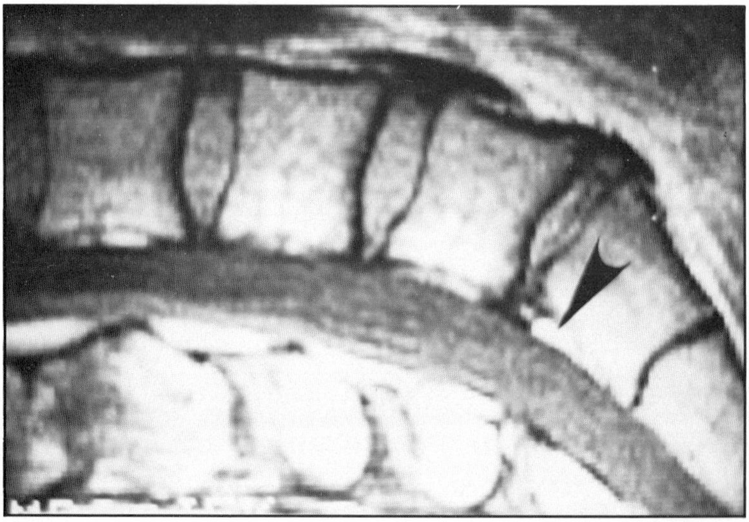

Figure 7-12A: Midline sagittal section. L5-S1 disc protrusion not indenting the theca in the midline, but there is a triangular high signal area ("fat wedge sign", arrowhead) inferior to L5-S1.

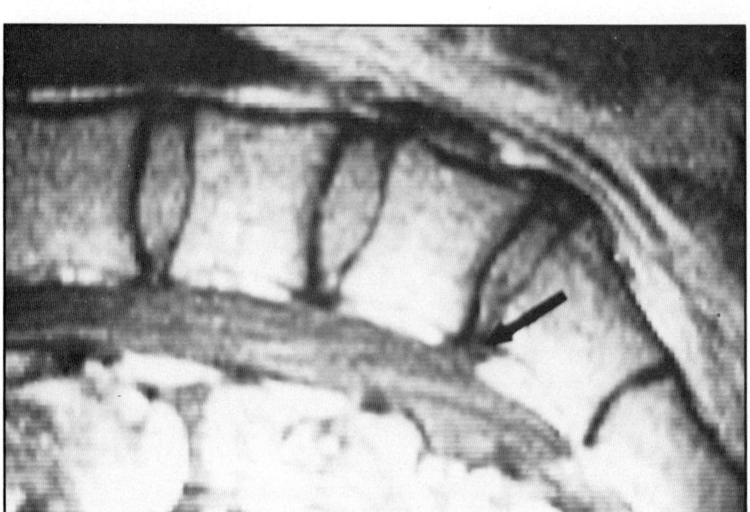

Figure 7-12B: Parasagittal section showing the L5-S1 disc herniation indenting the anterior theca.

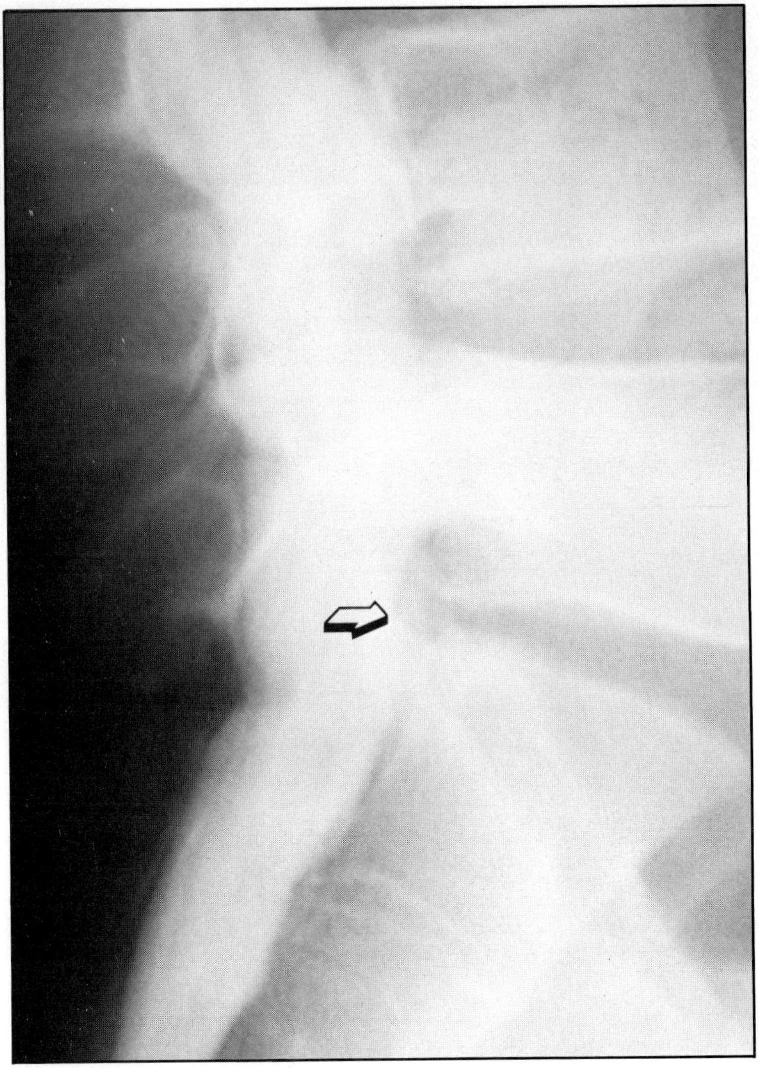

Figure 7-12C: Water soluble contrast myelography. Anterior extradural defect (open arrow) with double density sign.

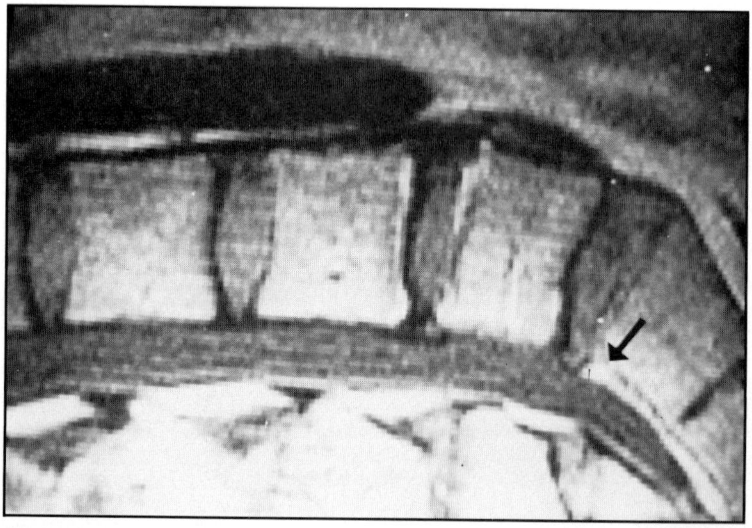

Figure 7-13A: Another central L5-S1 disc protrusion with "fat wedge sign" (arrow).

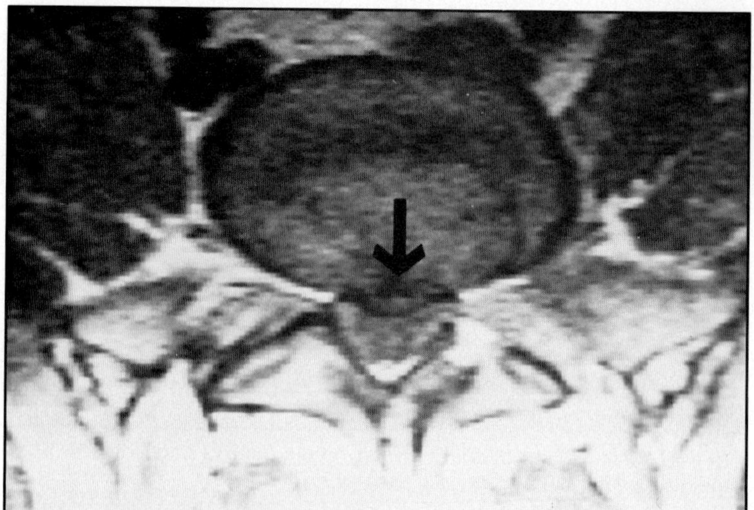

Figure 7-13B: Transaxial MR showing the central focal disc protrusion (arrow) indenting the theca.

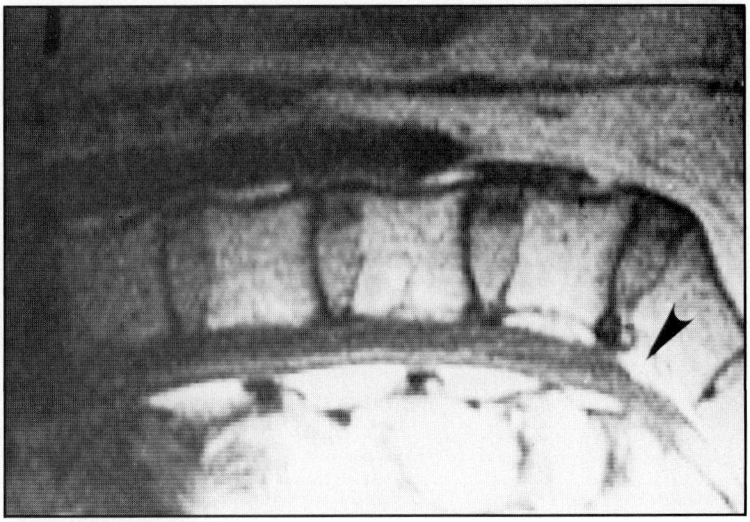

Figure 7-14A: Sagittal MR demonstrates another example of the "fat wedge" sign (arrowhead). There is slight pseudoretrolisthesis of L5 on S1. Little if any indentation of the theca.

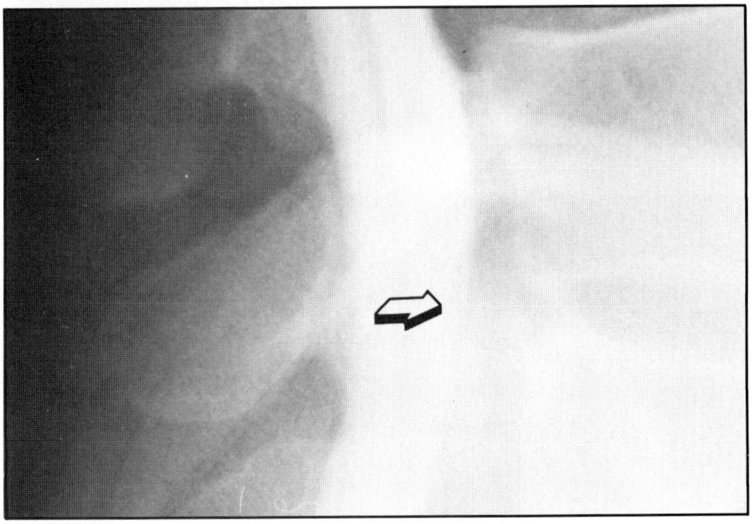

Figure 7-14B: Erect view from water soluble myelogram demonstrates subtle anterior extradural defect (open arrow).

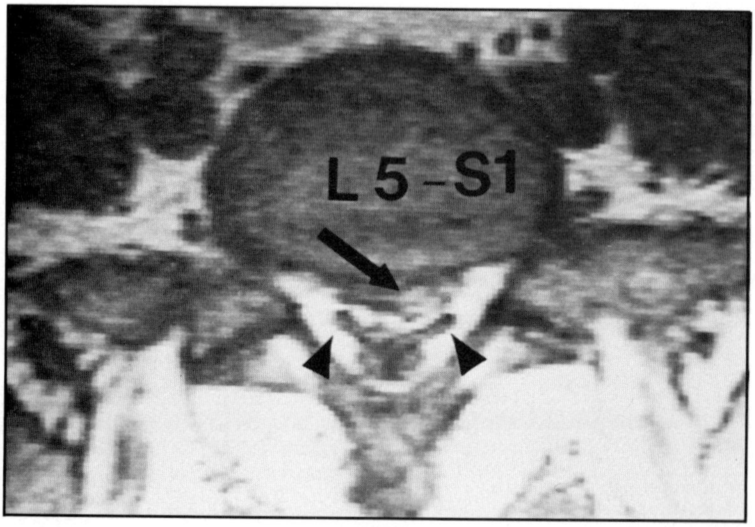

Figure 7-14C: Axial supine MR demonstrating the central disc protrusion (arrow). The S1 nerve roots (arrowheads) appear to be separated from the disc by a thin line of epidural fat in the supine view.

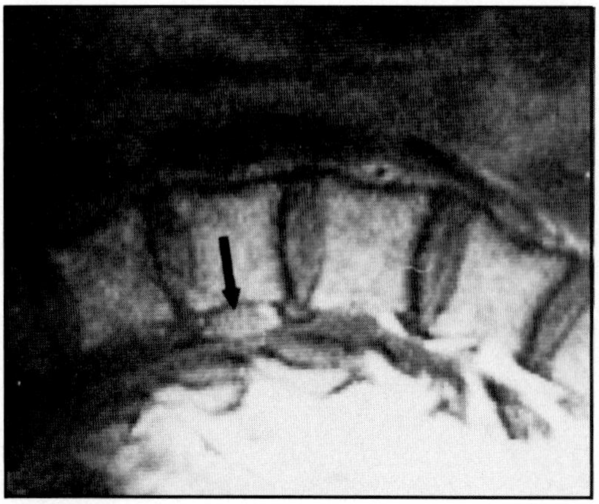

Figure 7-15A: Parasagittal MR demonstrating large free disc fragment (arrow).

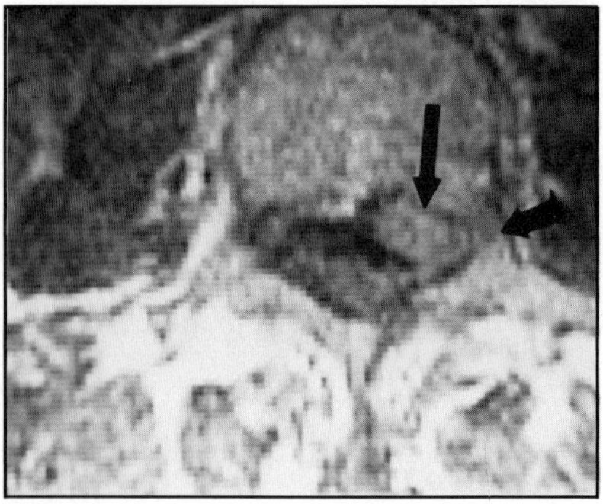

Figure 7-15B: Axial MR shows large free fragment (straight arrow) medial to the left L3 pedicle (curved arrow).

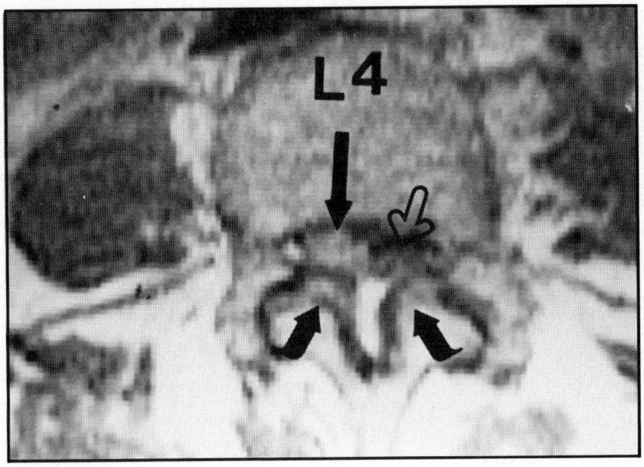

Figure 7-16A: Transaxial MR demonstrates free disc fragment in the spinal canal (solid arrow) medial to the right L4 pedicle. The theca (open arrow) is displaced. Mild central canal stenosis related to hypertrophy of the inferior articular facets of L3 (curved arrows).

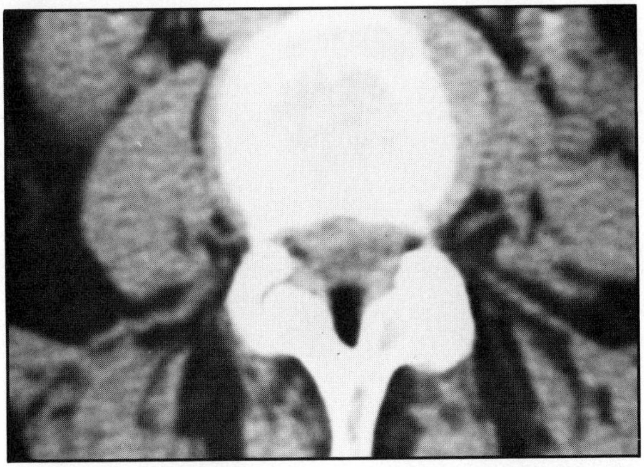

Figure 7-16B: CT scan through L4 level. The free fragment is seen with difficulty, if at all.

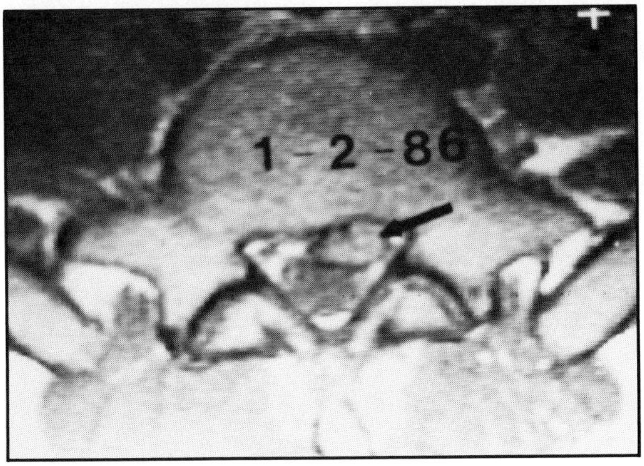

Figure 7-17: Free disc fragment (arrow) behind the right side of S1.

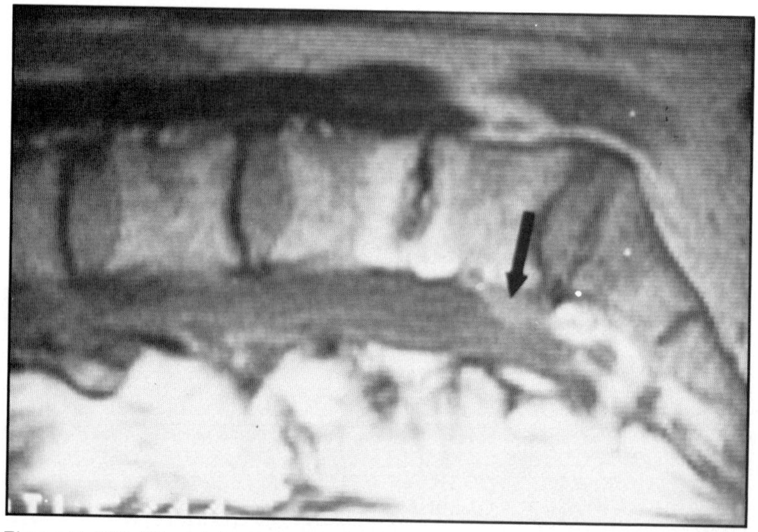

Figure 7-18A: T1 weighted sagittal MR. Extruded disc fragment posterior to L5 (arrow). Also present is high marrow signal adjacent to the degenerated L4-5 disc. This represents replacement of red marrow by yellow fatty marrow.

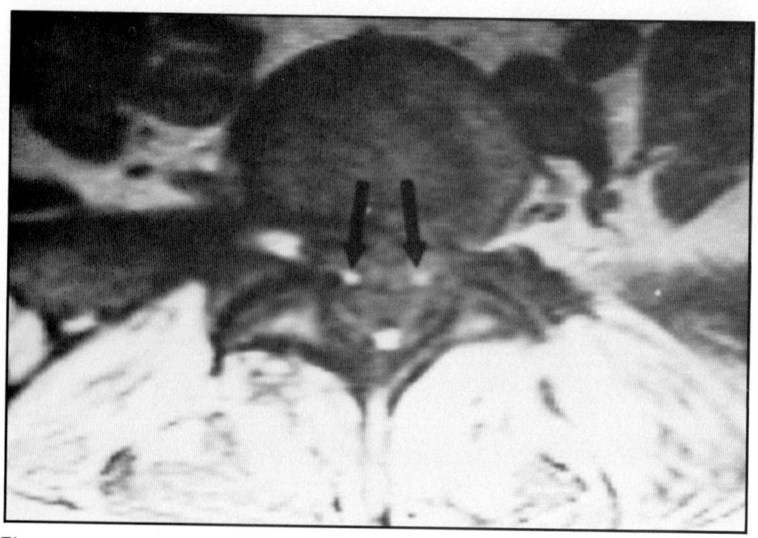

Figure 7-18B: Axial MR demonstrating the disc fragment posterior to L5 (arrows).

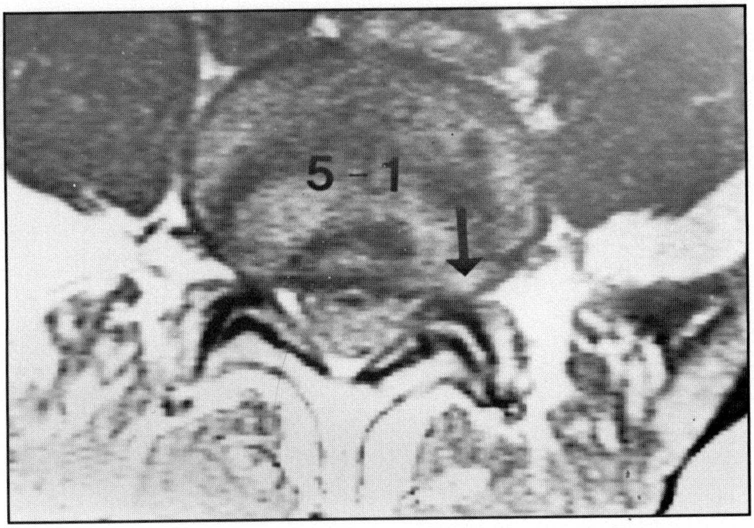

Figure 7-19A: Left lateral focal disc protrusion (arrow) impinging on intervertebral canal.

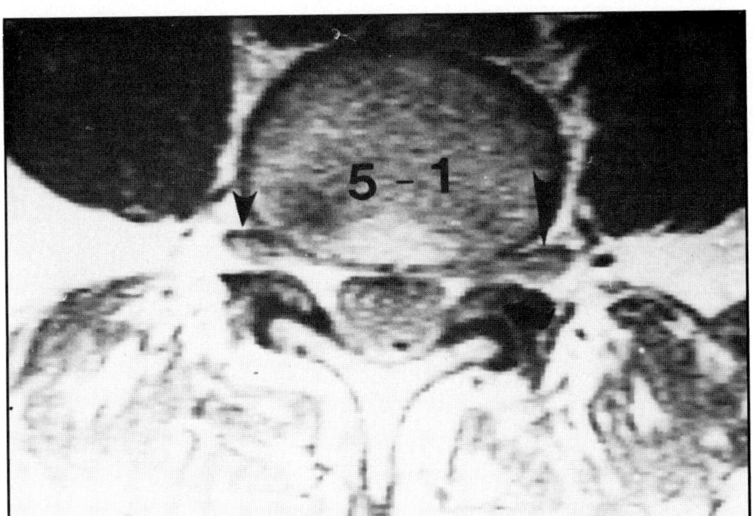

Figure 7-19B: There is mild swelling of the left L5 root (large arrow) as compared to the right (arrowhead).

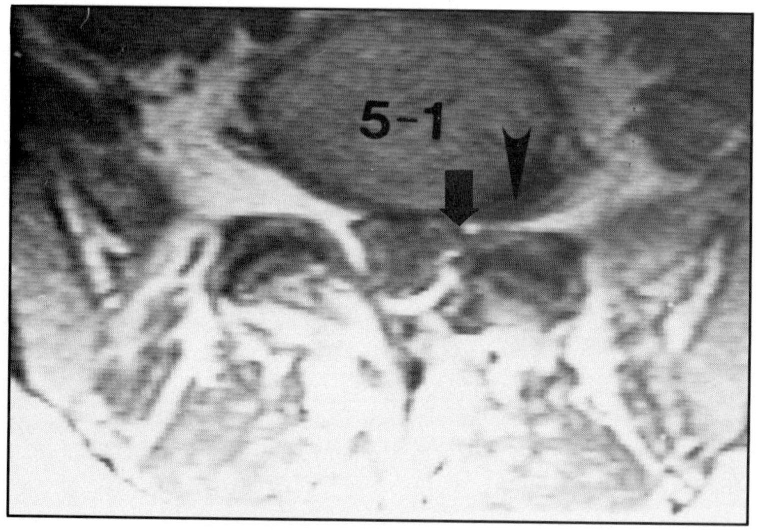

Figure 7-20A: Axial section through L5-S1. There is disc protrusion and/or osteophyte spurring impinging on the left L5-S1 intervertebral canal. Also indistinctness and loss of epidural fat about the left S1 nerve root (arrow).

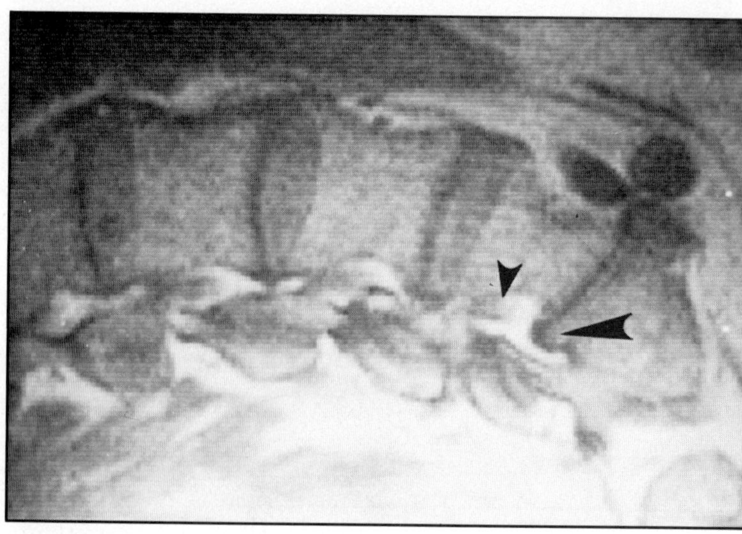

Figure 7-20B: Left parasagittal section. Disc protrusion and osteophyte spurring in the inferior half of the left L5-S1 intervertebral canal is confirmed (large arrowhead), but the left L5 nerve root (small arrowhead) is protected by abundant epidural fat and not significantly compressed.

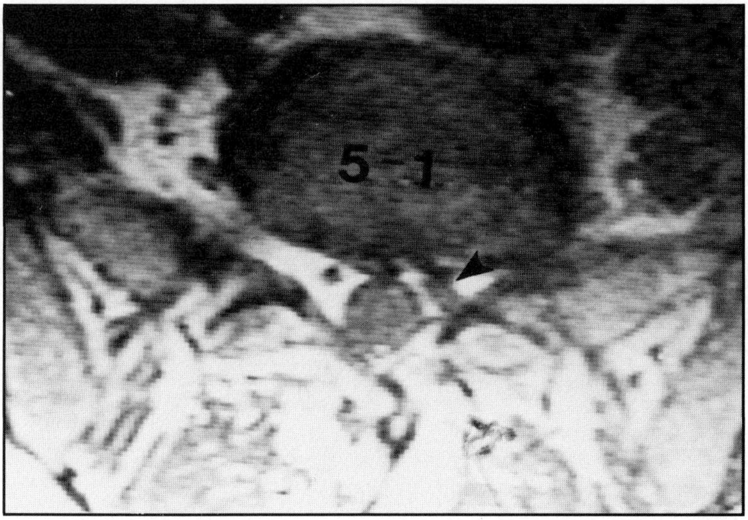

Figure 7-20C: Axial section more inferiorly through the L5-S1 disc does show abnormality related to the S1 root consistent with a disc fragment (arrowhead).

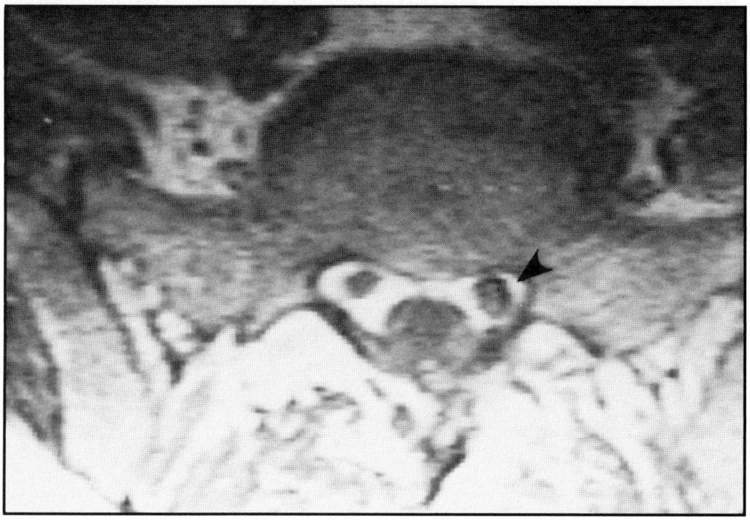

Figure 7-20D: Section slightly caudal to that in C demonstrates swelling of the left S1 root (arrowhead) confirming significant compression.

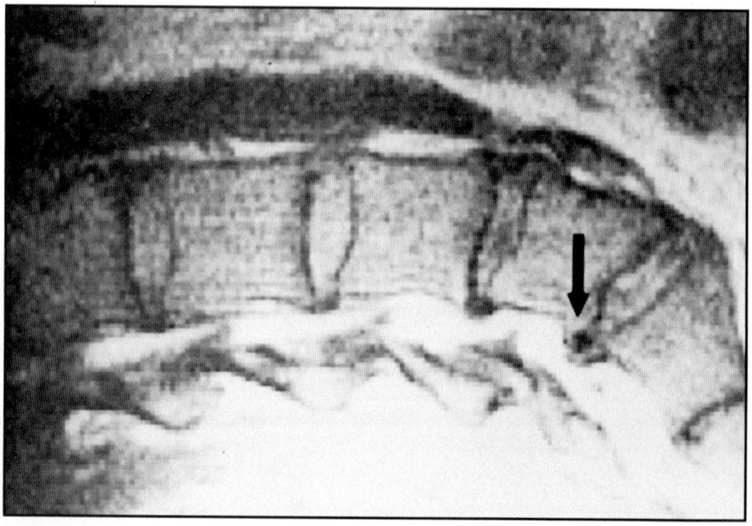

Figure 7-21A: Chronic disc degeneration of L5-S1 is accompanied by osteophyte spur which contains marrow (arrow), as compared to calcified spurs which produce decreased signal.

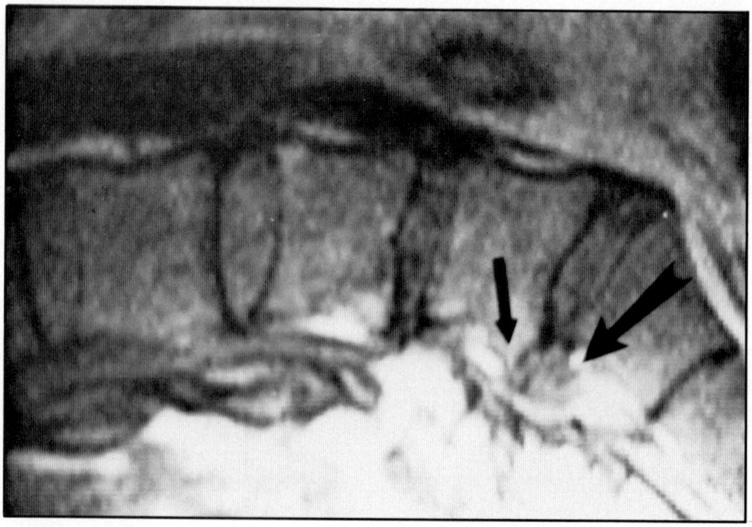

Figure 7-21B: Another example of chronic degenerative change with osteophyte spur (small arrow). This is associated with disc extrusion (large arrow).

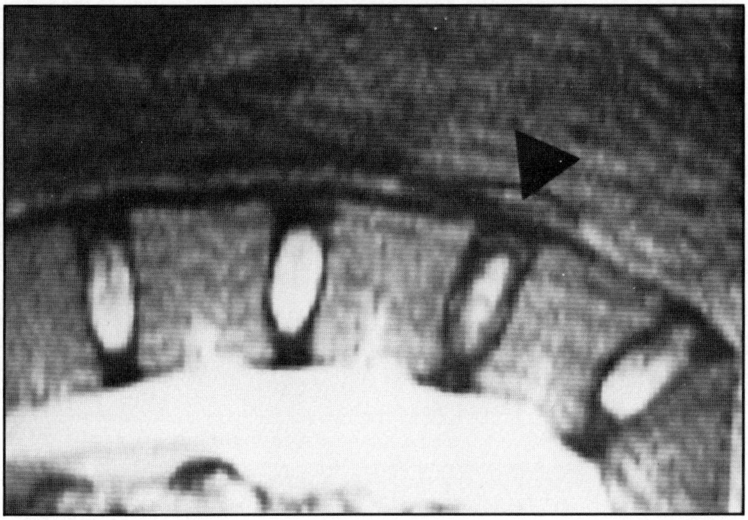

Figure 7-22: 23 year old female with back pain following injury. The only MR abnormality is very slight relative loss of the signal of L4-5 intervertebral disc. Significance is unknown.

Figure 7-23: Spinal evaluation by CT or MR relies largely on epidural fat (arrow). There is loss of the epidural fat detail on the postoperative right side following hemilaminectomy and discectomy with normal epidural fat on the left (arrows). A: CT B: MR.

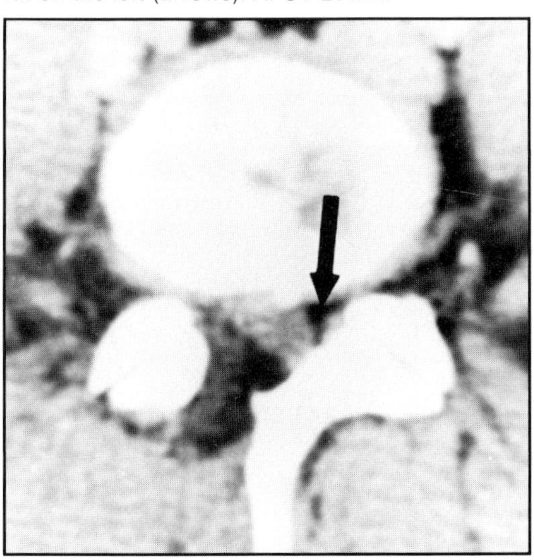

Figure 7-23A

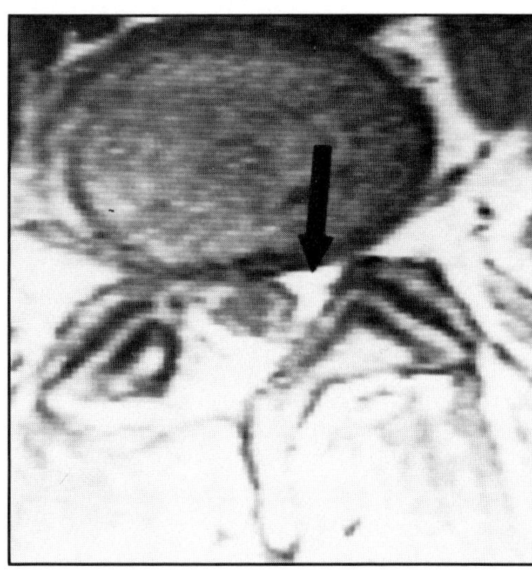

Figure 7-23B

Figure 7-24A: Sagittal MR demonstrating postoperative fat graft (arrow). There is relative decrease in the thecal signal at the operated level and poor detail and question of recurrent disc.

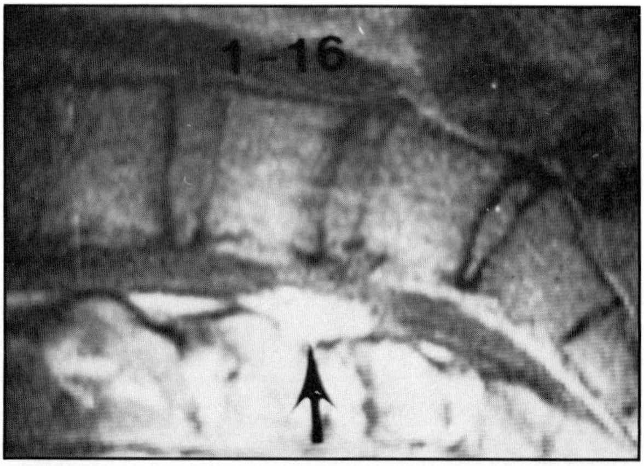

Figure 7-24B: Axial image showing the right hemilaminectomy and fat graft (arrow). The theca is deformed and compressed (arrowhead).

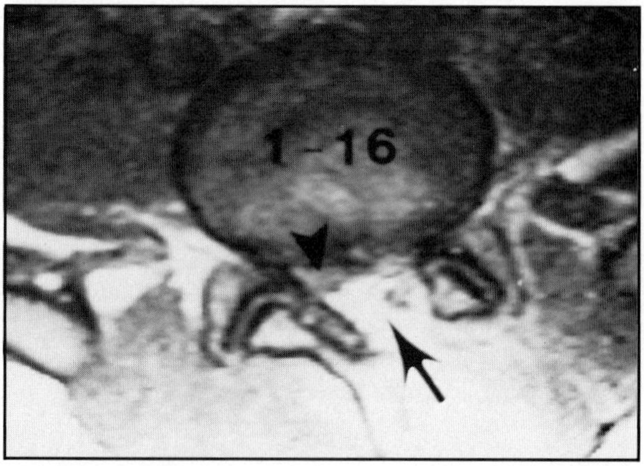

Figure 7-24C: Recurrent or residual disc herniation is evident (arrow) on a slightly more caudal slice.

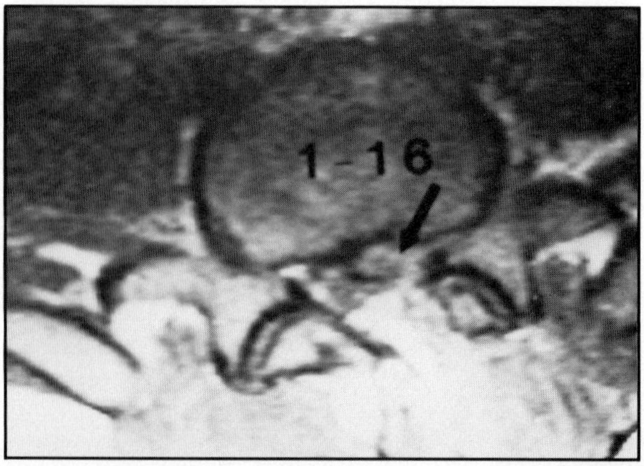

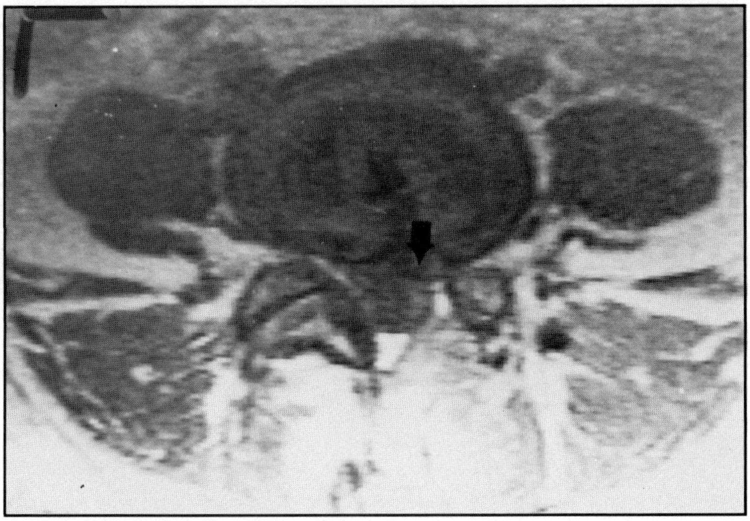

Figure 7-25A: Postoperative right hemilaminectomy at L4-5. The abnormal signal and loss of epidural fat in the right lateral recess (arrow) are visualized but not well characterized.

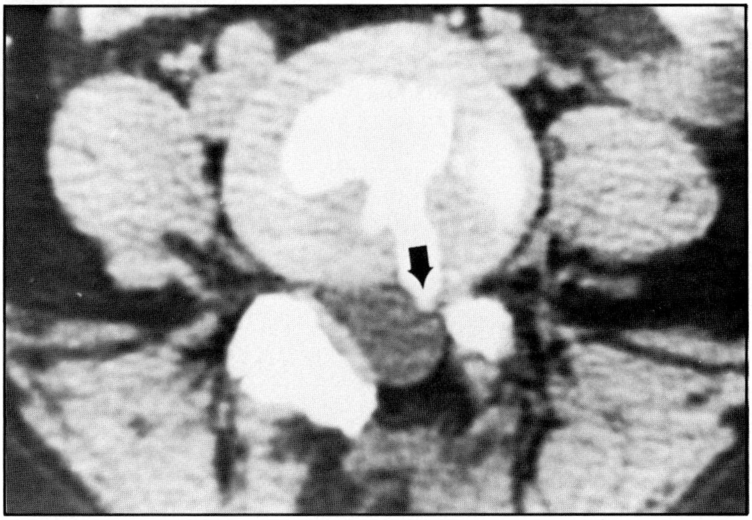

Figure 7-25B: Axial CT demonstrates extruding bone graft (arrow) following discectomy and posterior interbody fusion.

epidural fat, the presence of material in anatomic continuity with the disc space and iso-intense with the disc on various pulse sequences, helps distinguish extruded disc material from epidural fibrosis. Disc fragments not in continuity with the disc space remain difficult to identify.

Following successful chemonucleolysis with chymopapain the lumbar disc shows an accelerated degenerative response with a loss of height and hydration and a dissolution or retraction of previously protruding portions. This MRI response can be matched to clinical response with good correlation (Mikhael et al., 1985).

CHAPTER 8

Spinal Stenosis

Spinal Stenosis

Although Epstein (1976) described the plain film and myelographic criteria of central spinal stenosis and Kirkaldy-Willis and McIvor described the surgical findings of lateral spinal stenosis, the widespread recognition of lumbar spinal stenosis as a common and significant clinical entity awaited the advent of high resolution CT scanning as applied to the lumbar spine.

CT scanning, by providing direct visualization of the osseous and soft tissue anatomy of the lumbar spine, led to a rapid increase in our understanding of the various lumbar spinal stenosis syndromes. The CT features of the anatomy and pathophysiology of these syndromes has been well summarized by many authors including Heitoff and Ray (1984), Burton (1984), Dorwart (1984), and especially Rothman and Glenn (1985).

The features of lumbar spinal stenosis displayed on MR studies are in many ways analogous to those on CT. As compared to CT scanning magnetic resonance imaging has the advantage of allowing direct imaging not only in the axial but also in the sagittal plane with equal resolution. This is particularly helpful in evaluation of the intervertebral canals, for which reformatted sagittal CT studies offer only limited detail.

Lumbar spinal stenosis may be congenital, acquired, or both. Acquired spinal stenosis is most commonly on an idiopathic degenerative basis; narrowing of the spinal canal secondary to trauma, infection, or neoplasm (discussed in Chapter 9) are much less common.

Although measurements of the normal size of the spinal canal have been published (Lee et al., 1978), in practice the diagnosis of spinal stenosis by CT or MR depends less on measurement than on an assessment of the configuration of the spinal canal and the relative amount of space available for the thecal sac and nerve roots at various levels. This assessment must take into account the size of the spinal canal as it relates to the overall size of the vertebral bodies; in general a larger patient is expected to have larger vertebrae including a larger spinal canal. Smaller but normal patients with a smaller spinal canal will have a proportionately smaller thecal sac. The presence of normal epidural fat about the thecal sac and nerve roots is an important indicator in this regard.

Congenital Central Stenosis

The hallmark of congenital central spinal stenosis is a small but otherwise normal appearing spinal canal. Although absolute measurements have little value under most circumstances, with congenital spinal stenosis showing uniform diminution of canal size, an AP diameter of the spinal canal of less than 12mm is abnormal. These patients are usually not symptomatic until associated degenerative changes occur, but the diminished size of the spinal canal does increase the significance of even minor to moderate degenerative processes.

Acquired Spinal Stenosis

Anatomy

The *central spinal canal* contains the dural sac and its contents and surrounding epidural fat and vessels. It is bordered by the vertebral bodies, intervertebral discs, and posterior longitudinal ligament anteriorly; by the medial margins of the pedicles and articular processes laterally; by the lamina and ligamenta flava posterolaterally; and by the base of the spinous processes and junction of ligamenta flava posteriorly. The central canal is circular to oval at the upper lumbar levels (L1-3) and oval or triangular at the lower lumbar levels. In 10%-20% of the population, the configuration at the L5 osseous level is trefoil, not to be confused with the *pathologic* trefoil configuration related to facet hypertrophy (Dorwart, 1984).

The *subarticular recess* of the central canal is bordered anteriorly by the posterolateral vertebral body and disc, laterally by the medial margin of the pedicle, and posteriorly by the superior articular process. The upper portion of the subarticular recess behind the disc space has also been termed the "lateral recess."

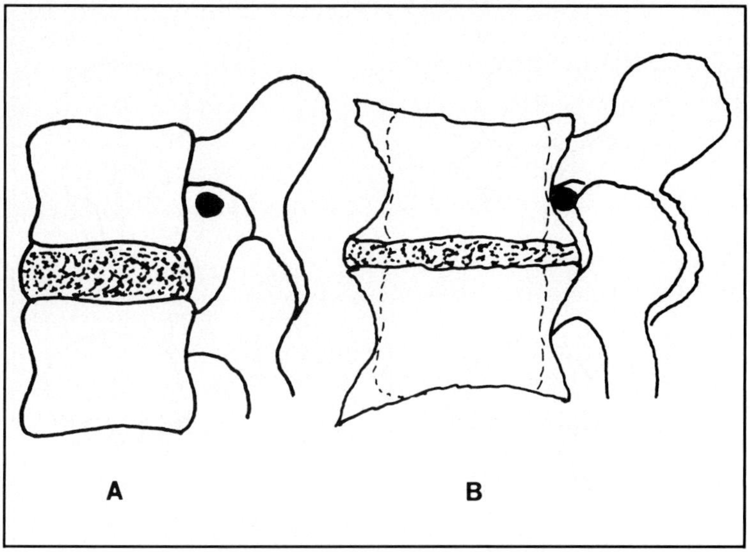

Figure 8-1A: Normal vertebral bodies, intervertebral disc, and articular processes. B. Severe degenerative change. There is loss of disc height, hypertrophy and osteophyte formation of the vertebral bodies and end plates, and hypertrophy of the articular processes, particularly the superior articular process.

The subarticular recess may be present normally at the osseous ring level in a trefoil shaped canal, but is also seen at the disc level when pathologic facet hypertrophy occurs. The term "subarticular recess" is used to indicate the position of this lateral extension of the central spinal canal beneath the facet articulation during posterior surgical approach to the spine.

The *intervertebral canal* (nerve exit canal) is bordered superiorly and inferiorly by the pedicles; anteriorly by the posterolateral aspect of vertebral bodies, end plates, and disc; and posteriorly by the superior articular process of the vertebra below. Medially it is continuous with the subarticular recess, with the intervertebral foramen indicating the lateral margin through which the spinal nerve exits. As noted in Chapter 5, the exiting spinal nerve root (e.g., L4 at L4-5) is located in the upper one-half of the lumbar intervertebral canal, although this relationship may be somewhat less constant at the L5-S1 level where the L5 nerve root is more vertically oriented and may exit lower within its foramen (Heitoff & Ray, 1984).

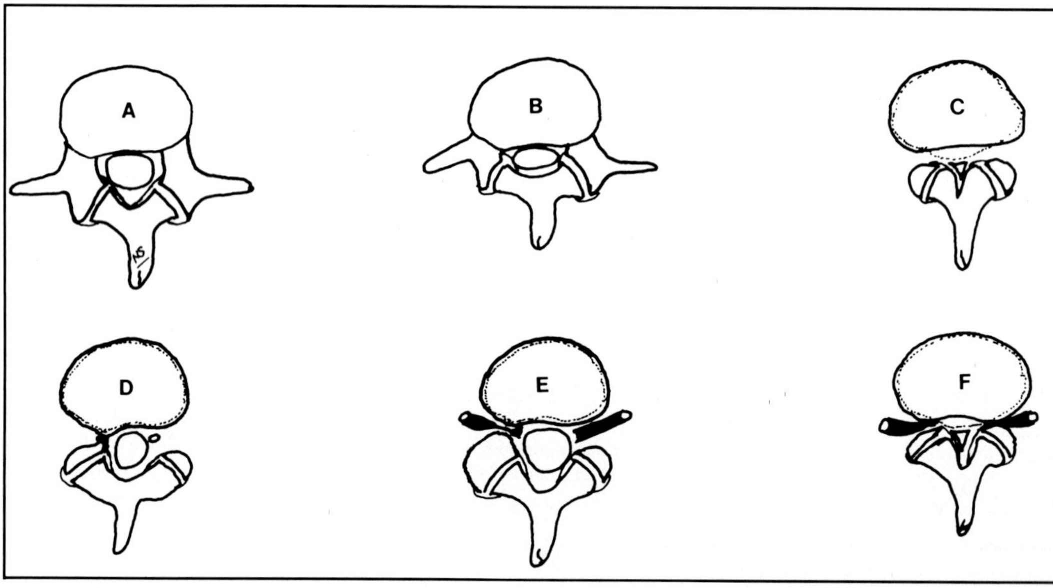

Figure 8-2: Spinal stenosis—types and pathologic mechanisms. A. Normal spinal canal. B. Congenital spinal stenosis with shortened pedicles. C. Central canal stenosis secondary to a combination of diffuse disc bulging and inferior articular process hypertrophy. D. Right subarticular (lateral) recess stenosis secondary to lateral disc protrusion and osteophyte of superior articular facet. E. Right intervertebral nerve root canal stenosis secondary to hypertrophy of the superior articular facet. F. Combined central, lateral recess, and exit canal stenosis.

Pathogenesis

The intervertebral disc and right and left facet joints between two vertebrae may be termed the "trijoint complex." These articulations are coupled mechanically in such a way that abnormality of the intervertebral disc may lead to secondary facet joint abnormalities, and vice versa (Figure 8-1).

Following acute and/or chronic injury the intervertebral disc may become desiccated and fragmented with resulting loss of disc height and function. Vertebral end plate hypertrophy and osteophytosis are often associated. Abnormal forces involving the zygoapophyseal joints lead to hypertrophy, particularly of the superior articular facets. Joint capsules and ligamenta flava become lax and/or hypertrophied.

Depending upon the particular pattern and combination of degenerative abnormalities, either compression of the thecal sac or of individual nerve roots predominates. Compression of the thecal sac causing direct compression of contained nerve roots or comprising their vascular supply may produce a clinical picture of multiple nerve root dysfunction (cauda equina syndrome). Compression of an individual nerve root in its subarticular recess or intervertebral canal may produce dysfunction of the nerve root involved.

Considering the frequency of spinal degenerative changes in an older population, the actual incidence of clinically significant lumbar spinal stenosis is remarkably low. The processes leading to degenerative spinal stenosis with bony overgrowth are clearly chronic, requiring years to develop. Factors determining the relationship of nerve root compression to nerve root dysfunction are not well understood.

Because of the differences in clinical presentation, and particularly in surgical approach, it is useful to divide acquired lumbar stenosis into three major types - central canal stenosis, subarticular recess stenosis, and intervertebral canal stenosis (Figure 8-2). Of course these types can, and often do, coexist.

Central Canal Stenosis

Adequacy of the diameter of the central spinal canal is best assessed by level to level comparison of cross-sectional images (Figure 8-3). Evaluation of sagittal and parasagittal images sometimes suggests the presence of AP diameter stenosis (Figure 8-4), but because of partial volume artifacts, axial studies are required for confirmation.

Significant narrowing of the central spinal canal is manifest as a reduction in cross section area of the involved level or levels as compared to those above and below. There is loss of the normal epidural fat, and compression of the thecal sac, frequently to only a few millimeters. Compression may be due to diffuse annular bulging, end plate hypertrophy and/or osteophytosis, hypertrophy and osteophytosis of the articular processes and facet joints, or hypertrophy of ligamenta flava. Most frequently a combination of these factors is present, causing a decreased sagittal diameter with a "flattened oval" configuration of the dural sac (Figure 8-5, 8-6). Pathologic trefoil configuration, related to hypertrophy of the articular processes, and concentric constriction of the dural sac are also common.

Surgical treatment of central canal stenosis consists of posterior decompression of the involved level or levels (Figure 8-7). This requires bilateral laminectomy with excision of hypertrophied ligamenta flava. Medial facetectomy is required when

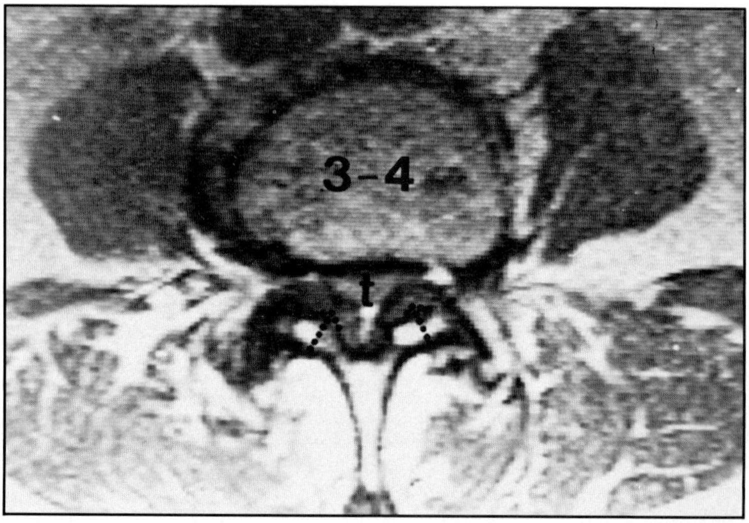

Figure 8-3A: Axial image through L3-4 shows central canal stenosis, with compression of the theca (T) by the hypertrophied inferior articular facets of L3 and hypertrophied ligamenta flava (dotted arrows).

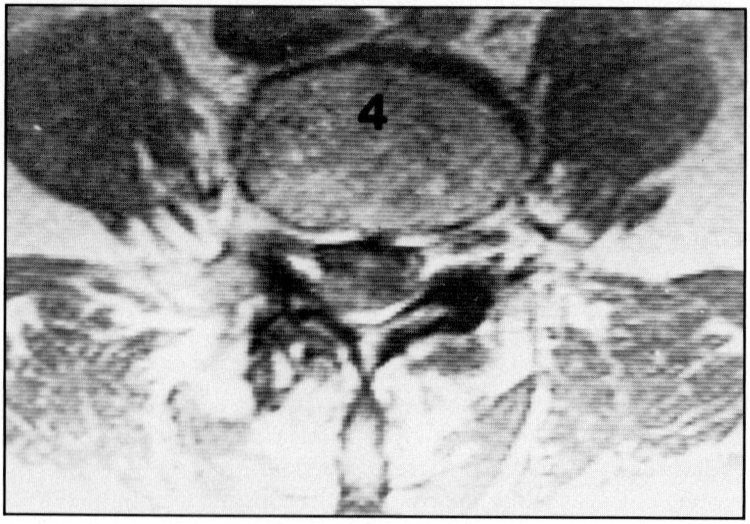

Figure 8-3B: Axial section through L4 shows normal cross-sectional area of the theca.

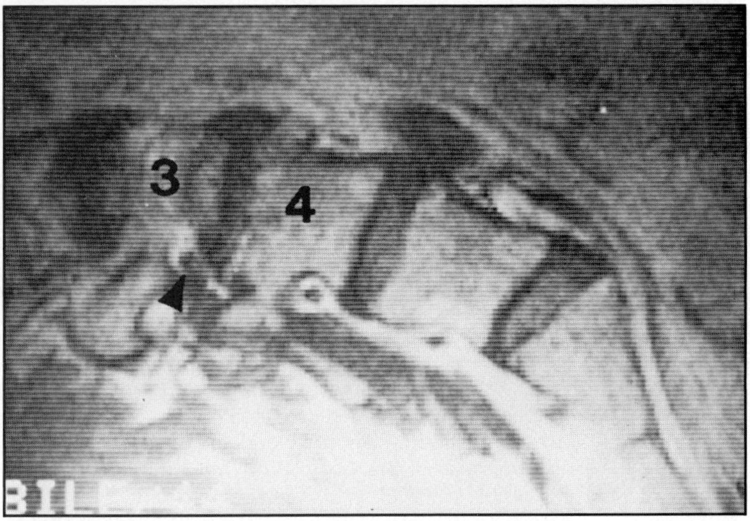

Figure 8-3C: Parasagittal section shows associated lateral stenosis with compression of the L3 nerve root (arrowhead).

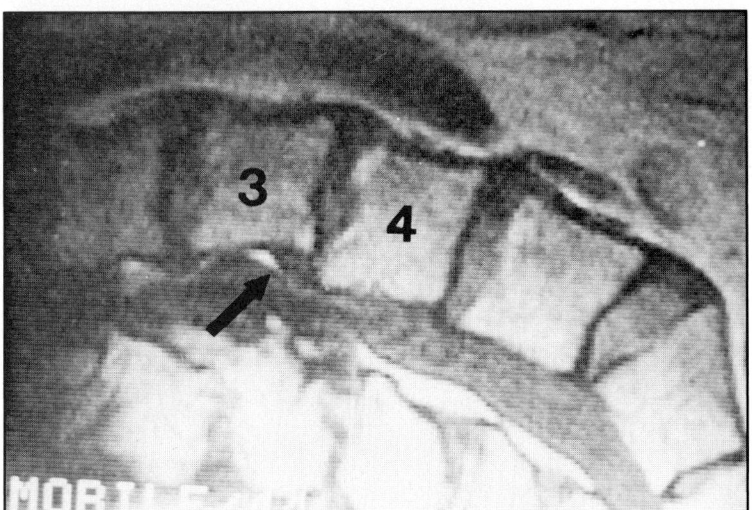

Figure 8-3D: There is associated degenerative spondylolisthesis at L3-4.

Figure 8-4: Central canal stenosis at L3-4.

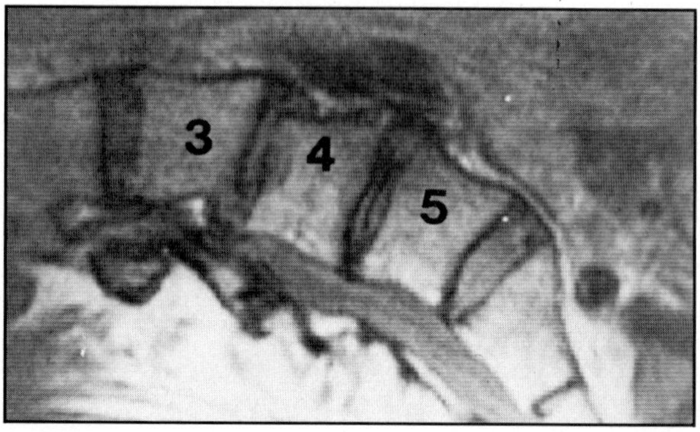

Figure 8-4A: Sagittal section showing degenerative spondylolisthesis of L3 with respect to L4. The section is slightly angled to the true sagittal plane so that the theca is sectioned posterior to L4 and L5 but not L3.

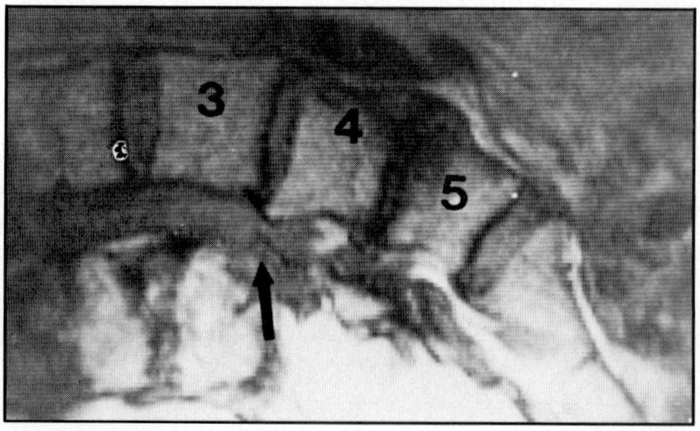

Figure 8-4B: Adjacent section now showing the theca at the upper lumbar levels. Narrowing posterior to the L3-4 is demonstrated.

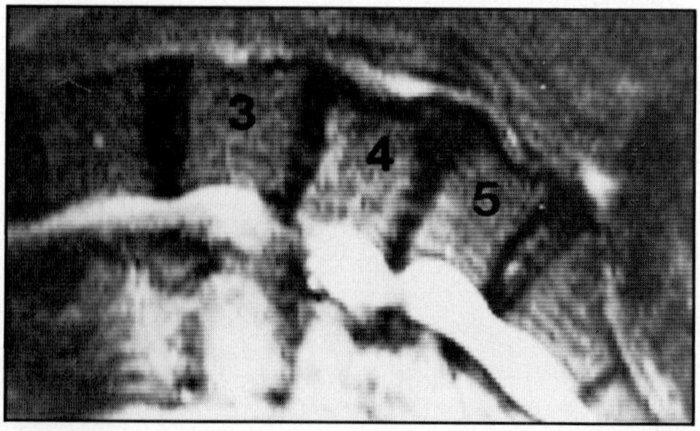

Figure 8-4C: T2 weighted image showing L3-4 spinal stenosis on the myelogram-like picture.

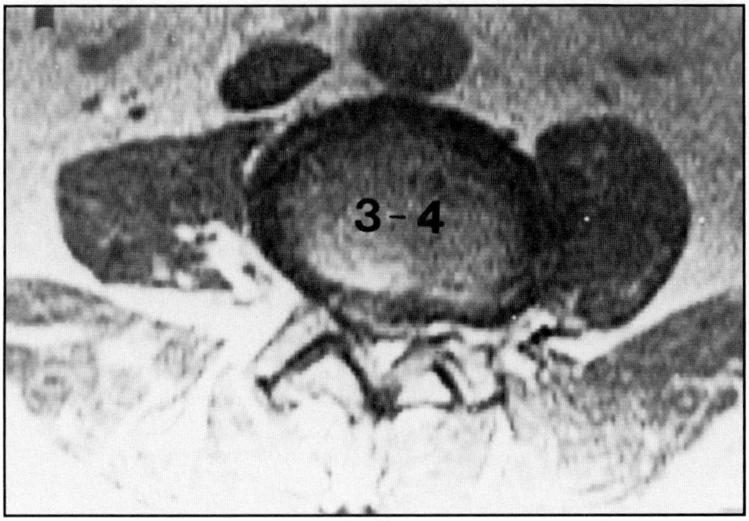

Figure 8-5: Axial section through L3-4 demonstrating narrowed central canal with compressed theca.

hypertrophied inferior articular facets impinge on the central canal.

Subarticular Recess Stenosis

The subarticular or lateral recess is bounded anteriorly by the intervertebral disc, end plates, and vertebral bodies; laterally by the pedicle; and posteriorly by the superior articular facet. Hypertrophy of any of these structures may entrap and compress the nerve root as it passes medial to the pedicle prior to exiting through the intervertebral canal. The most common offending element is a hypertrophied superior articular facet (Figures 8-8 through 8-10), but focal disc protrusions or end plate osteophytes may also contribute (Figure 8-11). Central canal stenosis often co-exists. Surgical decompression of the lateral recess depends on partial resection of the superior articular facet, preserving as much of the facet joint as possible in order to preserve stability.

Intervertebral Canal Stenosis

Diagnosis of stenosis of the intervertebral canal, sometimes called *lateral* or *foraminal* stenosis, depends on high quality sectional images such as obtained with high resolution CT or MR. In

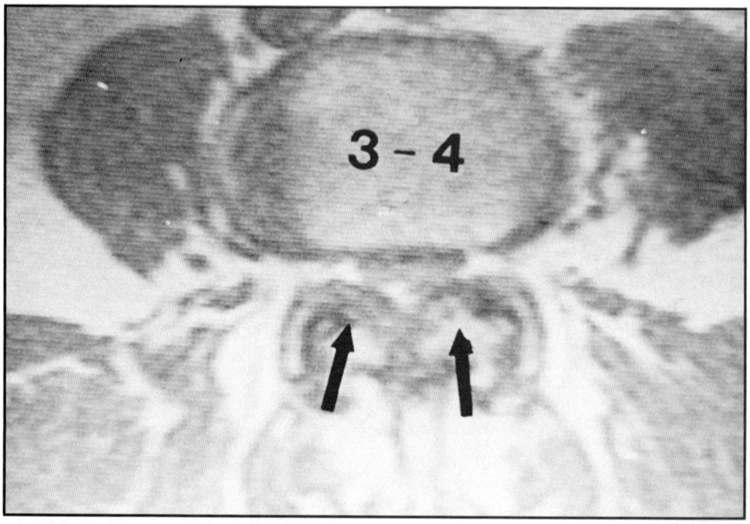

Figure 8-6A: Central canal stenosis at L3-4 associated with hypertrophied inferior articular processes of L3 (arrows).

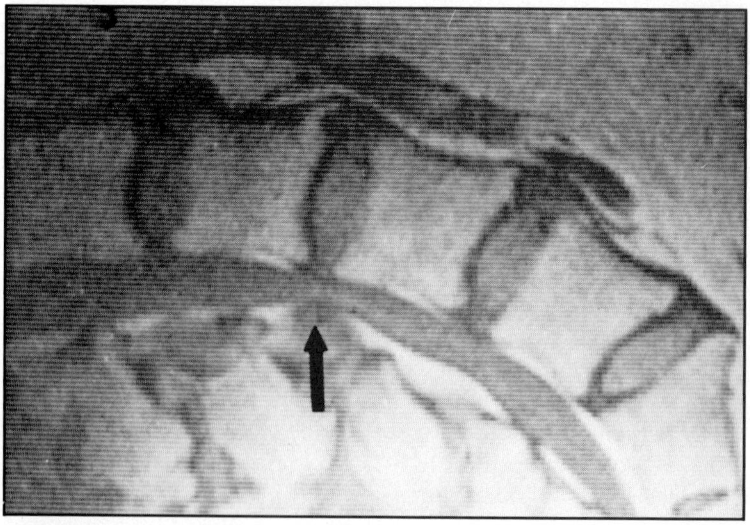

Figure 8-6B: Sagittal MR showing the posterior indentation of the theca (arrows).

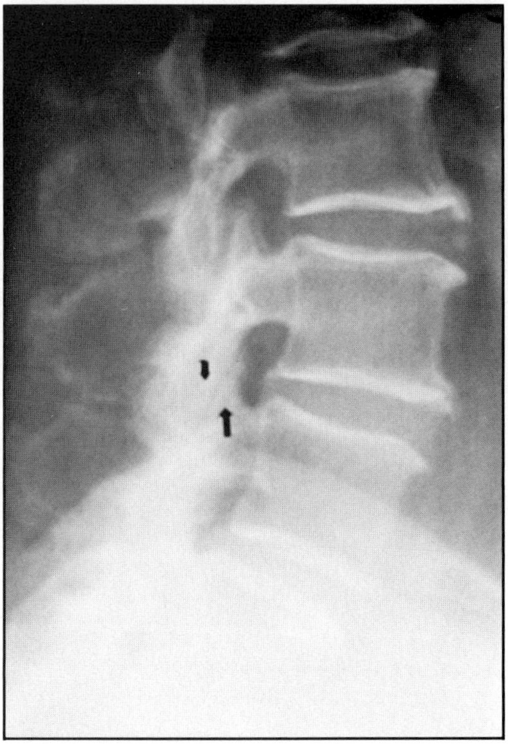

Figure 8-6C: Lateral radiograph demonstrates the hypertrophy of the inferior articular processes of L3 (curved arrow).

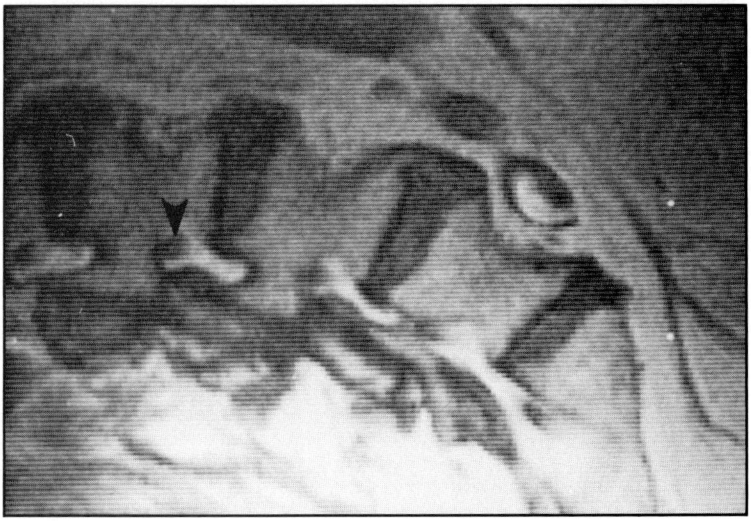

Figure 8-6D: Parasagittal image shows no significant lateral stenosis, with the L3 nerve root (arrowhead) surrounded by epidural fat.

Figure 8-7: Postoperative decompression at L4-5.

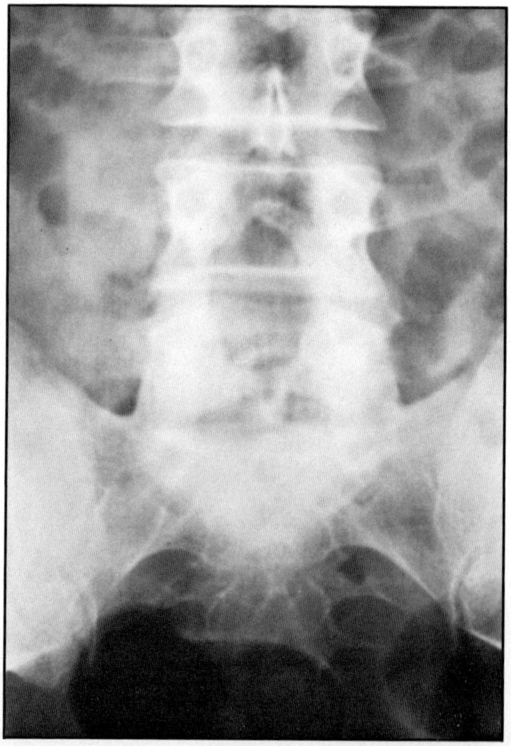

Figure 8-7A: AP radiograph.

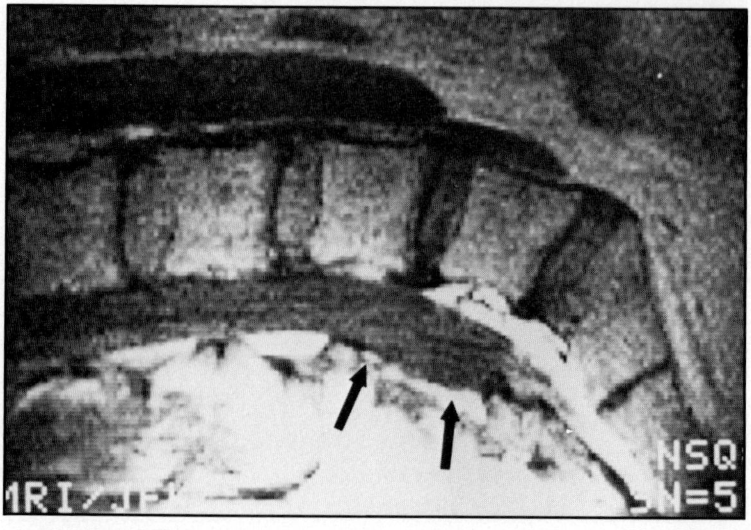

Figure 8-7B: Sagittal MR. The theca bulges posteriorly into the laminectomy site (arrows).

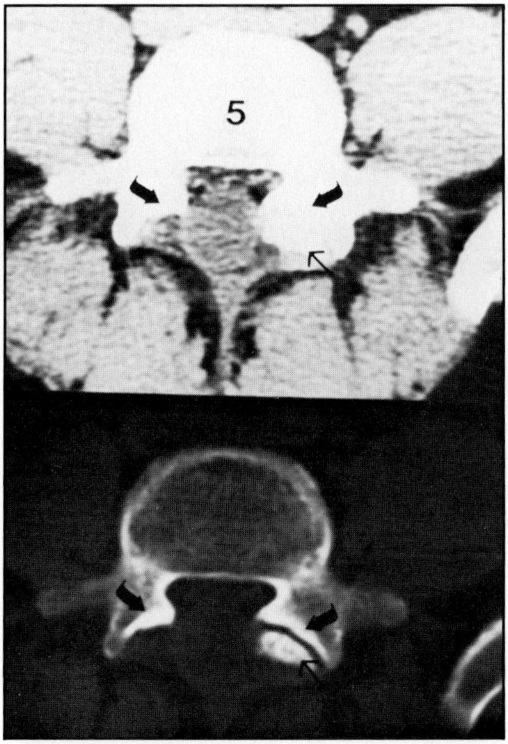

Figure 8-7C: CT scan through L5 vertebral body at the level of the pedicles. The theca is displaced slightly posteriorly. Superior articular processes of L5 (curved arrows) are displayed. The left inferior articular facet of L4 is demonstrated; the right has been excised.

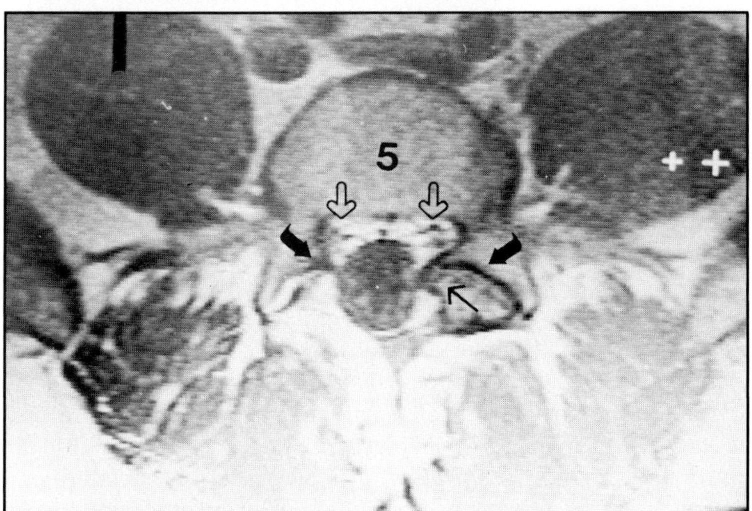

Figure 8-7D: Corresponding axial MR study through L5. Epidural veins can be seen running within the epidural fat (open arrows). Superior articular processes of L5 (curved arrows) as well as the left inferior articular process of L4 (straight arrow) are well demonstrated. Osteophyte of this articular process displaces the theca towards the right.

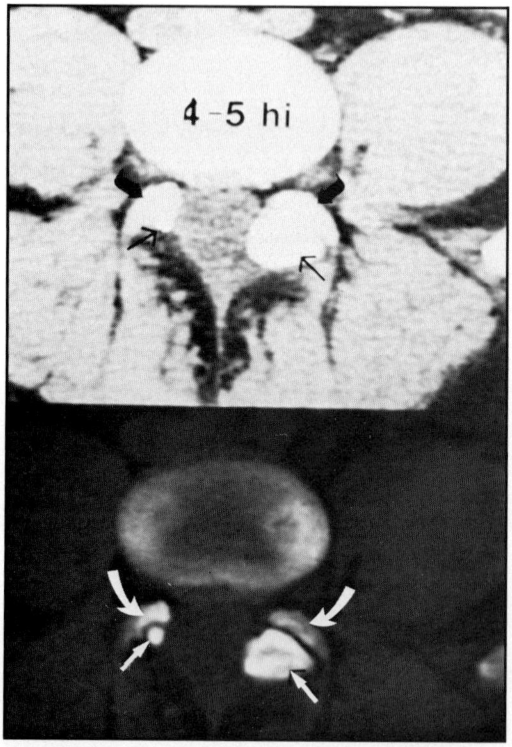

Figure 8-7E: CT section through the L4-5 disc and inferior end plate of L4. Articular processes are again demonstrated including small residual portion of the right inferior process of L4 (straight arrow) following the extensive medial facetectomy.

the past several years there has been a marked increase in our understanding of the diagnosis and treatment of lateral spinal stenosis, particularly as it relates to the "failed back surgery syndrome" (Burton, 1984). The importance of diagnosing lateral stenosis is emphasized by a multi-institutional survey (Burton et al., 1981) demonstrating unrecognized lateral spinal stenosis as the cause of more than one half the cases of failed back surgery studied.

Factors causing nerve entrapment within the intervertebral canal (Figure 8-12) include vertebral or facet joint osteophytes, diffuse annular bulging or focal disc protrusion, and hypertrophy of the superior articular facet. Narrowing of the intervertebral disc is associated with narrowing of the intervertebral canal in an up/down direction. Overriding articular facets associated with retrolisthesis and/or spondylolisthesis also contribute to narrowing of the intervertebral canal. Most commonly neural compression results from a combination of these factors rather from an

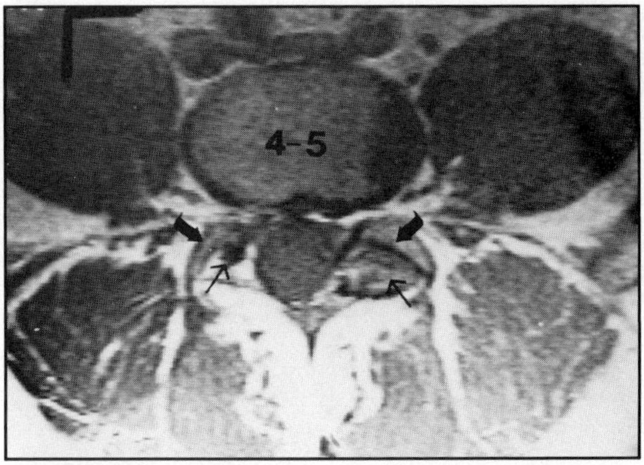

Figure 8-7F: Corresponding axial MR section shows similar anatomy.

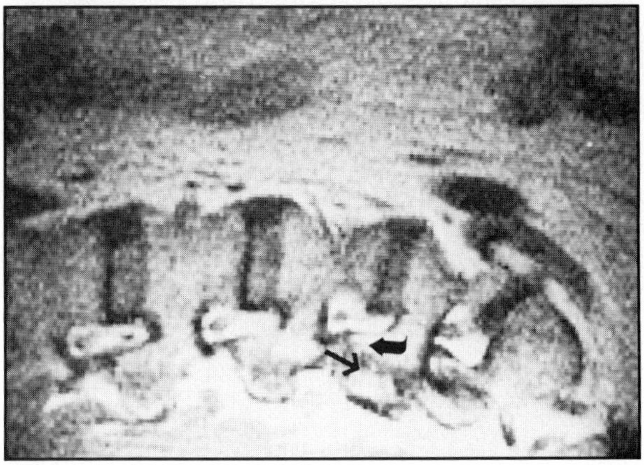

Figure 8-7G: Right parasagittal MR section showing the normal relationship of the superior articular process of L5 (curved arrow) and the inferior articular process of L4 (straight arrow).

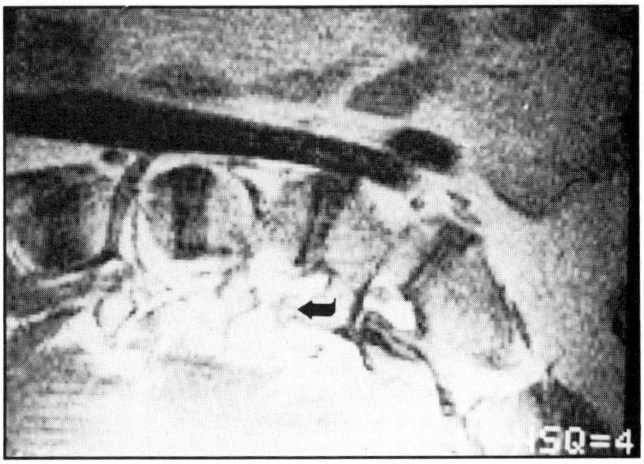

Figure 8-7H: Left parasagittal MR. The superior articular process of L5 (curved arrow) is visualized but the corresponding inferior articular process is surgically absent ("naked facet").

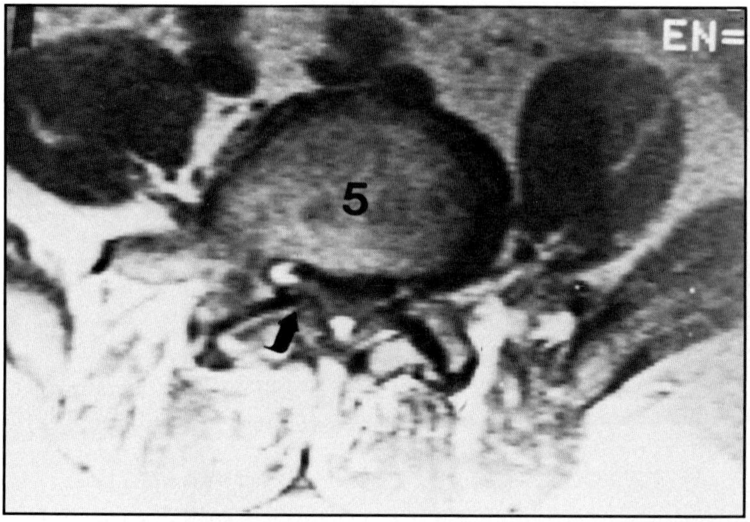

Figure 8-8: Axial sections through pedicles of L5. Osteophyte formation at the right L4-5 facet joint (arrow) is causing subarticular lateral recess stenosis with compression of the right L5 nerve root.

isolated abnormality. In severe cases combined bony hypertrophy of vertebral bodies, pedicles, and superior articular processes along with degenerative disc narrowing are present leading to severe concentric boney stenosis in both the up/down and front/back directions.

Although both high resolution CT and MR scanning provide an adequate demonstration of the anatomy of the intervertebral canal in the axial plane, the ability of magnetic resonance to provide sagittal sections is particularly helpful in assessment of the up/down component of a lateral stenosis. The direct visualization of the exiting nerve root, intervertebral disc, epidural fat and bony components allows a precise 3-dimensional understanding of anatomic relationships (Figures 8-13 through 8-17).

Surgical treatment of lateral spinal stenosis involves the conflicting goals of decompressing neural structures while avoiding segmental instability. This requires removal of adequate bone from the anteromedial aspect of the superior articular facet of the vertebra below, along with removal of offending disc fragments or vertebral end plate osteophytes where appropriate (Burton, 1984).

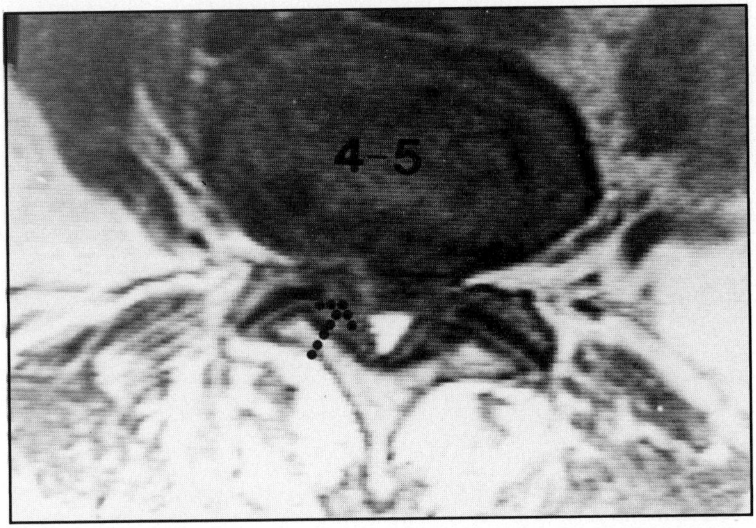

Figure 8-9A: Axial section through L4-5. The ligamentum flavum about the right facet joint is markedly hypertrophied, (dotted arrow) with encroachment on the right lateral recess.

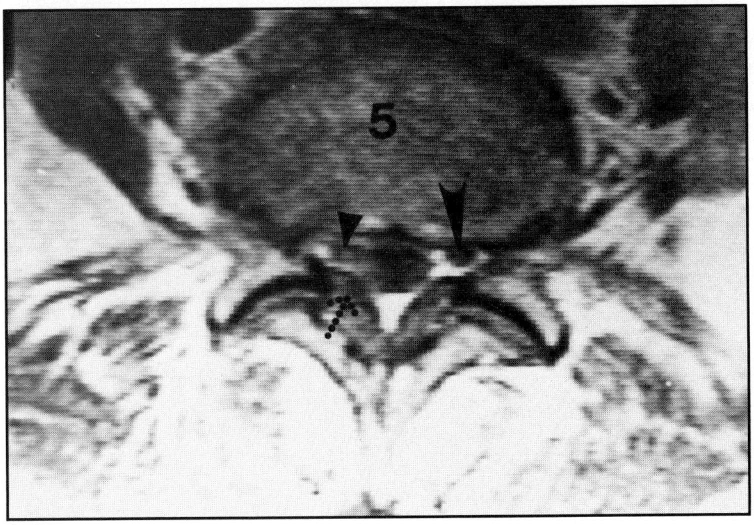

Figure 8-9B: Section through L5 demonstrates distortion of the right L5 nerve root (arrowhead) by the hypertrophied ligamentum flavum (dotted arrow). The left L5 nerve root (large arrowhead) is normal.

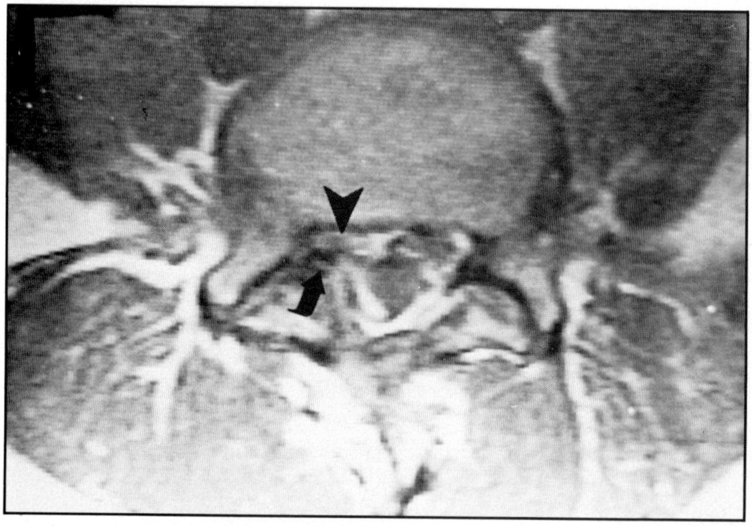

Figure 8-10A: Right subarticular recess stenosis with facet joint hypertrophy (curved arrow) causing compression of the right L5 nerve root (arrowhead) medial to the pedicle of L5.

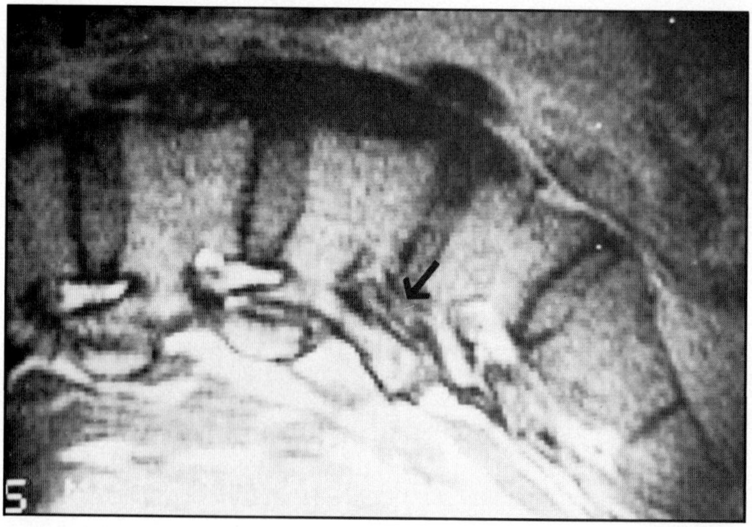

Figure 8-10B: Parasagittal section demonstrating concomitant lateral disc protrusion (arrow) and intervertebral canal stenosis.

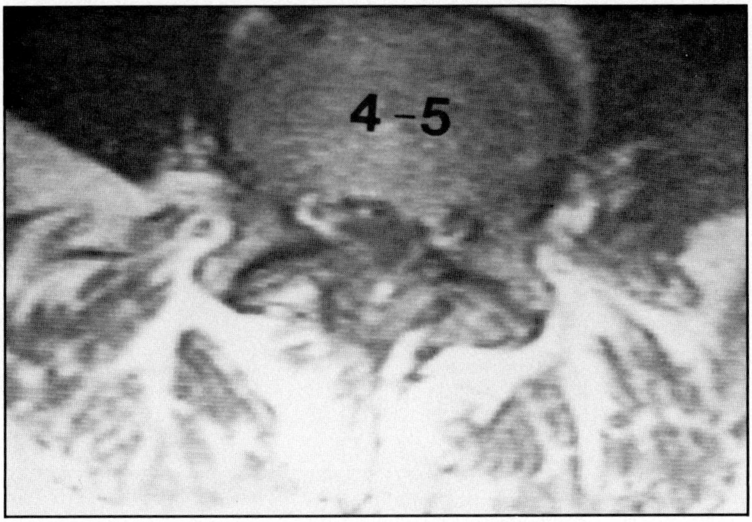

Figure 8-11: Left subarticular recess stenosis is related to end plate osteophytosis as well as articular process hypertrophy.

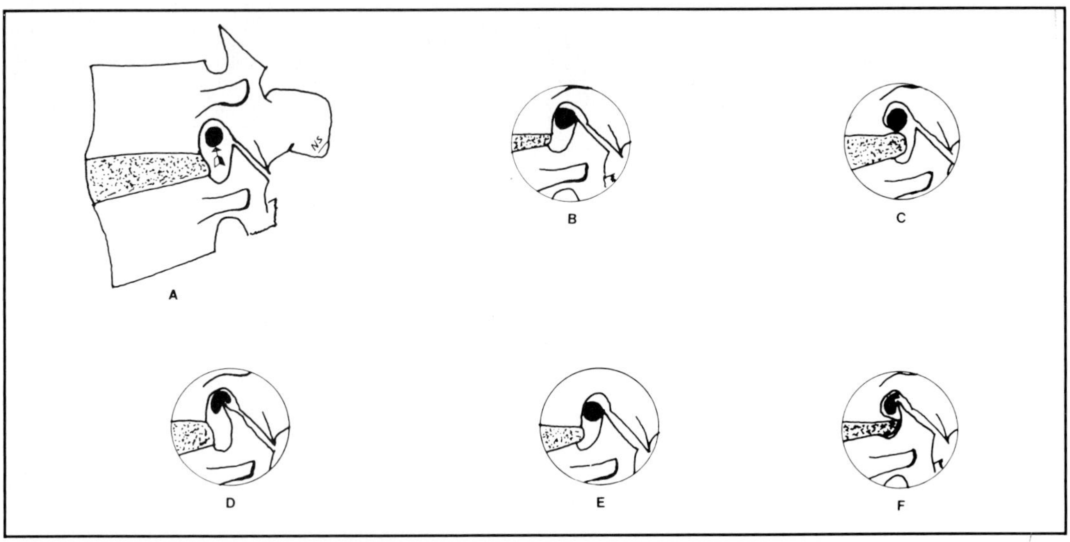

Figure 8-12: Factors contributing to stenosis of the intervertebral nerve exit canal. A: Normal. The exiting nerve root (arrow) is surrounded by abundant epidural fat in upper one-half of the intervertebral canal. B: Loss of disc height contributes to an "up-down" stenosis. C: Disc protrusion and/or end plate osteophytosis impinging on the intervertebral canal. D: Hypertrophy of the superior articular process and/or facet joint osteophytosis narrows the intervertebral canal in a "front-back" direction. E: Degenerative retrolisthesis trapping the nerve root between the superior articular process of the vertebra below and the vertebral body above. F: Combination of the factors above causing a severe concentric stenosis of the intervertebral canal.

Figure 8-13: L4-5 intervertebral canal stenosis due primarily to hypertrophy of the superior articular process of L5 (curved arrow).

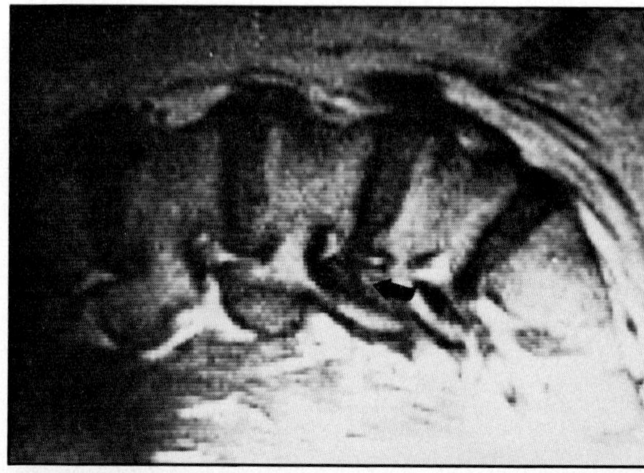

Figure 8-14A: Right L5-S1 intervertebral canal stenosis with compression of the right L5 nerve root (arrowhead).

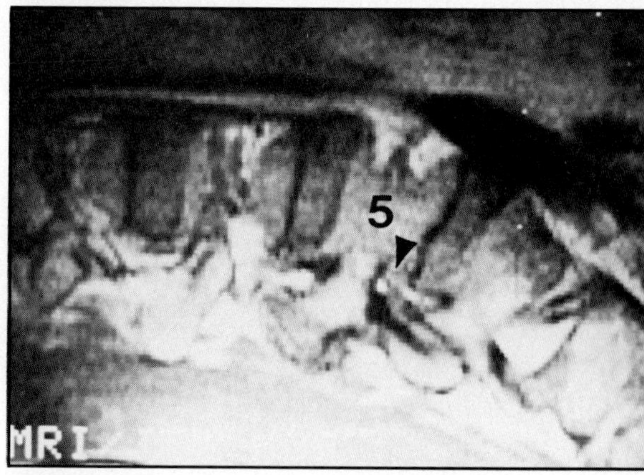

Figure 8-14B: Left parasagittal section in the same patient. The inferior half of the L5-S1 intervertebral canal is compromised by a protruding disc (straight arrow) extending back almost to the superior articular process of L5 (curved arrow). The left L5 nerve root (arrowhead) remains protected by epidural fat.

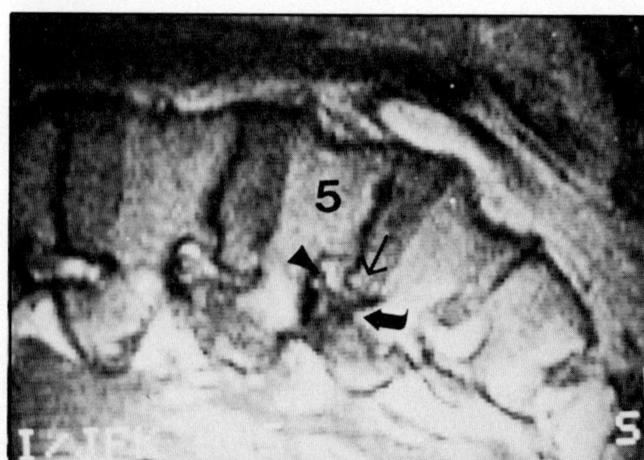

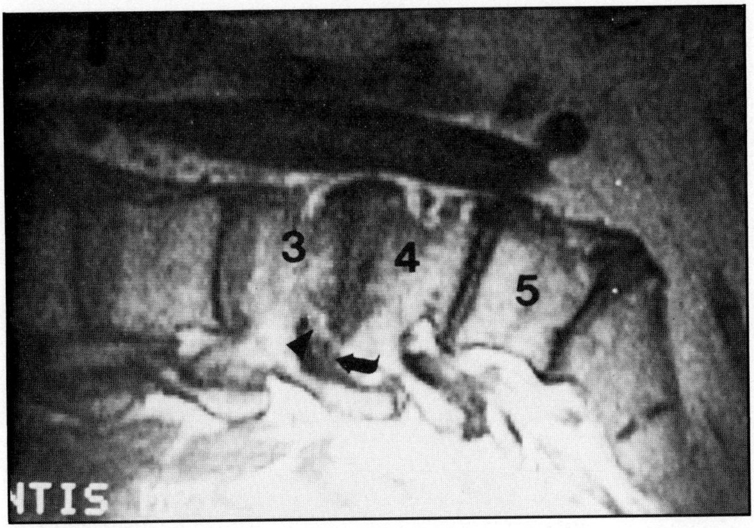

Figure 8-15: Severe concentric stenosis of the L3-4 intervertebral canal. There is almost no epidural fat about the exiting L3 nerve root (arrowhead).

Far Lateral Stenosis

Occasionally nerve root entrapment is caused by disc, osseous, or other pathology occurring just lateral to the intervertebral canal. This most commonly occurs at the lumbo sacral level, where the iliolumbar ligament (Figure 8-18) creates a closed space in which the exiting nerve root may become entrapped.

Far lateral stenosis may be caused by osseous abnormality (Figure 8-19), or far lateral disc herniation, or less commonly by infection or neoplasm.

Dynamic Spinal Stenosis

Routine CT and MR studies of the lumbar spine are performed with the patient supine and the knees flexed. This is the least provocative position for narrowing of the intervertebral canal and for disc protrusion. Thus in a patient with facet disease and symptoms referable to the nerve root exiting the intervertebral canal bordered by the abnormal facet, there is a possibility of dynamic nerve root compression despite an absence of compression in the supine views. However, to date this concept of dynamic stenosis has received only limited evaluation by CT scanning (Heitoff & Ray, 1984), and has not yet been evaluated by MR.

Figure 8-16A: Severe concentric stenosis of the L5-S1 intervertebral canal compromising the L5 root (arrowhead). Hypertrophy of the superior nerve articular process of S1 (straight arrow) contributes to the stenosis. Note that the inferior articular process of L5 (curved arrow) plays no role in the intervertebral canal stenosis.

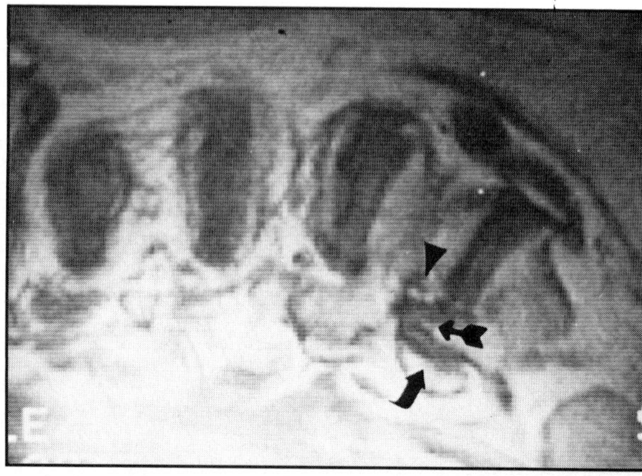

Figure 8-16B: Transverse image through the L5-S1 level showing the hypertrophied S1 superior articular processes (arrows) bilaterally. These are impinging on the lower one-half of the intervertebral canal.

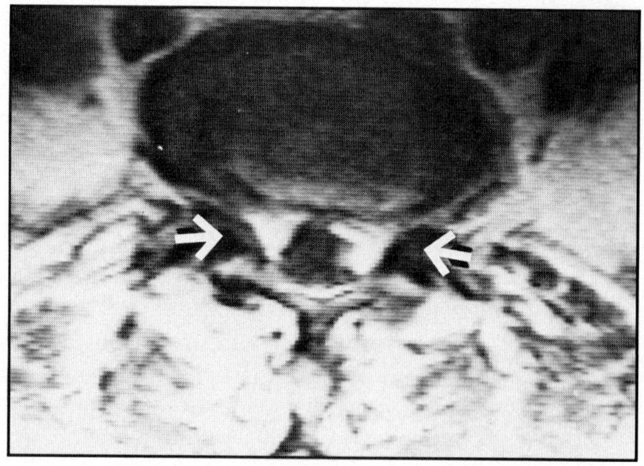

Figure 8-16C: Section cephalad to that in B. Increased AP diameter of the exiting L5 nerve roots (arrowheads) related to compression in the up-down direction and/or nerve root swelling.

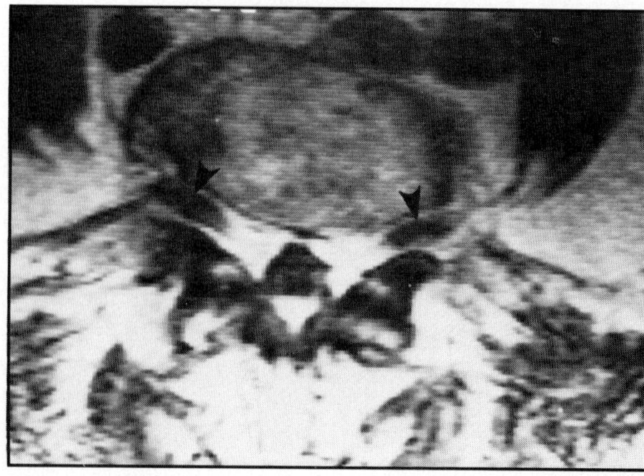

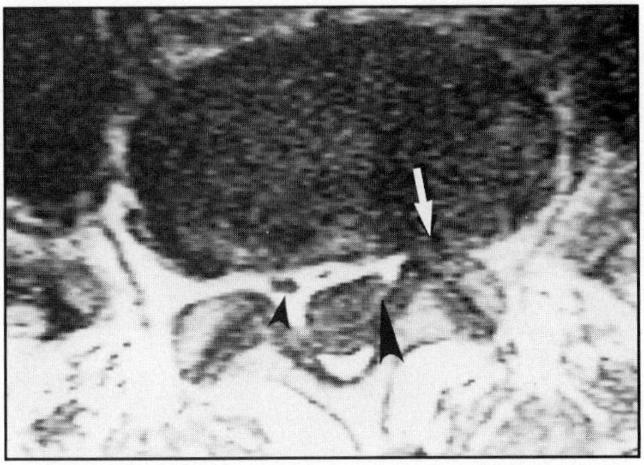

Figure 8-17A: Axial MR through the L5-S1 disc level. There is encroachment on the left intervertebral canal (arrow). Asymmetrical origin of the right (small arrowhead) and left (large arrowhead) S1 roots.

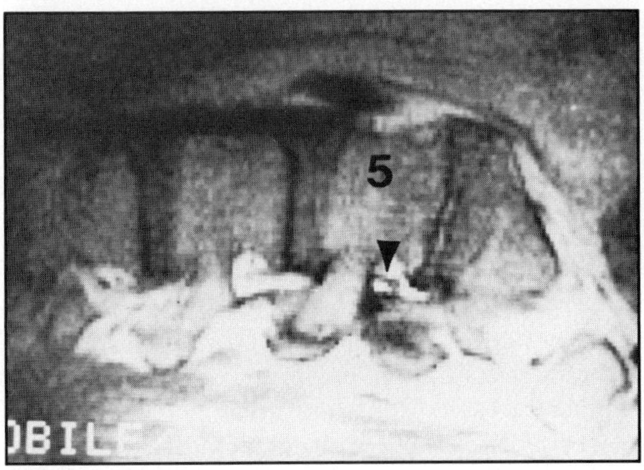

Figure 8-17B: Right parasagittal section. There is degenerative loss of height of the L5-S1 intervertebral disc. Only mild narrowing of the L5-S1 intervertebral canal. The L5 nerve root (arrowhead) is surrounded by abundant epidural fat.

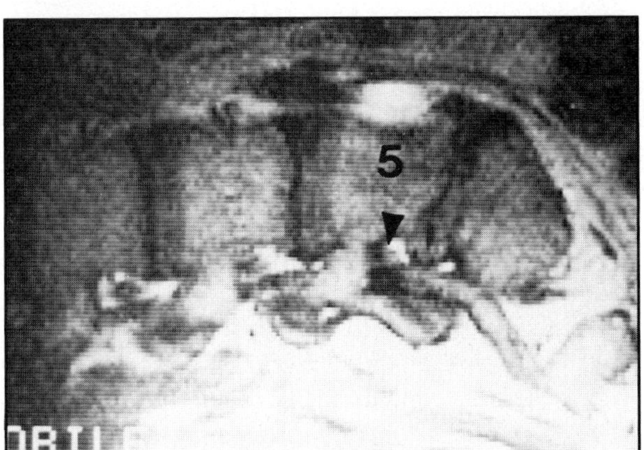

Figure 8-17C: Right parasagittal section. L5-S1 degenerative narrowing with osteophyte formation encroaching on the caudal aspect of the intervertebral canal. The right S1 nerve root (arrowhead) is seen passing through the narrowed canal.

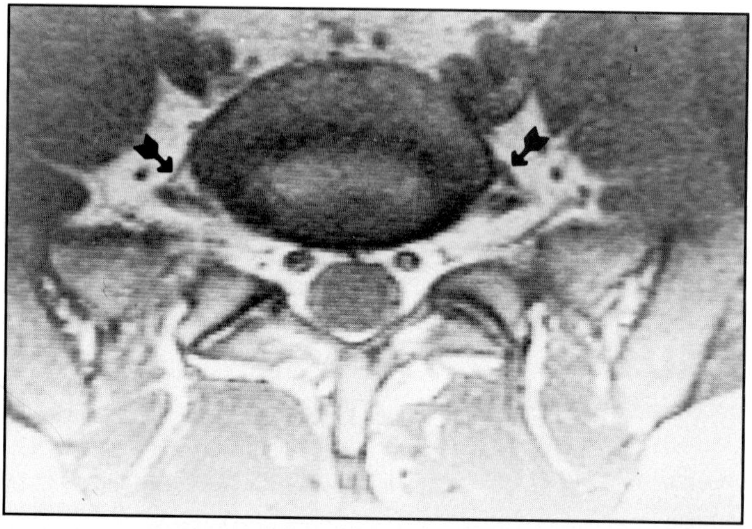

Figure 8-18: Transverse sections through L5-S1 intervertebral disc demonstrating the ilio-lumbar ligaments (arrows).

Summary

Initial suspicion of lumbar spinal stenosis depends on clinical findings. Sectional imaging with either CT or MR confirms the diagnosis, permitting identification of the sites and levels of spinal stenosis present and classification into central, subarticular, lateral, or combined stenoses. MR has the advantage of providing high quality, direct images in multiple planes including the sagittal.

The need for surgical decompression of lumbar spinal stenosis is determined primarily on a clinical basis. However, the thorough understanding of the underlying anatomic abnormality and neural compression provided by sectional imaging methods is essential to rational preoperative planning of appropriate decompression, and helps avoid the costly failed back surgery syndrome.

The diagnosis of spinal stenosis by MR scanning, like that by CT, depends more on the visual assessment of compression of neural structures than it does on actual measurements. Due to the complex anatomy and pathophysiology involved, interpretation of these studies by those with limited knowledge or only casual interest in the spine leads to frequent observer error. Because of the precise anatomic images provided, any discrepancy between the MR diagnosis of spinal stenosis and the surgical findings represents either misinterpretation of images by the radi-

Figure 8-19: "Far lateral" stenosis.

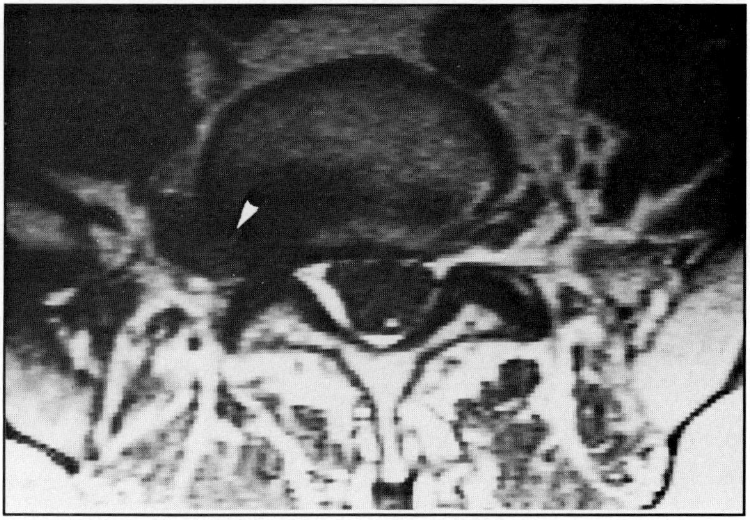

Figure 8-19A: Axial MR demonstrates obliteration of the right S1 nerve root and paraspinal fat in the far lateral region (arrowhead) by material of low to intermediate signal intensity extending from the intervertebral canal.

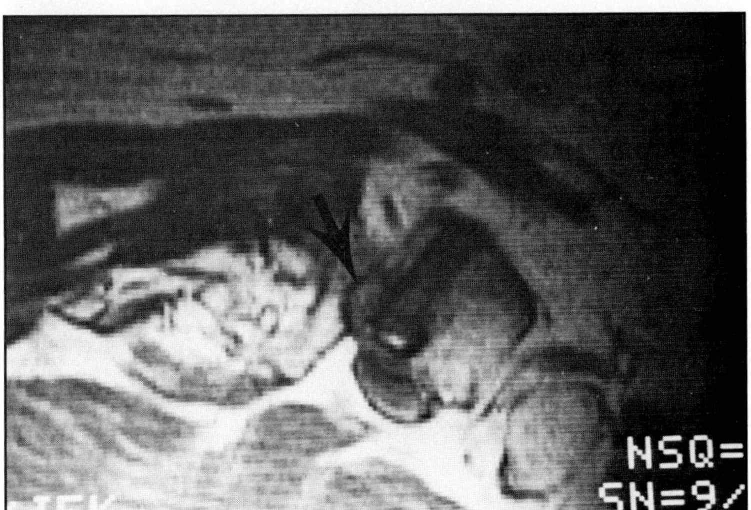

Figure 8-19B: Sagittal MR through the lateral margin of the right L5 pedicle. The lateral aspect of the intervertebral canal (arrow) is almost devoid of epidural fat.

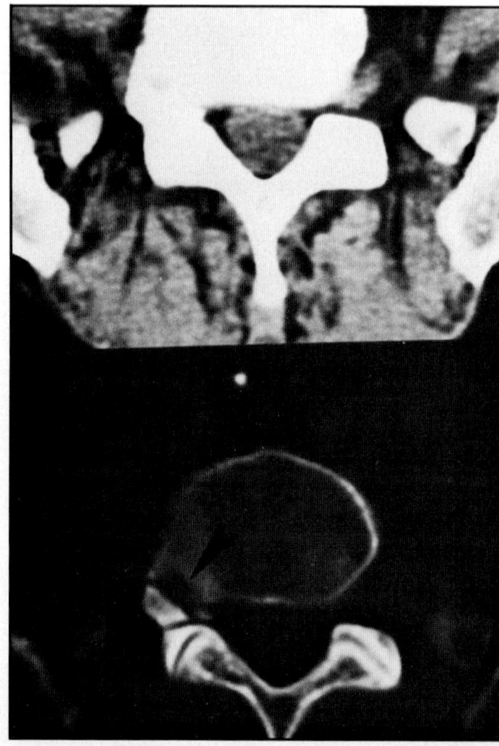

Figure 8-19C: Axial CT demonstrates abnormal bony density (arrowhead) in the far lateral region.

ologist or of operative findings by the surgeon. Either may occur, and in many respects the MR study provides a more complete spinal evaluation than is possible utilizing the limited field of view available surgically.

A final caveat is in order. As stressed by Rothman and Glenn (1985) discussing spinal CT, one must avoid the tendency to overread spinal stenosis. The same principle applies to interpretation of MR scans:

> *"The main problem when evaluating a spine CT for spinal stenosis is the tendency for people with limited experience to overcall the diagnosis. Not all narrow spinal canals are stenotic . . . One should reserve diagnosis of stenosis for those patients who have asymmetrical developmental deformity—mainly pedicles that are* disproportionately *short or*

facets that are disproportionaly *large . . . Simply stating that a patient has "spinal stenosis: on a CT report produces a specific reaction in the mind of a surgeon: He will think about radical laminectomy, facetectomy, and possibly foramenotomy. It is inappropriate to perform that much surgery when it is not absolutely necessary."*

CHAPTER 9

Miscellaneous Conditions

Miscellaneous Conditions

Although low back pain syndrome is the most common cause leading to referral for lumbar MR scan, a variety of other conditions may be studied. These may either be suspected beforehand, or encountered unexpectedly during evaluation for possible lumbar disc disease.

Spondylolisthesis

Spondylolisthesis secondary to facet joint degenerative changes may be seen as a component of lumbar spinal stenosis and has been discussed in Chapter 8.

Magnetic resonance imaging also aids in the evaluation of spondylolisthesis associated with pars interarticularis defect (spondylolysis). Cross-sectional images through the level of a spondylisthesis, whether by CT or MR, often lead to a false impression of disc herniation due to partial volume effect (Figure 9-1). The direct sagittal views available with MR are helpful to clarify the anatomy under these circumstances (Figure 9-2).

Perhaps an even more important role for MR imaging in lytic spondylolisthesis is in assessment of the hydration state of the disc above the level of the spondylolisthesis. Thus in a patient with an obvious L5-S1 spondylolisthesis, known from plain films, the presence of a normally hydrated L4-5 disc may be an indication to limit spinal fusion from L5 to the sacrum, whereas an abnormal L4-5 disc may lead to fusion from L4 to the sacrum (Mark Brown, personal communication).

Trauma

Although high resolution CT with multiplanar reformatting remains the imaging modality of choice for demonstrating the

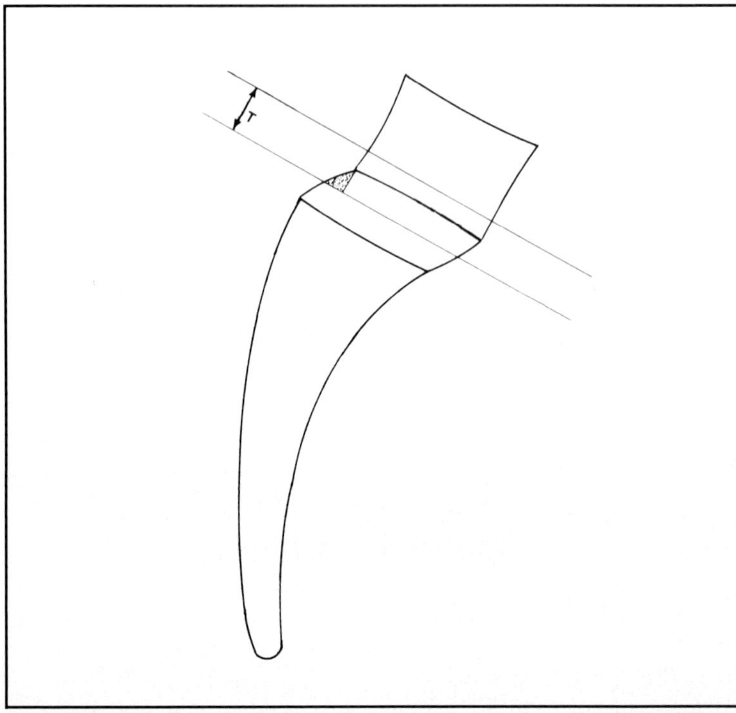

Figure 9-1: Spondylolisthesis causing artifactual appearance of disc protrusion. An axial slice of finite thickness T will show disc material (stippled area) projecting posterior to the inferior end plate of L5 (partial volume effect).

detailed bony abnormalities in lumbar spine fractures, magnetic resonance imaging is also helpful in assessing impingements on the spinal canal (Figure 9-3). In the upper lumbar and thoracic region MR also helps in evaluation of the spinal cord.

Traumatic injuries of the vertebral end plates and intervertebral discs, including anterior disc herniation, are well imaged by MR (Figure 9-4).

Radiation Effects

The MR appearance of the previously irradiated lumbar spine is easily recognizable (Ramsey et al., 1985). On T1-weighted images the irradiated region shows a brighter signal intensity than normal marrow (Figure 9-5). This distinction tends to be sharply margi-

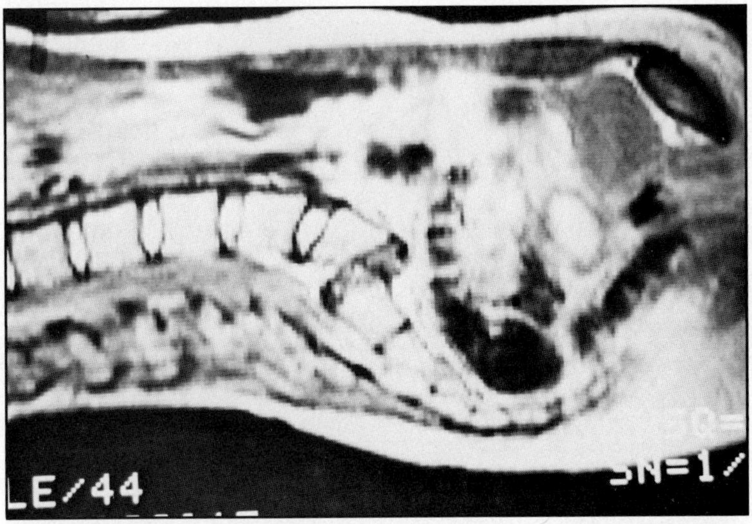

Figure 9-2A: Spondylolisthesis of L5 on S1 (proton density weighted).

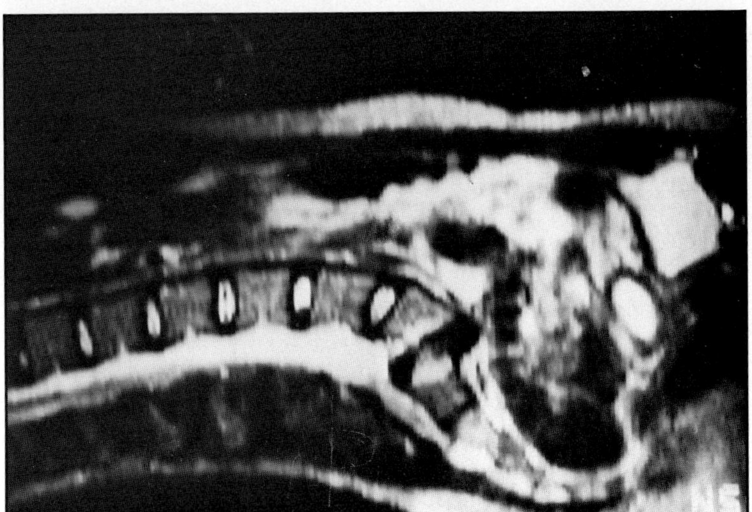

Figure 9-2B: Image with T2 weighting shows the marrow changes associated with the disc degeneration at the L5-S1 level. The L4-5 disc maintains normal hydration.

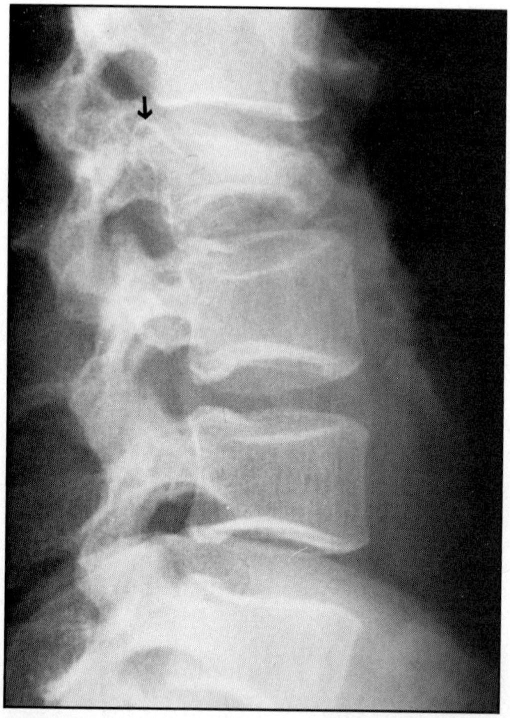

Figure 9-3A: L2 compression fracture with retropulsed fragment (arrow).

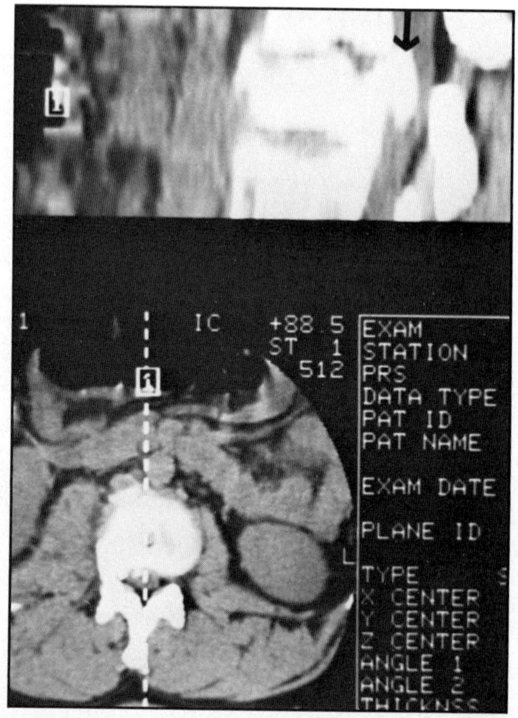

Figure 9-3B: CT scan with sagittal reformatting shows the retropulsed fragment (arrow) in the spinal canal.

nated, corresponding to the radiation portal. This effect occurs over the generally utilized dose range for therapeutic radiation, developing within weeks to months and lasting many years, and probably permanently. The appearance is due to fatty replacement of bone marrow following irradiation, with the MR signal of the irradiated vertebral bodies approximating that of fat.

Although recognition is usually straight forward when normal and irradiated vertebral bodies are included within the image, replacement of the non-irradiated vertebral bodies by tumor (Figure 9-6) complicates evaluation.

Infection

Magnetic resonance imaging is helpful in the evaluation of

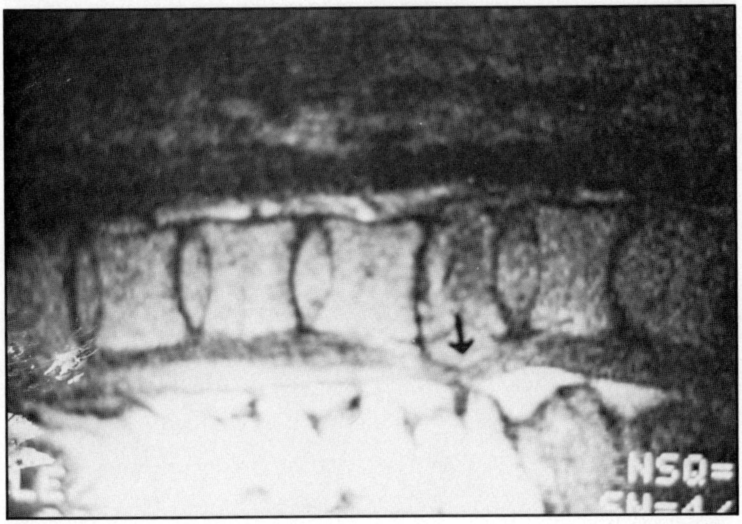

Figure 9-3C: Sagittal MR shows the compression of L2 with the retropulsed fragment (arrow) in the spinal canal. Spinal cord is seen ending posterior to L1.

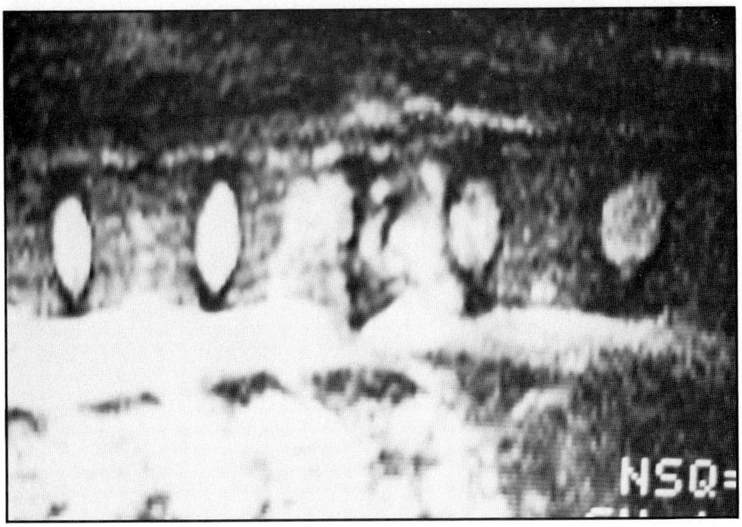

Figure 9-3D: T2 weighted MR shows the associated injury of L1-2 disc. Also, abnormal signal of the L1 vertebral body indicated subtle evidence of L1 injury or reaction as well.

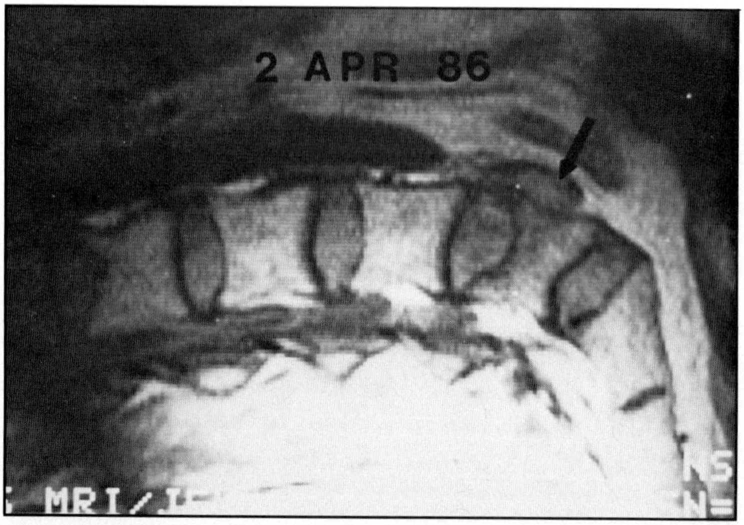

Figure 9-4A: Compression fracture of L5 associated with anterior herniation (arrow) of the L4-5 disc as seen in the left parasagittal plane.

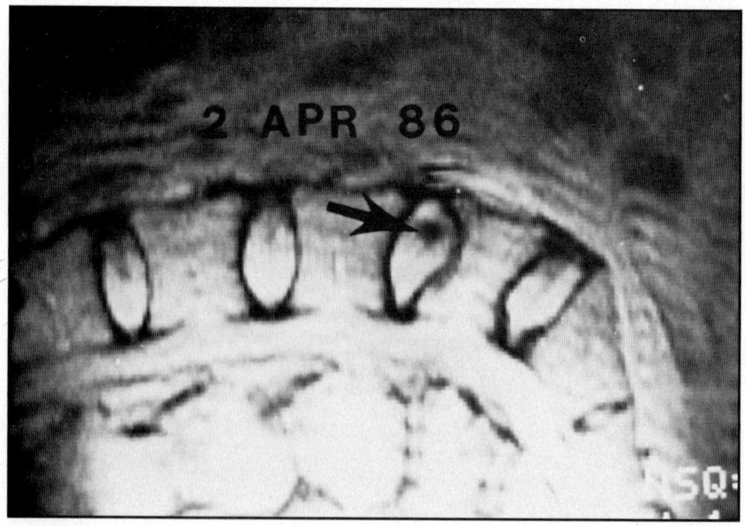

Figure 9-4B: T2 weighted study in the midline shows a localized region of decreased signal (arrow) in the L4-5 disc with the remainder of the disc signal maintained on this study obtained several days following injury.

Figure 9-5: On T1 weighted images radiation produces characteristic bright signal from the vertebral bodies due to replacement of red marrow by fatty yellow marrow.

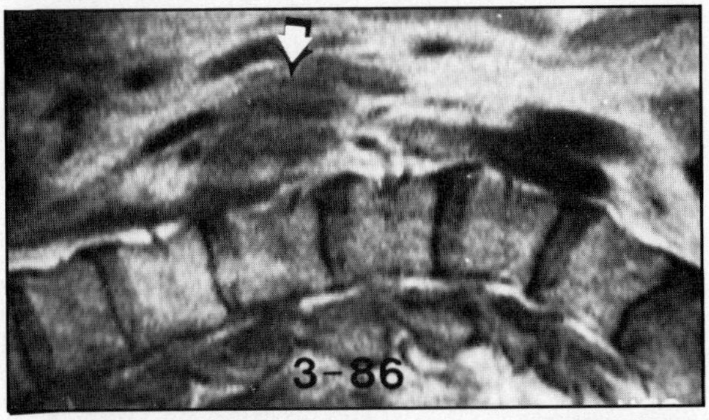

Figure 9-5A: T1 weighted image prior to radiation. Note tumor mass (arrow) anterior to spine. Vertebral body signals are normal.

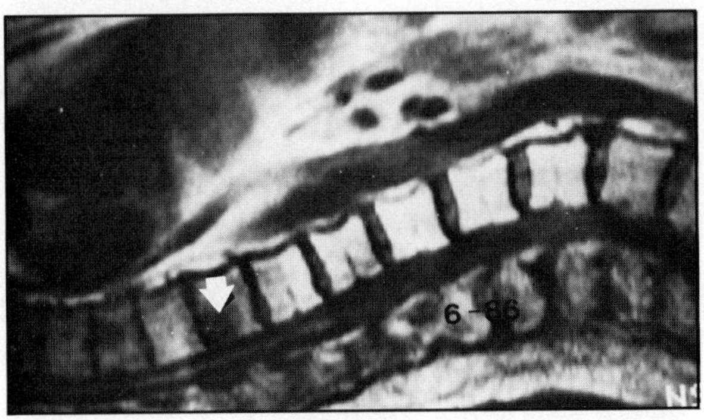

Figure 9-5B: T1 weighted image three months later. Radiation effect manifest as bright marrow signal within the radiation port. Low signal intensity lesion (arrow) is a vertebral metastasis outside the radiation field.

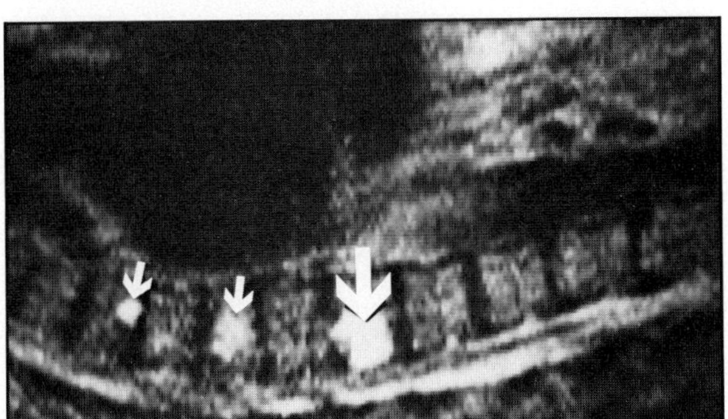

Figure 9-5C: T2 weighted image following radiation. Vertebral metastases (arrows) shown as areas of bright signal. Radiation effect is much less apparent with T2 weighting.

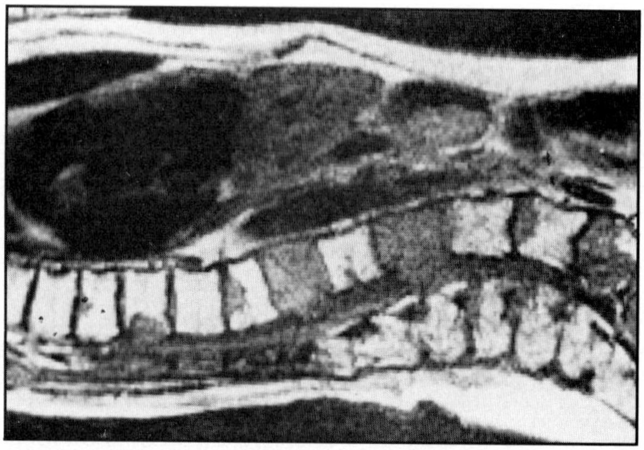

Figure 9-6: Combination of radiation effect and metasteses. The bright signal of the thoracic bodies is due to prior radiation. Vertebral bodies at L1, 3 and 4 show relatively normal signal. Loss of signal at multiple levels indicates metastatic involvement.

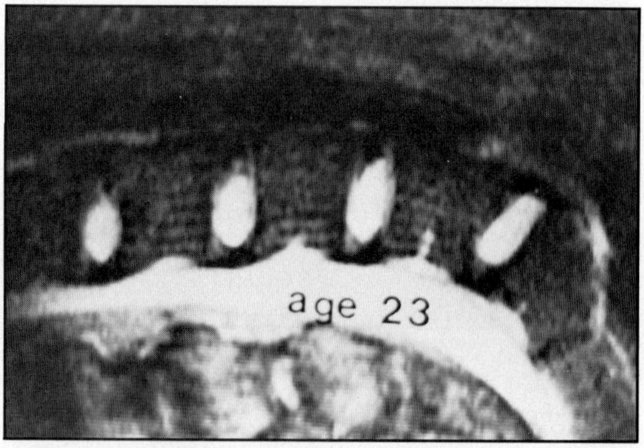

Figure 9-7A: 23 year old female demonstrating bright disc signal. Lack of intranuclear cleft is normal under age 30.

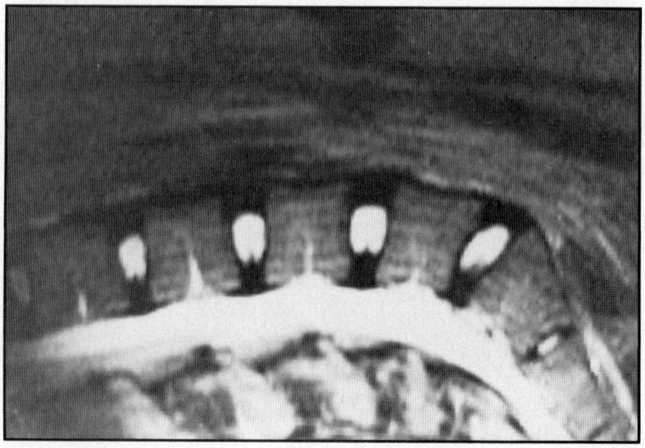

Figure 9-7B: Normal bright discs including the MR finding of "intranuclear cleft".

Figure 9-8: Infectious discitis (staph. aureus) with delayed diagnosis.

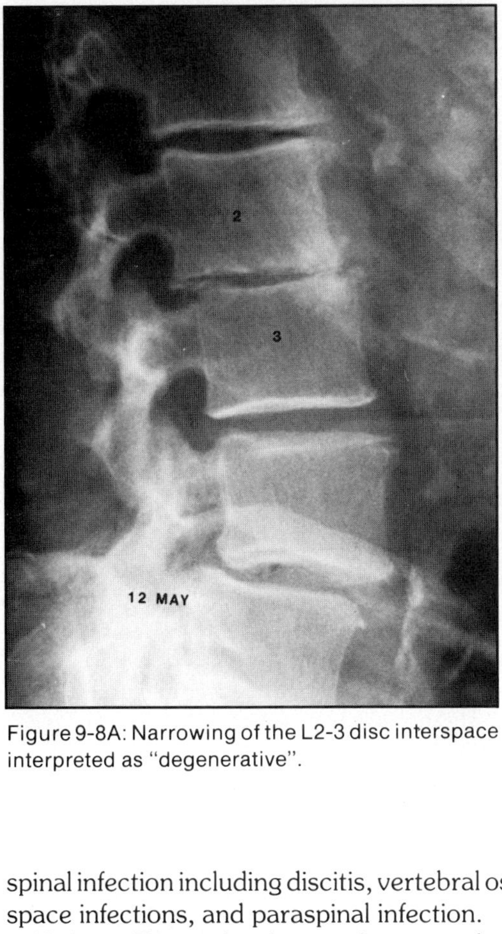

Figure 9-8A: Narrowing of the L2-3 disc interspace interpreted as "degenerative".

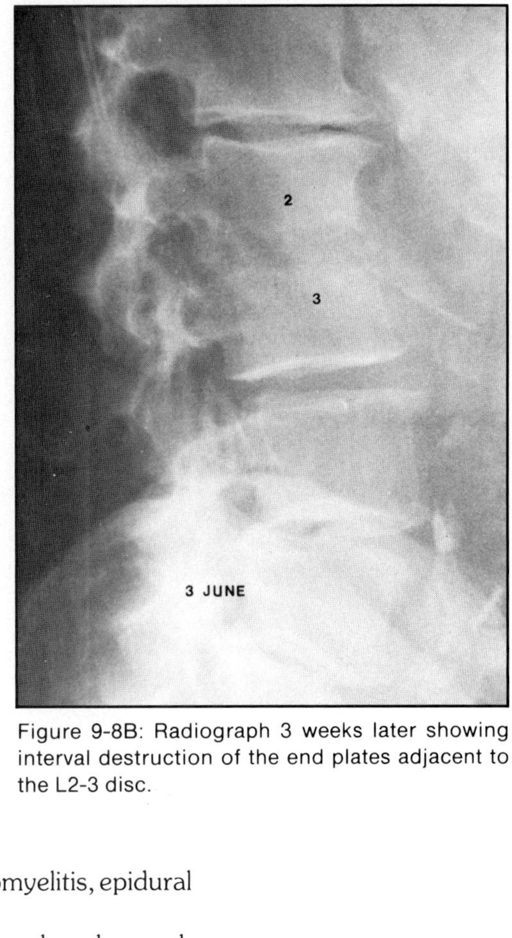

Figure 9-8B: Radiograph 3 weeks later showing interval destruction of the end plates adjacent to the L2-3 disc.

spinal infection including discitis, vertebral osteomyelitis, epidural space infections, and paraspinal infection.

Utilizing T2-weighted sagittal images, the normal nucleus pulposus in a young patient is seen as an area of uniformly increased signal intensity within the disc space (Figure 9-7). By the age of 30 most patients will develop a characteristic intranuclear cleft within the nucleus pulposus.

Not all bright discs are normal. As noted previously, the high signal intensity of the normal nucleus pulposus on T2-weighted images is related to its water content. Disc space infection, whether characterized by frank pus or inflamed, edematous, granulation tissue, also has high water content and may produce a bright disc signal. The presence of an unexpectedly bright signal within a narrowed disc, or of a bright disc signal which is poorly

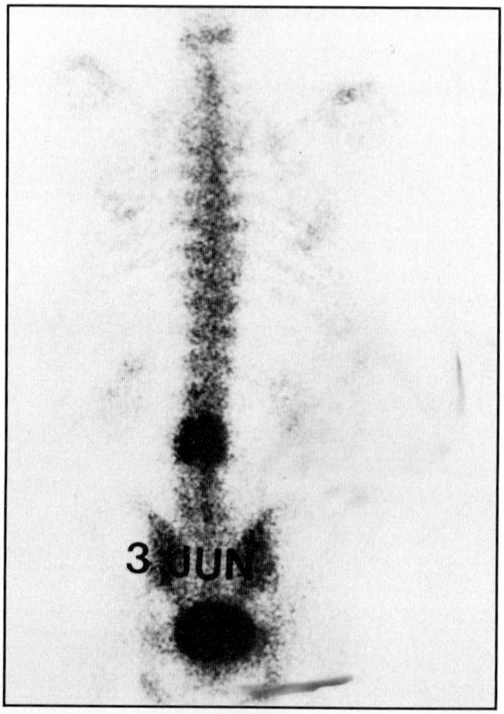

Figure 9-8C: Nuclear bone scan demonstrates the increased uptake of isotope in the L2 and L3 vertebral bodies.

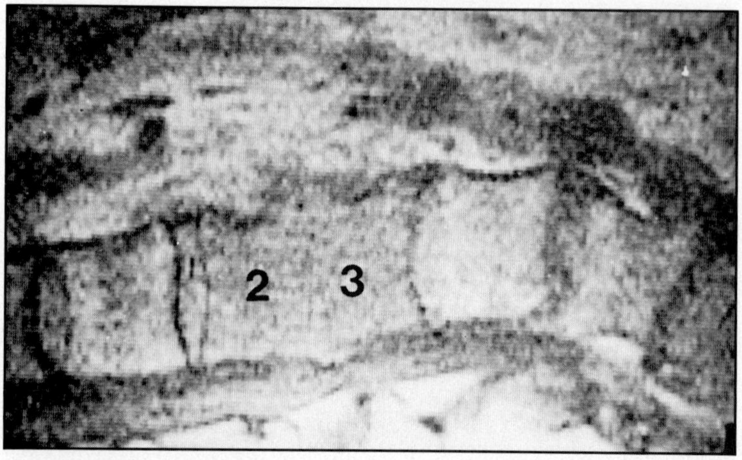

Figure 9-8D: T1 weighted MR shows diffuse loss of signal of the L2 and L3 vertebral bodies. The bodies are iso-intense with the L2-3 disc on this sequence.

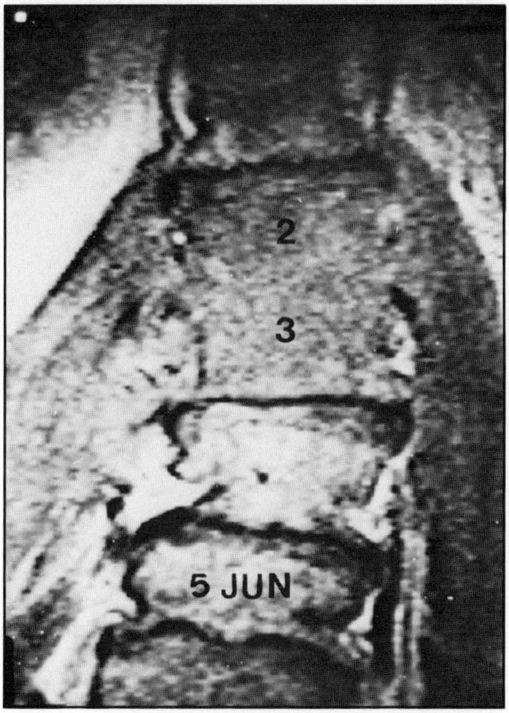

Figure 9-8E: Similar findings demonstrated in coronal view.

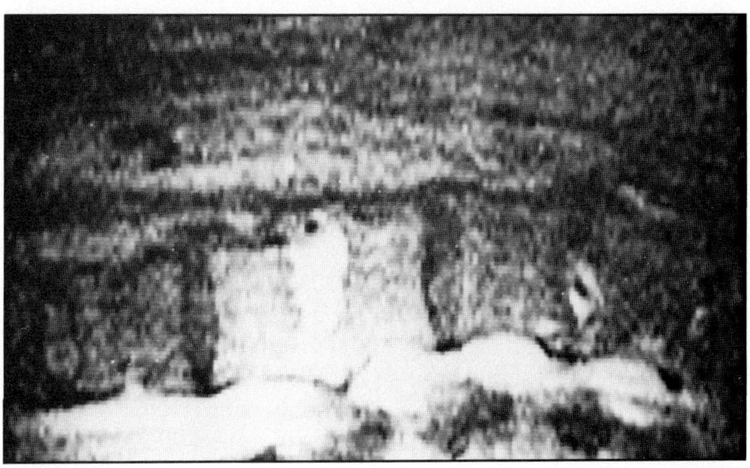

Figure 9-8F: T2 weighted MR (TR2000,TE160) shows dramatic abnormal bright signal of L2-3 disc, with mildly increased signal of the L2 and L3 vertebral bodies.

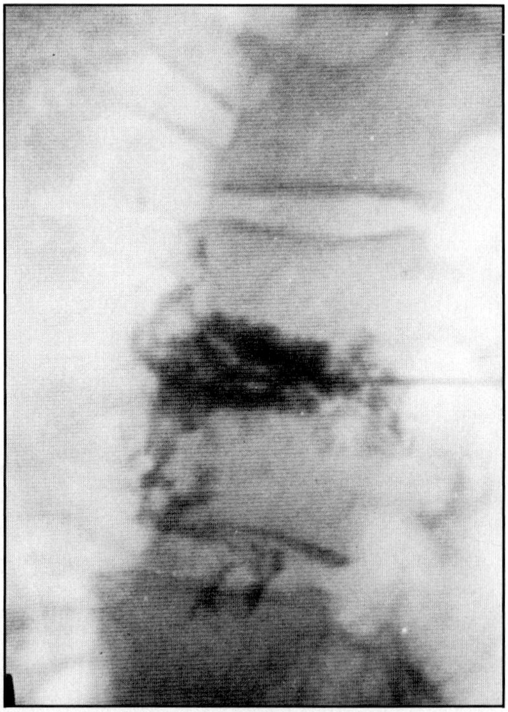

Figure 9-8G: Contrast discogram. Several cc's of thin purulent material were aspirated and cultured staph aureus.

formed and lacking an intranuclear cleft in a patient over the age of 30, suggests discitis (Aguilla, et al., 1985). Such an abnormal bright disc signal may be associated with irregularity or loss of detail of the subjacent vertebral body end plates (Figure 9-8). Infectious discitis may be present within a narrowed disc (Figure 9-9a,b) or may actually cause disc space widening (Figure 9-9c,d).

Vertebral body osteomyelitis in association with disc space infection is indicated by a loss of the normal marrow appearance, with a diminished signal intensity on T1-weighted sequences and increased intensity on T2-weighted sequences (Figure 9-8).

Not all inappropriately bright intervertebral discs represent active infection; non-infectious discitis (Figure 9-10) may also yield a bright signal so that clinical correlation and bacteriologic study are required to fully evaluate the inappropriately bright disc. With

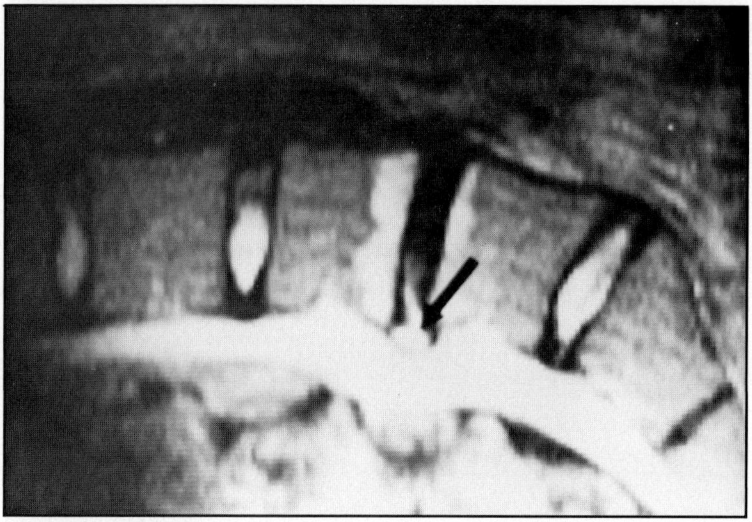

Figure 9-9A: Postoperative discitis with narrowed disc space. There is protruding disc material (arrow) as well as inflammatory end plate change.

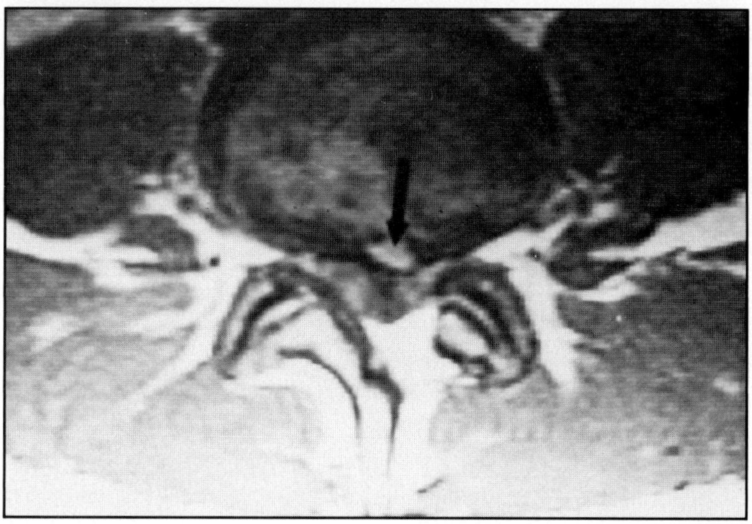

Figure 9-9B: Axial image in the same postoperative case showing the recurrent central protrusion with bright signal.

Figure 9-9C & D: Infectious discitis with disc space widening and end plate erosion (Figures 9-9 C & D courtesy of Dr. Ruth Ramsey, Rush-Presbyterian-St. Luke's Medical Center).

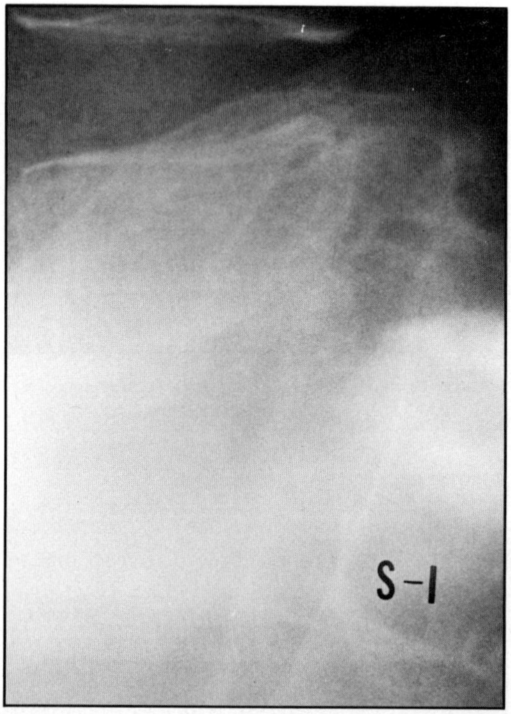

Figure 9-9C

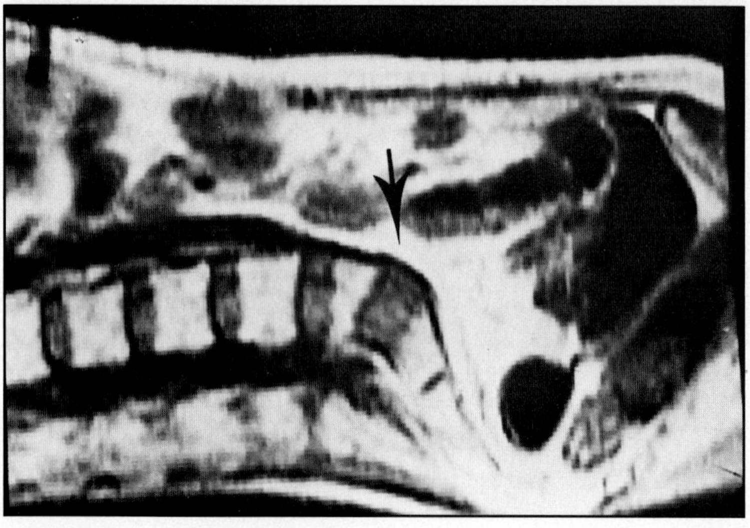

Figure 9-9D

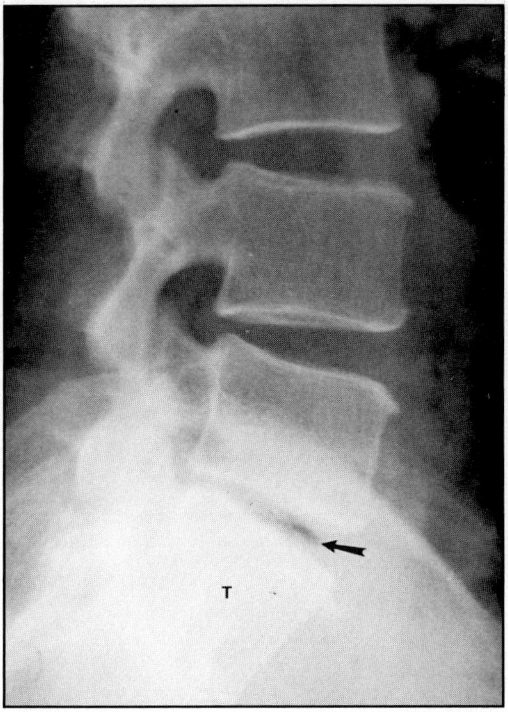

Figure 9-10A: Degenerative disc with vacuum lucency (arrow).

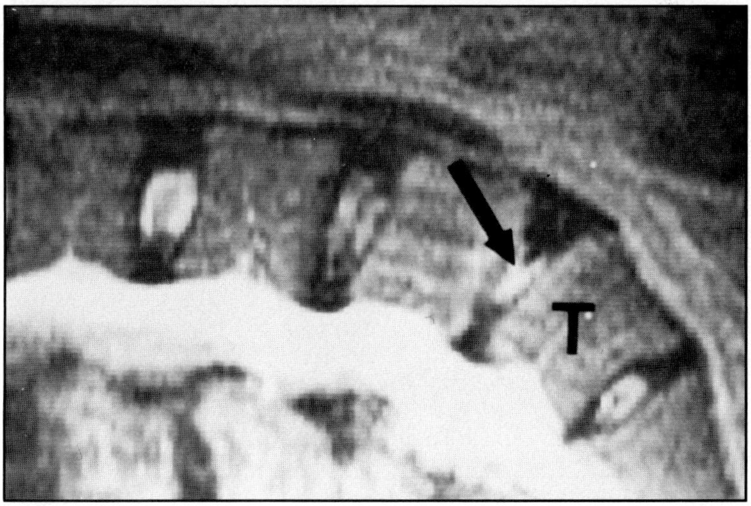

Figure 9-10B: T2 weighted MR showing inappropriate bright signal in the narrowed disc (arrow). No clinical evidence of infection.

Figure 9-11: Treated E-coli discitis. MR examination after three weeks of antibiotic treatment for positive blood culture. Disc space culture at time of MR is negative.

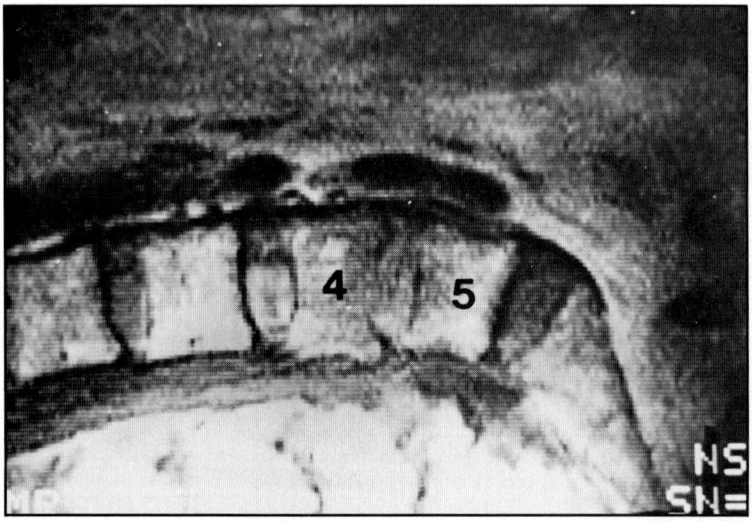

Figure 9-11A: T1 weighted sagittal MR. Loss of signal with disc space and vertebral bodies blending together.

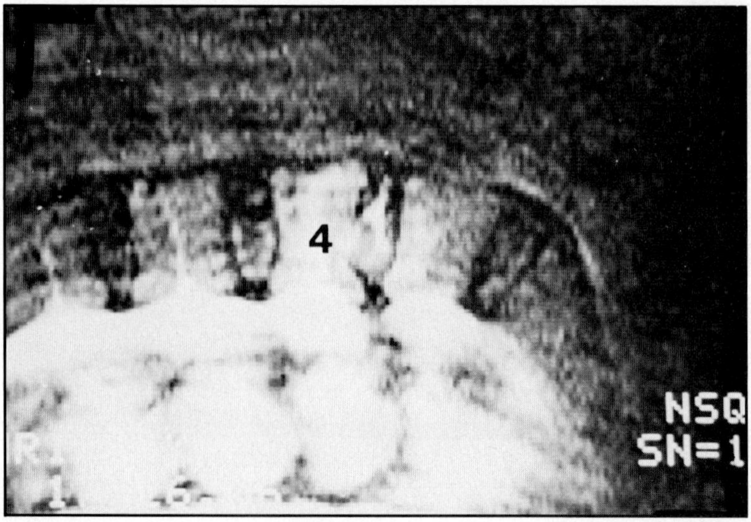

Figure 9-11B: T2 weighted sagittal MR. There is increased signal of the L4 vertebral body and the upper half of the L5 body as well as increased L4-5 disc space signal with an abnormal configuration.

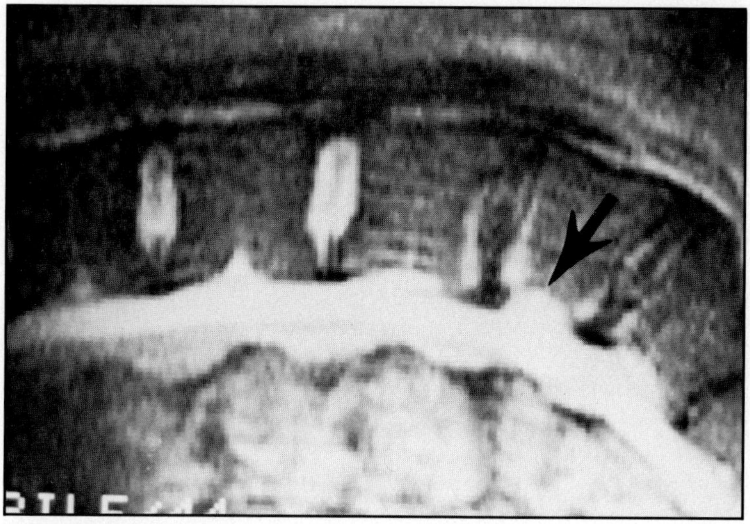

Figure 9-12A: T2 weighted MR. The discs cephalad and caudal to transitional lumbo-sacral vertebra (arrow) showed decreased disc signal with a line of bright signal of the end plate indicating inflammatory type change.

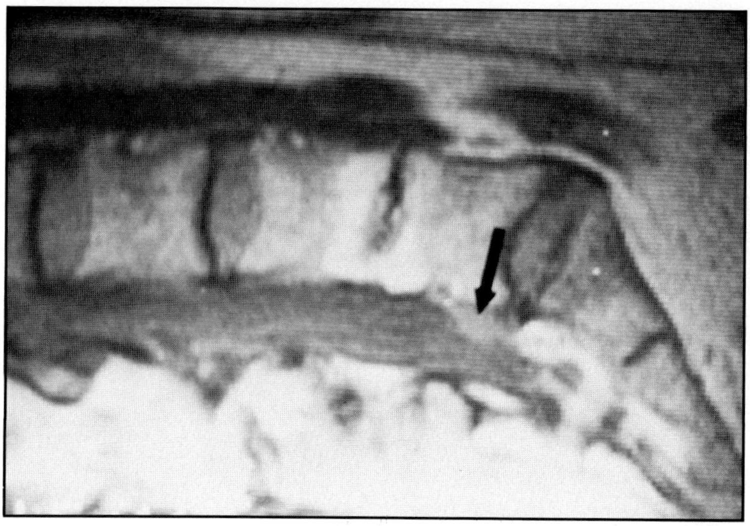

Figure 9-12B: T1 weighted image. Degenerative narrowing of the L4-5 disc. The bright marrow signal adjacent to the narrowed L4-5 disc indicates yellow fatty marrow replacing red marrow (ref). There is also an extruded L5-S1 disc (arrow).

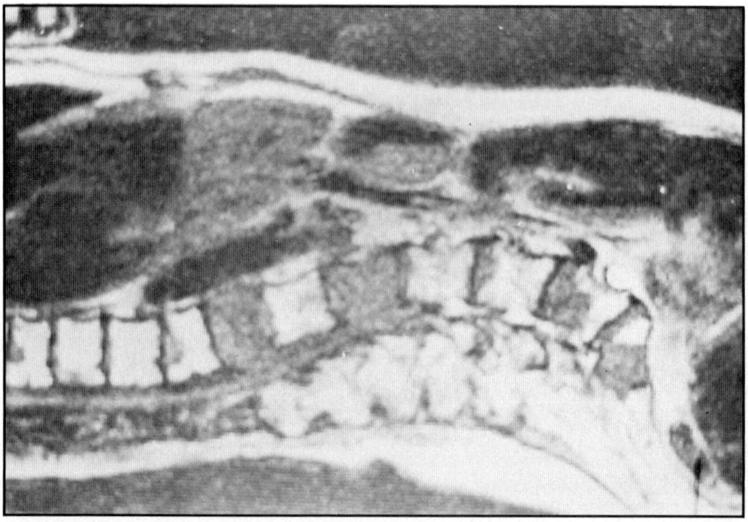

Figure 9-13A: Metastatic lesions to multiple vertebral bodies are shown as decreased signal on T1 weighted image. No hepatic lesions seen.

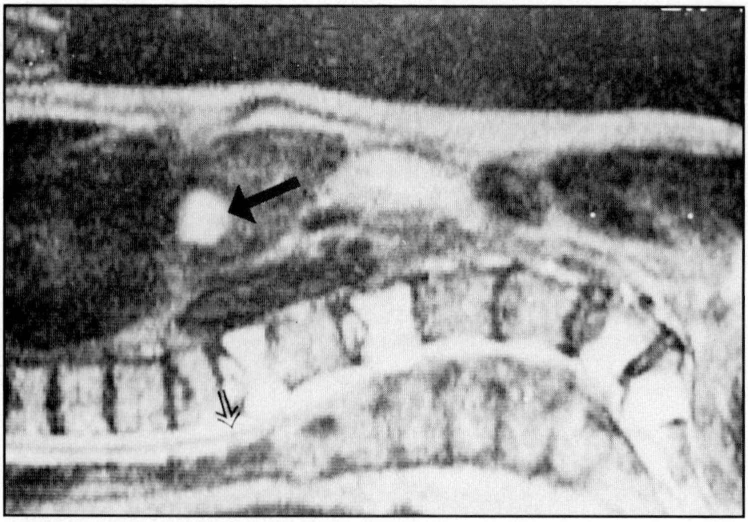

Figure 9-13B: T2 weighted image. Metastatic lesions now have bright signal intensity. A hepatic lesion is clearly delineated (solid arrow). Relationship of the spinal cord (arrow) to the expanding metastatic lesion at T12 is defined.

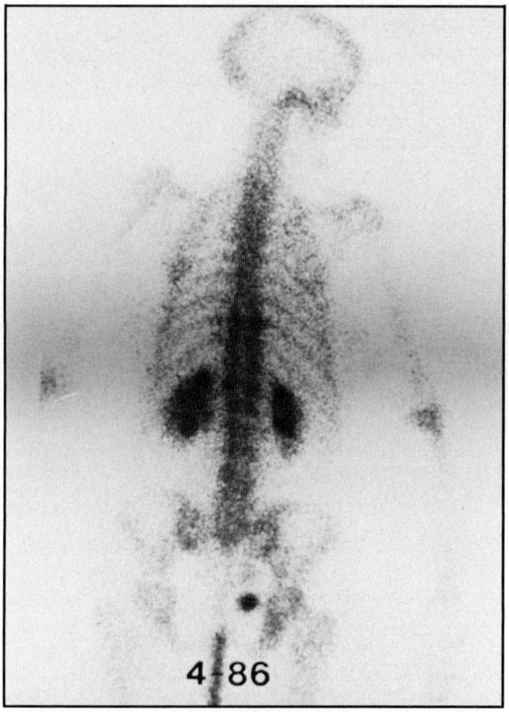

Figure 9-13C: Nuclear bone scan showing no definite abnormality (metastatic parotid carcinoma).

treated infection MR abnormalities persist for some time following bacteriologic cure (Figure 9-11).

On T2-weighted images the finding of increased signal intensity involving the region of the vertebral end plates adjacent to a degenerated disc is not uncommon (Figure 9-12); this region of bright intensity may involve the end plate region itself or up to about one-third of the vertebral body. It is not known whether this finding represents secondary reactive change to the underlying disc abnormality, or whether the end plate abnormality is primary, interfering with disc nutrition and thus causing secondary disc degenerative change.

Neoplasm

Magnetic resonance imaging is valuable in the evaluation of both primary and secondary neoplasm involving the lumbar

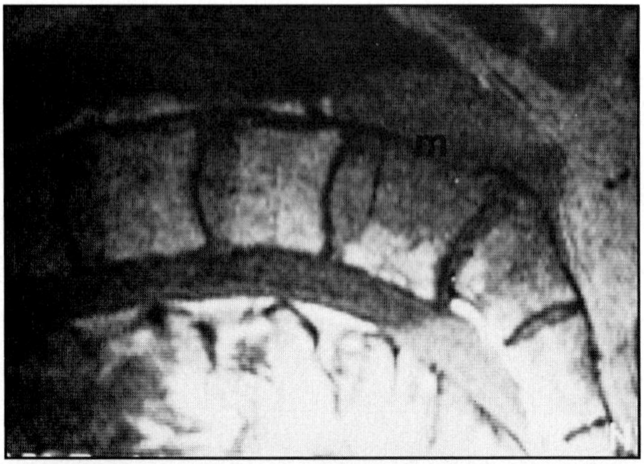

Figure 9-14A: 75 year old man referred for right sided sciatica, "R/O HNP". Tumor involving L5 and S1 and extending anteriorly (M) is seen, as well as tumor within the sacral spinal canal. The brighter signal of the tumor within the spinal canal is due to the sensitivity response pattern of the surface coil (see Figure 2-5).

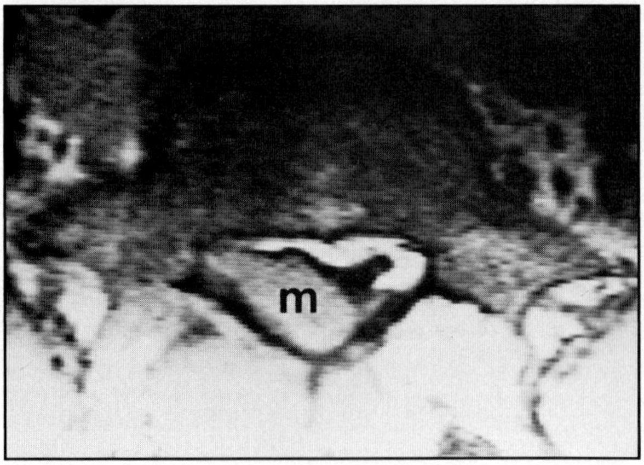

Figure 9-14B: Axial image demonstrates the mass within the spinal canal (M) to better advantage.

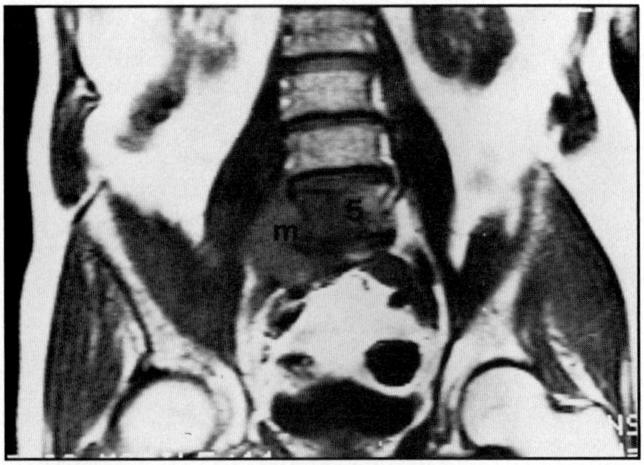

Figure 9-14C: Coronal view showing the mass involving L5 and extending to the right paraspinal region (M) beneath the psoas muscle (P).

Figure 9-15: Chordoma presenting clinically as sciatica.

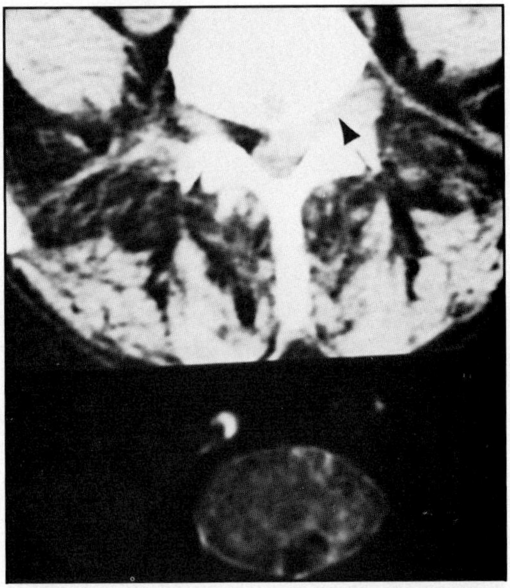

Figure 9-15A: CT scan at time of presentation shows soft tissue mass filling the right lateral recess and intervertebral nerve exit canal at L5-S1 (arrowhead).

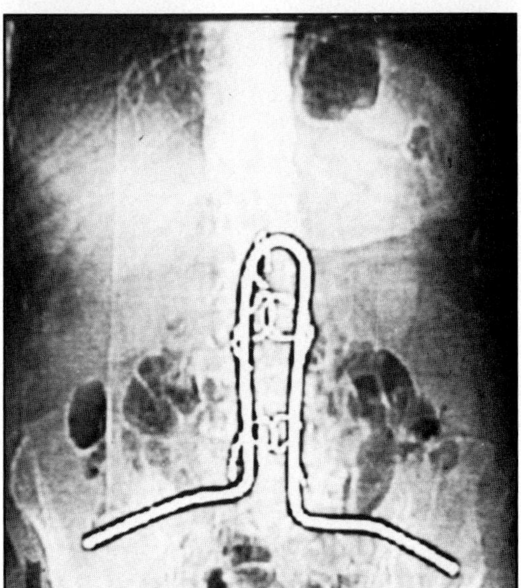

Figure 9-15B: AP radiograph following surgical excision and fusion at L5. Note the large metallic fixation rod.

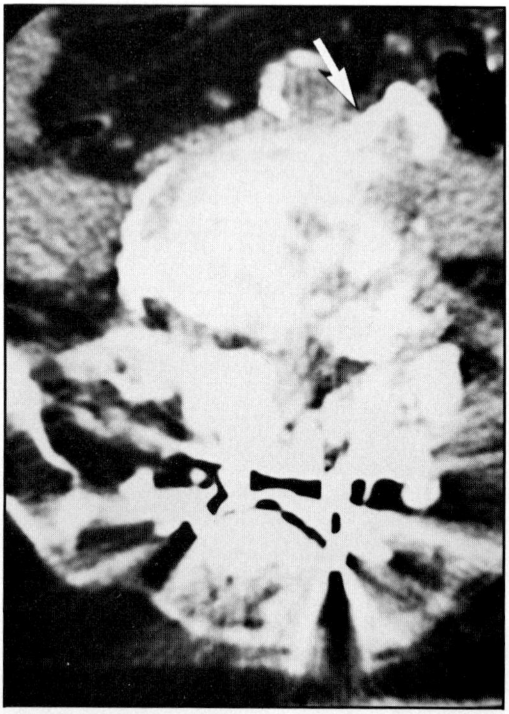

Figure 9-15C: Postoperative CT scan. Extensive artifact from the metallic rod. Portion of the anterior fusion bone (white arrow) identifies slice location for correlation to the MR.

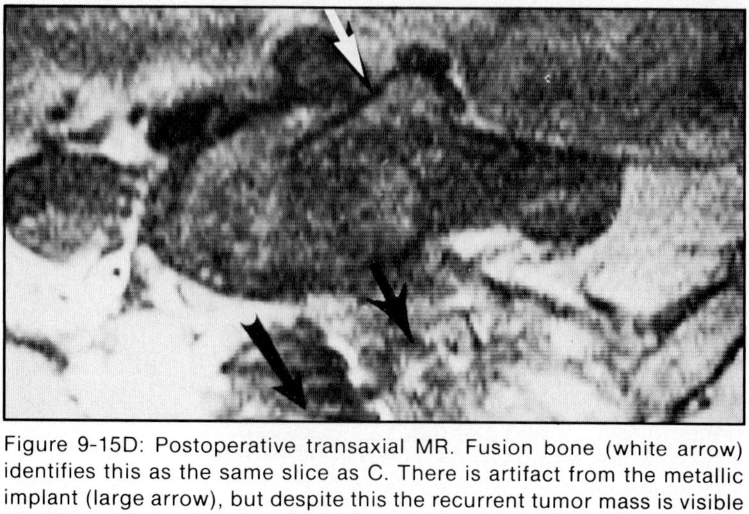

Figure 9-15D: Postoperative transaxial MR. Fusion bone (white arrow) identifies this as the same slice as C. There is artifact from the metallic implant (large arrow), but despite this the recurrent tumor mass is visible (small arrow).

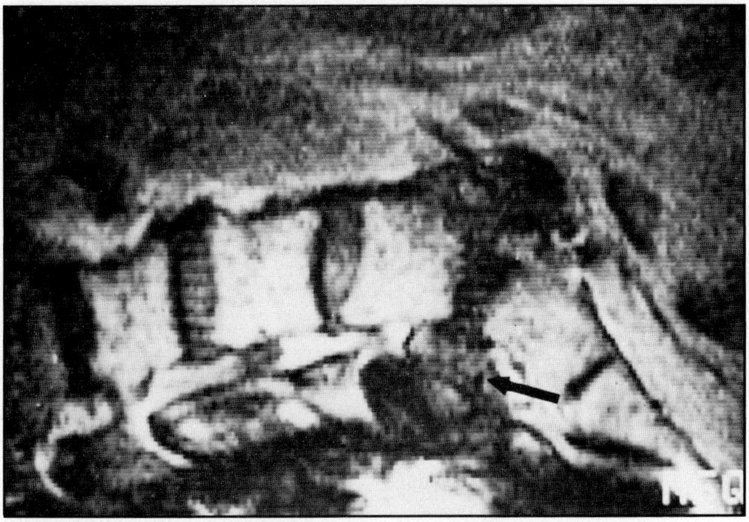

Figure 9-15E: Sagittal MR again showing the recurrent tumor (arrow).

spine. For the detection of abnormalities involving bone marrow, including metastatic neoplasm, MR has a sensitivity exceeding the nuclear bone scan (Daffner et al., 1986). Sites of metastatic involvement are easily demonstrated (Figure 9-13), including sites outside the skeleton. The effect of metastases on the spinal cord and cauda equina are demonstrated, and myelography may be obviated.

Both metastatic (Figure 9-14) and primary (Figure 9-15) neoplasms may masquerade clinically as lumbar disc syndrome; the destructive nature of these processes is readily apparent on the MR study. Sacral lesions are well visualized (Figure 9-15).

Vertebral body hemangiomas are commonly encountered on MR studies. These benign tumors may involve part or all of a vertebral body; they are among very few lesions causing an appearance of increased signal on T1-weighted images (Figure 9-16). Although vertebral hemagiomas are usually innocent, more aggressive hemangiomatous lesions may expand the vertebral body and compromise the spinal canal (Figure 9-17).

Intradural neoplasms are well visualized, and their relationship to the spinal cord and cauda equina in the lumbar and lower thoracic region ascertained with detail comparable to or exceeding that of water soluble myelography (Figure 9-18).

Figure 9-16: Vertebral body hemangioma.

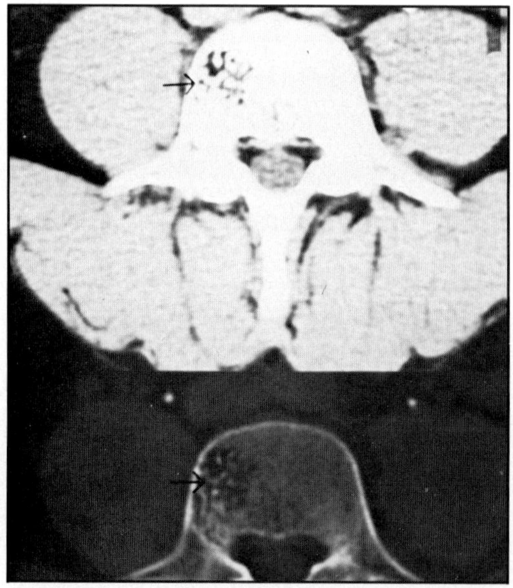

Figure 9-16A: CT showing an area of decreased overall density with coarsened trabeculae (arrow).

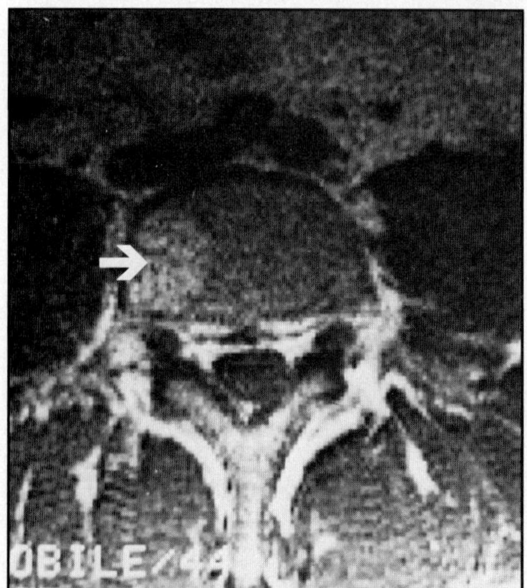

Figure 9-16B: MR shows the hemangioma as a lesion of increased signal intensity (arrow) on T1 weighted study.

Figure 9-17: Hemangiomatous lesion of T12.

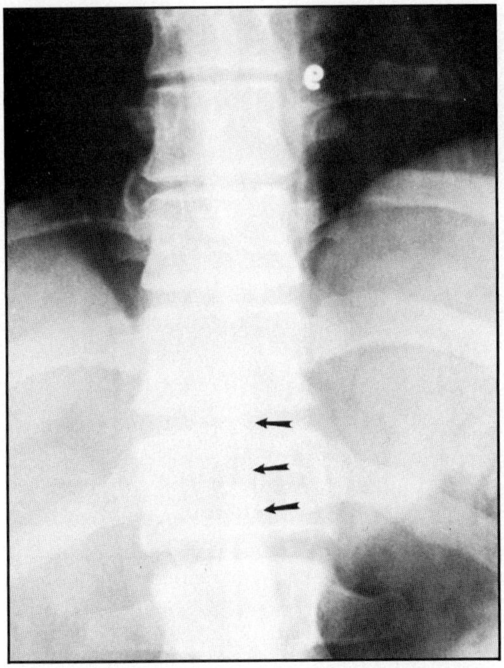

Figure 9-17A: AP view from myelogram with water soluble contrast. The striated, expanding lesion of T12 is seen. There is subtle extradural defect on the contrast column at the T12 level (arrows).

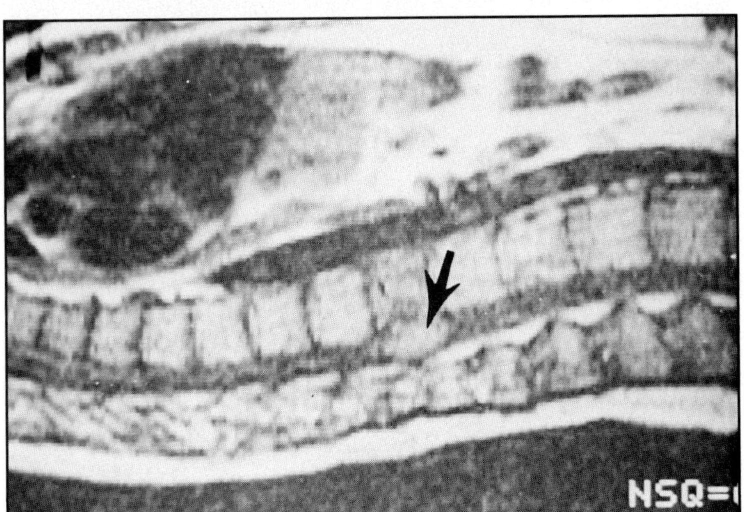

Figure 9-17B: T1 weighted sagittal MR demonstrates the expanding lesion extending into the spinal canal.

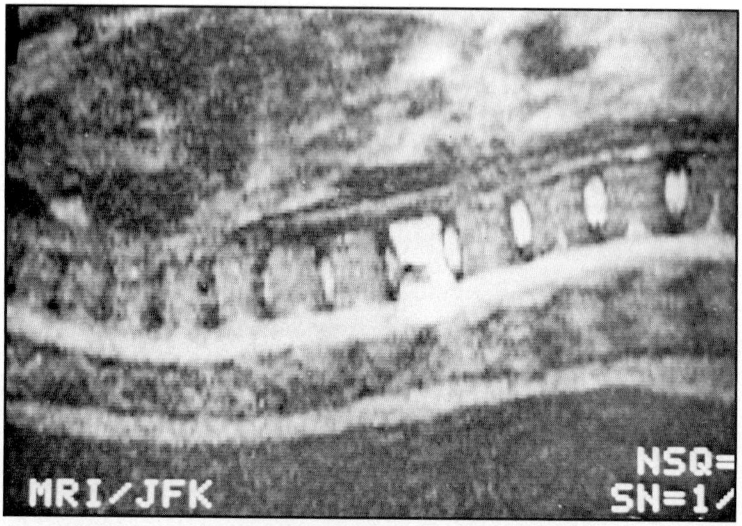

Figure 9-17C: T2 weighted sagittal MR again demonstrates the expanding lesion of T12 extending into the spinal canal, and demonstrates the relationship to the spinal cord.

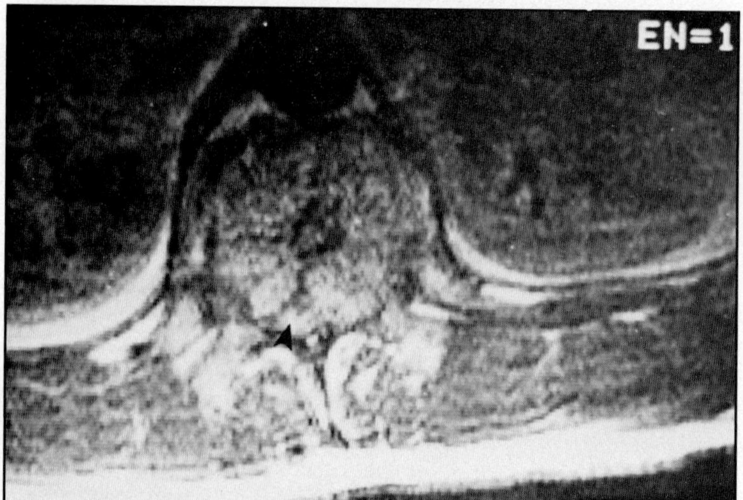

Figure 9-17D: Transverse MR shows the compressed cord (arrowhead) with the expanded vertebral body impinging on the spinal canal.

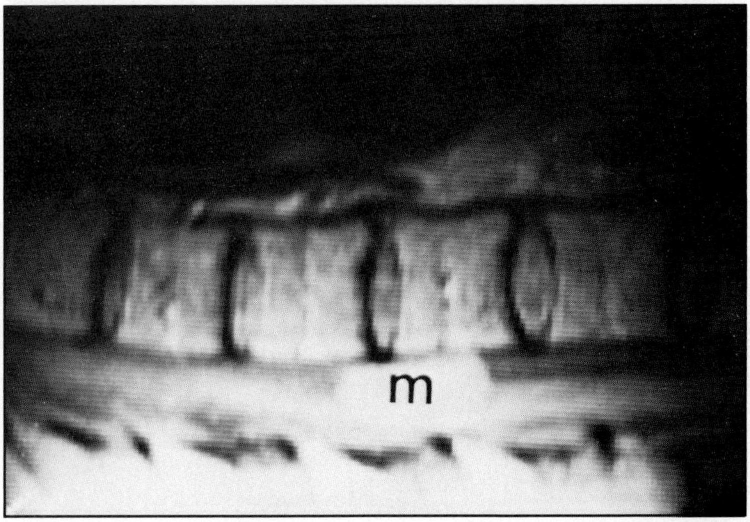

Figure 9-18A: Meningioma (M) at the level of T10 shown with signal greater than CSF on proton density weighted image (TR2000,TE32).

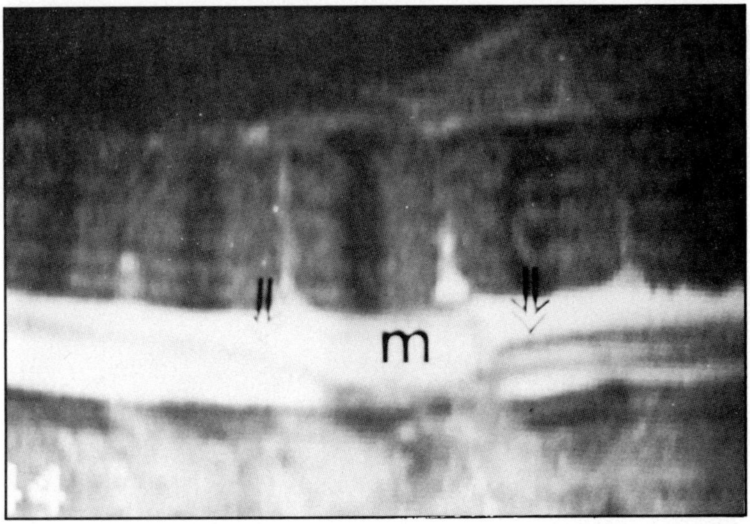

Figure 9-18B: T2 weighted image (TR2000, TE192) shows the meningioma (M) as less intense as CSF. Displacement of the spinal cord (open arrows) by the intradural, extradural medullary tumor is demonstrated.

Figure 9-19: Diffuse marrow involvement in leukemia.

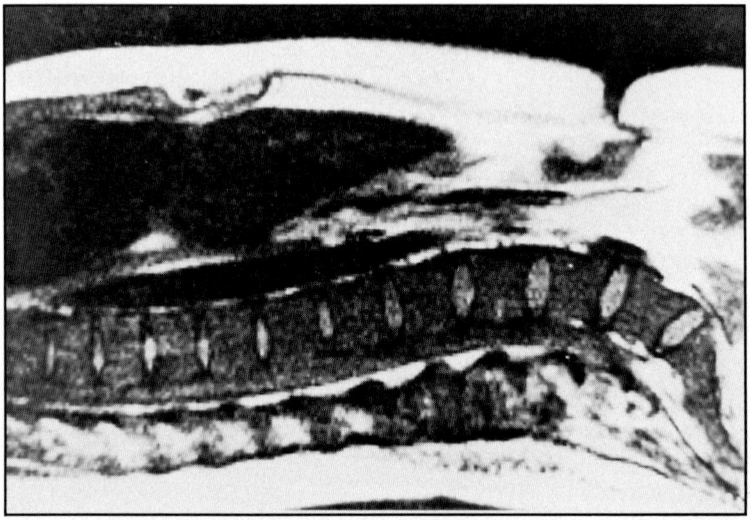

Figure 9-19A: T1 weighted image shows vertebral body signal iso-intense with CSF and less than the intervertebral discs.

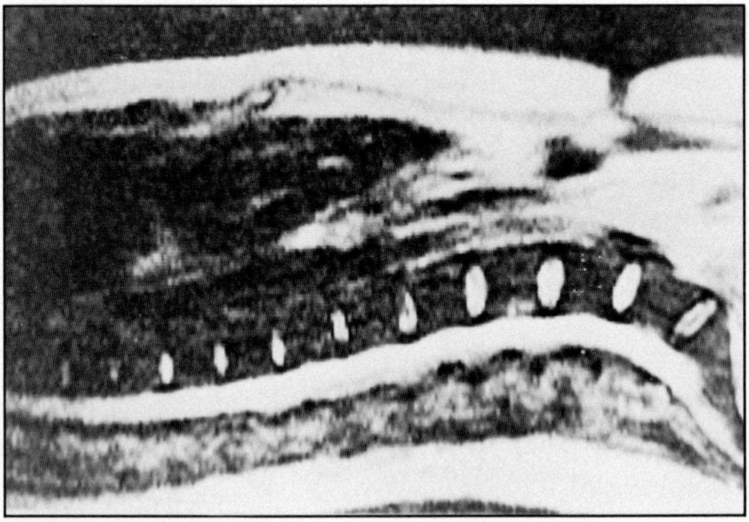

Figure 9-19B: T2 weighted image (TR2000, TE192) shows the meningioma (M) as less intense as CSF. Displacement of the spinal cord (open arrows) by the intradural, extradural medullary tumor is demonstrated.

Diffuse bone marrow abnormality such as leukemia may be manifest as a generalized abnormality of marrow signal (Figure 9-19) without focal lesion. This is appreciated by comparison of the marrow signal to that of the adjacent intervertral discs and CSF. This finding is not specific for leukemia; other processes of marrow replacement, or of iron deposition in the marrow, may cause similar appearance.

CHAPTER 10

Pitfalls; Artifacts and Limitations; Legal Implications; Future Directions

Pitfalls

Transitional Vertebrae

Operating at the wrong level is one of the most serious errors in spinal surgery. As discussed previously in Chapter 6, the identification of transitional vertebrae may be difficult on MR images, and requires a conscious search. Although the precise terminology to describe a transitional vertebra is unimportant, proper correlation of levels between the MR study and radiographs is essential to avoid surgical misadventure.

Scoliosis and Partial Volume Effects

Scoliosis complicates evaluation of lumbar MR images by two basically different, although related, mechanisms (Figure 10-1).

First of all, the routine sagittal and angled axial planes utilized to image the lumbar spine are chosen because they lie parallel to or perpendicular to key anatomic structures. In the scoliotic spine, axial images will pass obliquely through the intervertebral discs, and sagittal sections obliquely through the intervertebral nerve exit canals. These oblique sections distort the anatomy displayed, and also make the images more susceptible to partial volume artifact.

Secondly, in addition to distorting individual anatomic structures, scoliosis produces a loss of normally expected symmetry. This loss of symmetry complicates the routine side-to-side and level-to-level comparison of anatomic structures. For example, on sagittal images sections through the concavity of the scoliosis will have no exact counterpart on the convexity, and no single parasagittal section will include all of the intervertebral canals in a single section (Figure 10-1, 10-2). A sagittal section through the midline of the thecal sac above and below the apex of the scoliotic curve may section the theca tangentially at the apex of the curve

Figure 10-1: Schematic representation of coronal projection of a levoscoliosis. A sagittal section through plane A passes through the right pedicle of L4, but medial to the pedicles at L3 and L5. The theca is sectioned at L3 and L5, but not at L4. This has the potential to create spurious appearance of AP diameter stenosis. Sections through sagittal plane B include the pedicles at L3 and L5 but pass medial to the L4 pedicle, sectioning the theca tangentially at the L4 level. Right parasagittal images have no exact counterpart on the left.

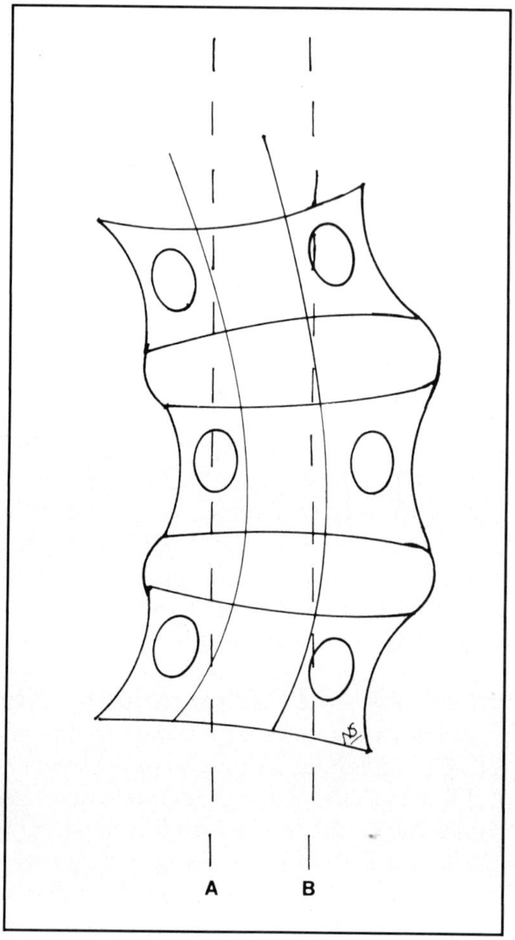

leading to a false impression of an AP diameter spinal stenosis. Similarly a section through the nucleus pulposus of a disc at the apex of a scoliosis and through the annulus fibrosis at levels above and below the scoliosis (Figure 10-1) may create a false impression of abnormal variation in disc signal intensities.

Despite these difficulties, the scoliotic spine can be evaluated by MR. The key to correct interpretation is careful evaluation of *each anatomic region individually*. In difficult cases, the addition of coronal and/or angled oblique sections is helpful.

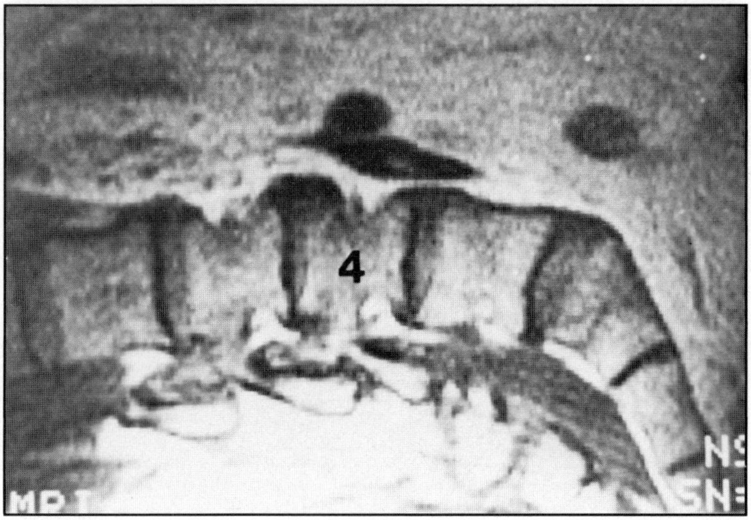

Figure 10-2A: Effect of scoliosis on sagittal MR image. Section through the right pedicle of L4 passes through the theca at more cranial and caudal levels.

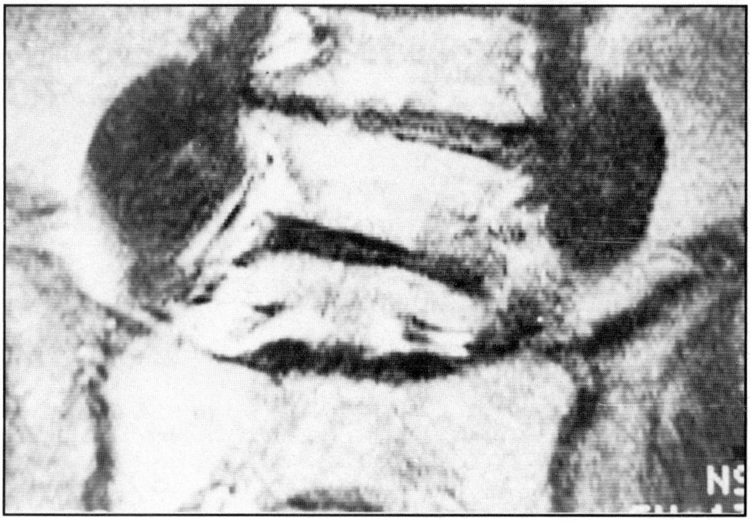

Figure 10-2B: Coronal view showing the vertebral body and disc relationships.

Figure 10-3: Congenital asymmetry of laminae.

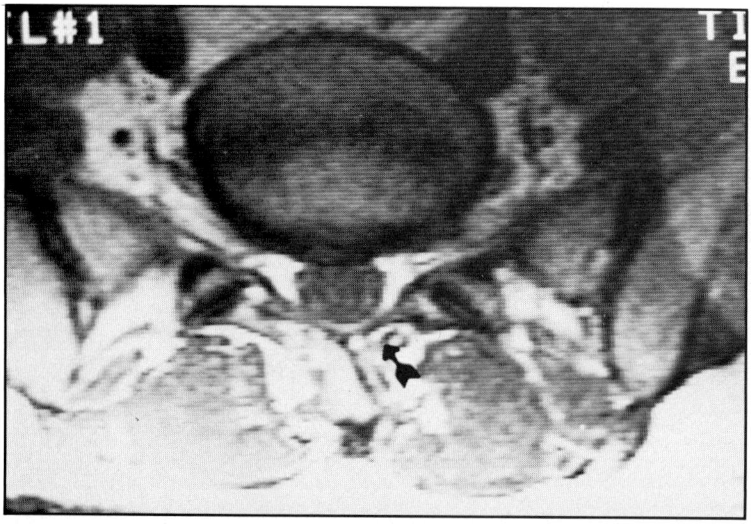

Figure 10-3A: There is thinning of the left laminae (arrow) as compared to the right.

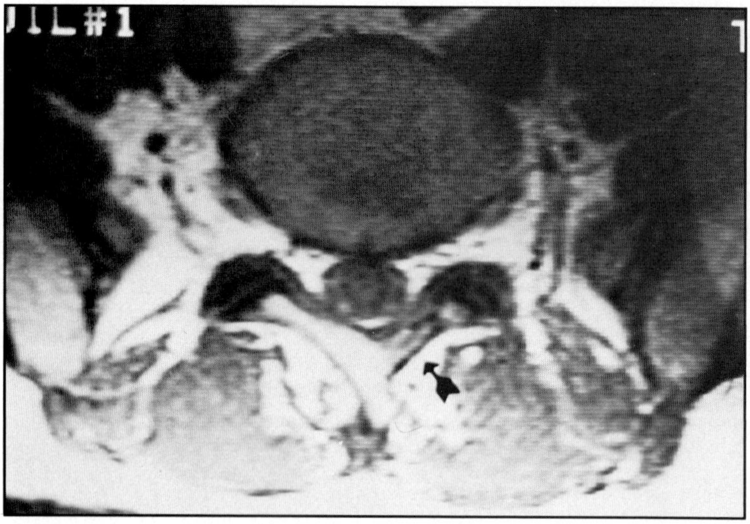

Figure 10-3B: Section slightly cephalad to A shows intact lamina and slight asymmetry of spinous process.

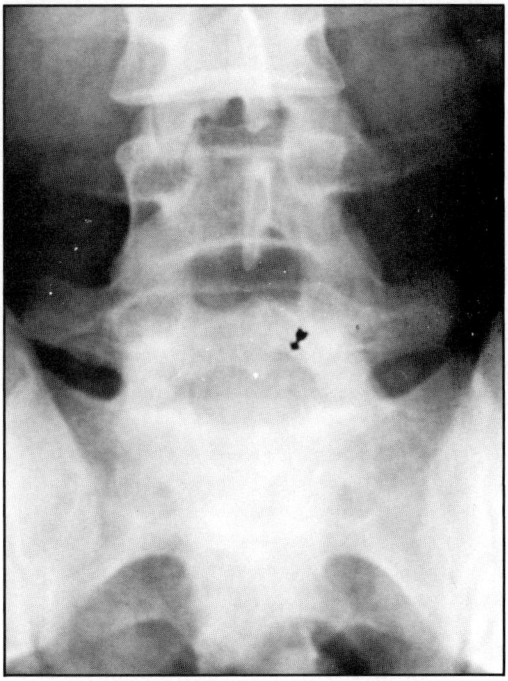

Figure 10-3C: AP radiograph showing the congenital variation with a "notch" in the inferior margin of the left lamina of L5 (arrow).

The *Pseudowashboard* Spine

On myelography, the appearance of multiple anterior extradural defects producing a scalloped appearance to the anterior border of the contrast column in lateral view has been referred to as a *washboard spine*. This is usually indicative of severe degenerative changes at multiple disc levels.

Sagittal T2-weighted MR images may show a similar appearance (Figure 10-4). This MR myelogram must be interpreted with caution. With certain pulse sequences, the CSF becomes isointense with epidural fat, so that the scalloped appearance of the anterior margin of the bright signal within the spinal canal actually represents a combination of the theca and the normal epidural fat posterior to the vertebral bodies, and not true pathologic indentiation of the theca. Careful scrutiny of the multi-echo sequence prevents misinterpretation.

Figure 10-4: "Pseudowashboard appearance of the spine.

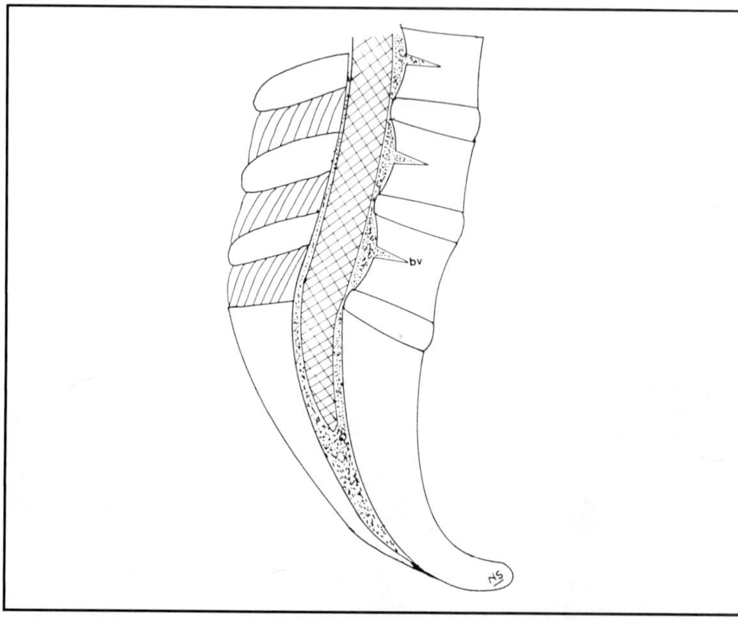

Figure 10-4A: Schematic of a T1 weighted pulse sequence on which the CSF (crosshatched) is distinguished from the epidural fat (stippled). Note the epidural fat about the basivertebral vein (BV) as it pierces the posterior vertebral body.

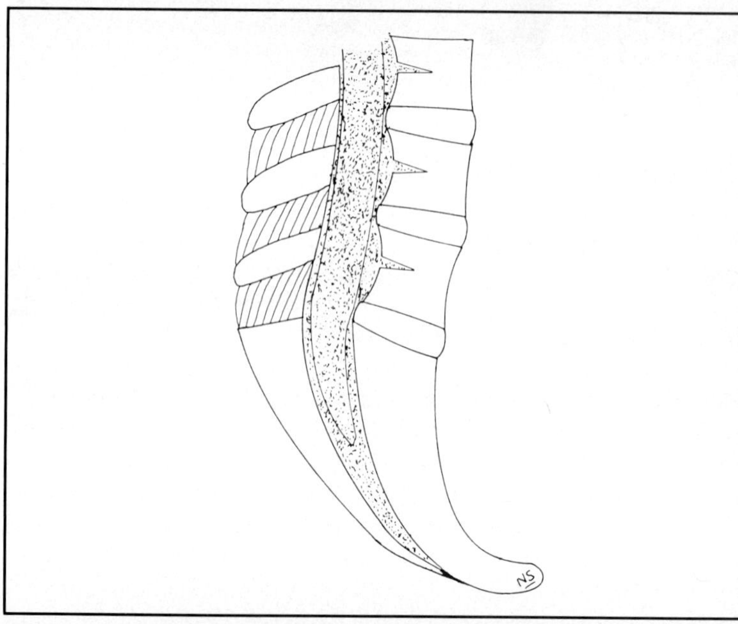

Figure 10-4B: With T2 weighting the CSF and epidural fat are iso-intense (stippled). This creates the false appearance of a "washboard" spine.

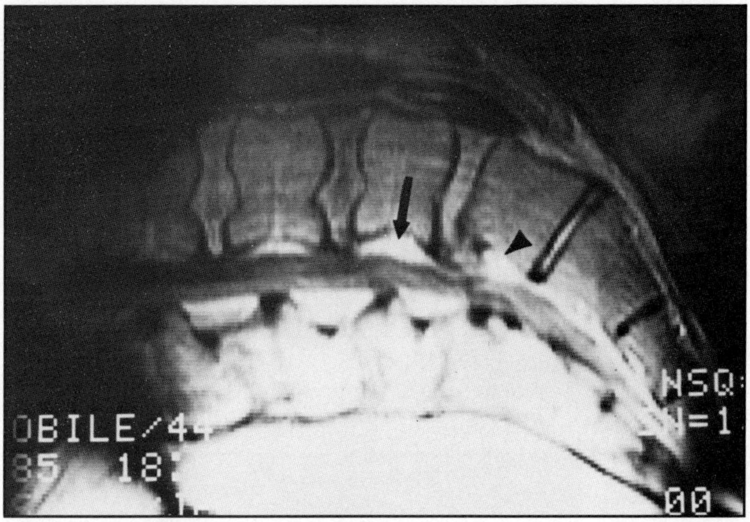

Figure 10-4C: Sagittal T1 weighted MR. There is a fat posterior to the L4 vertebral body (arrow) as well as a "fat wedge" beneath an L5-S1 disc protrusion associated with pseudoretrolisthesis.

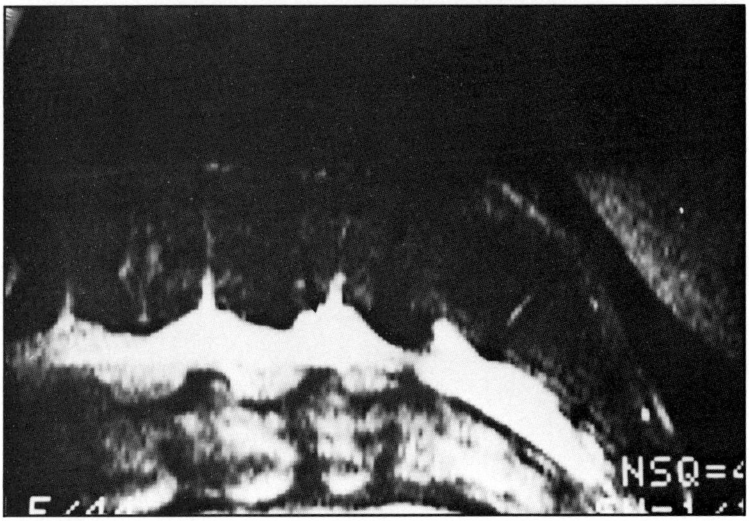

Figure 10-4D: T2 weighted (TR2000,TE250) sagittal MR. CSF and epidural fat are iso-intense, exaggerating the washboard appearance of the spine.

Figure 10-5: MR appearance of Pantopaque.

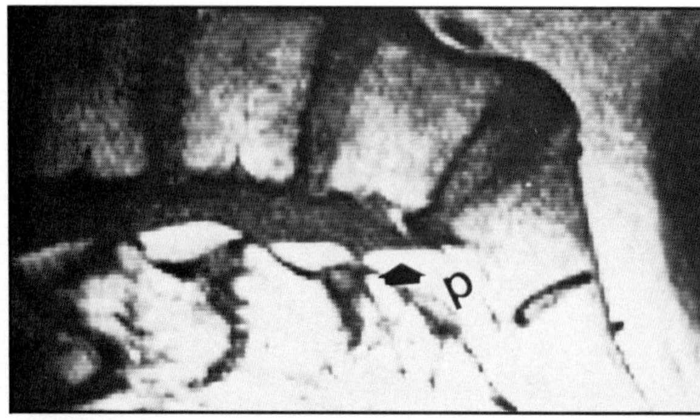

Figure 10-5A: T1 weighted image showing the Pantopaque (P) with bright signal and a contrast-CSF level (arrow).

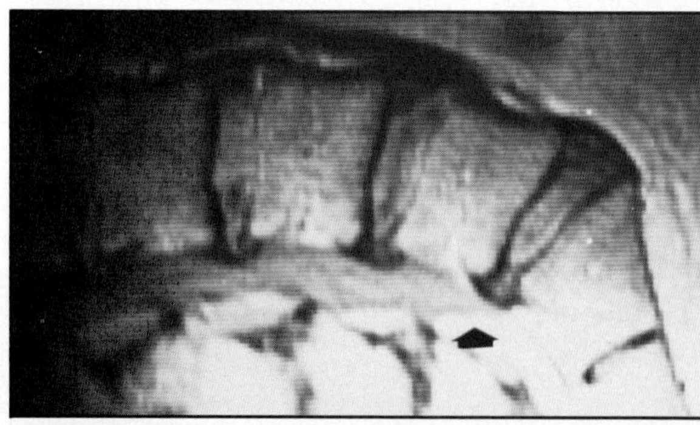

Figure 10-5B: Proton density weighted image (TR2000, TE30) again shows the contrast-CSF level with the dependent contrast showing increased signal intensity.

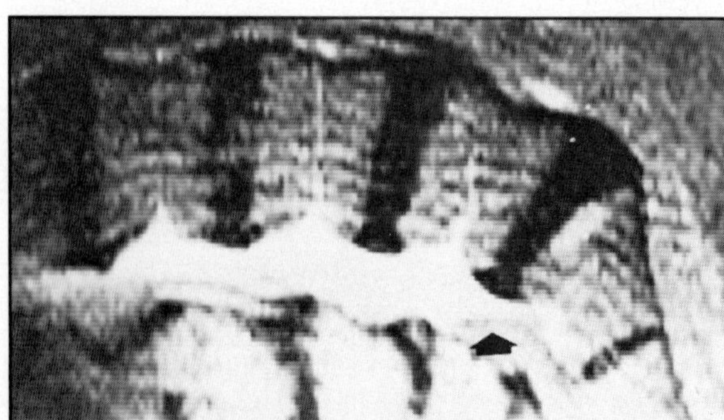

Figure 10-5C: T2 weighted image (TR2000, TE180) shows the dependent Pantopaque with intermediate signal less than the bright CSF. CSF-Pantopaque interface (arrow).

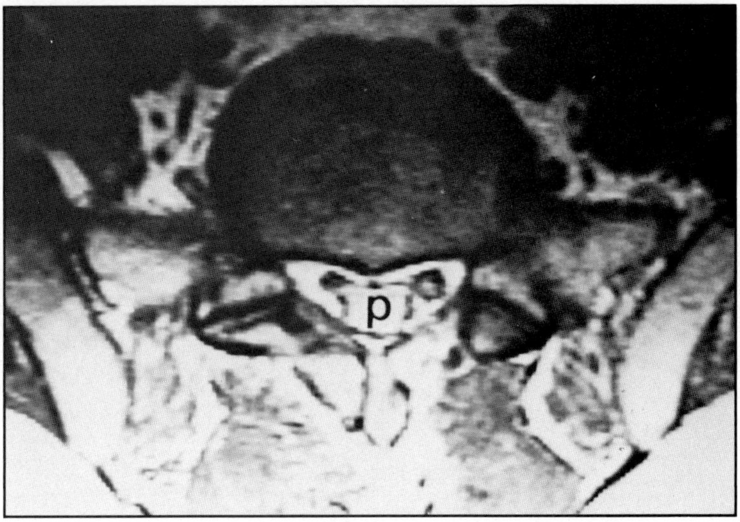

Figure 10-5D: Transverse moderately T1 weighted image. The Pantopaque (P) has relatively bright signal only slightly less than epidural fat.

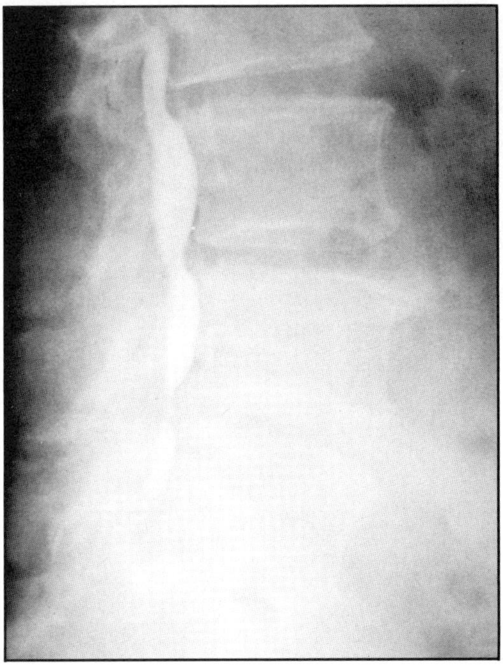

Figure 10-5E: Lateral lumbar radiograph showing Pantopaque.

Figure 10-6: Artifact from tiny metallic particles following surgery.

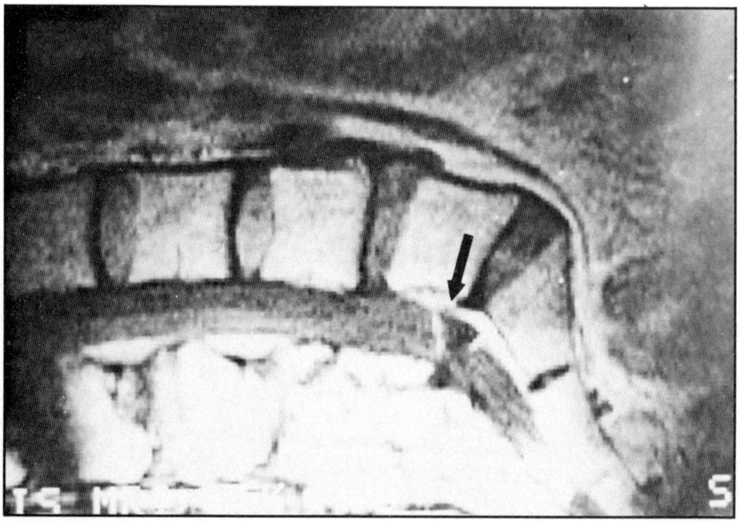

Figure 10-6A: Sagittal MR demonstrating artifactual appearing areas of linear bright signal posterior to L5-S1 in a postoperative case.

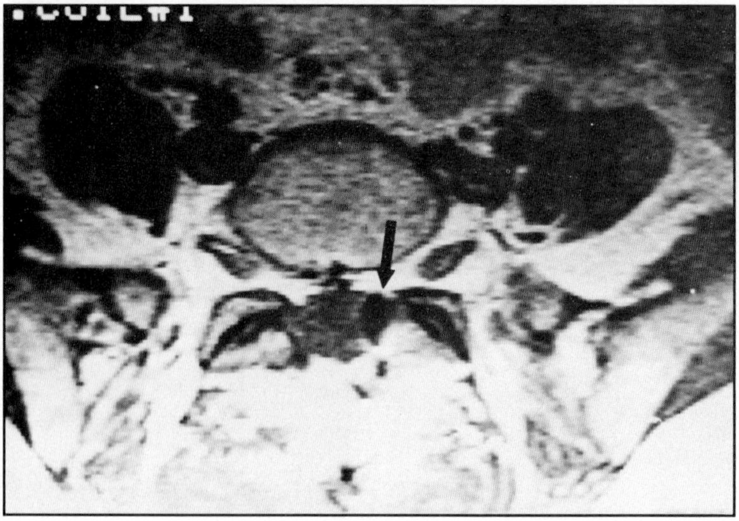

Figure 10-6B: Corresponding axial MR showing artifact at similar location. CT scan was negative for metallic particle or other abnormality at this location.

Figure 10-6C & D: Another patient demonstrating a more striking example of this artifact.

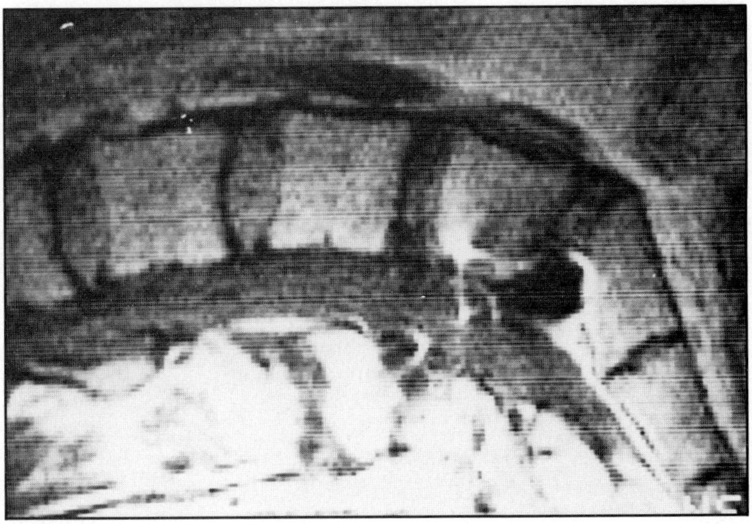

Figure 10-6C.

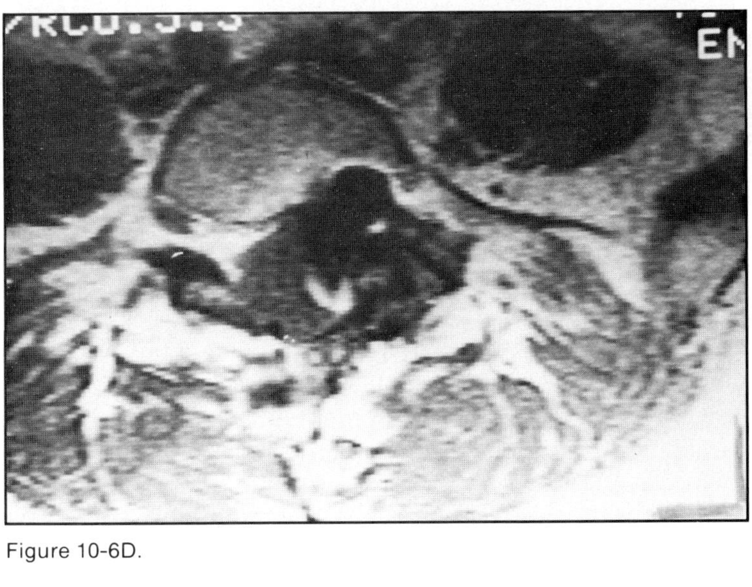

Figure 10-6D.

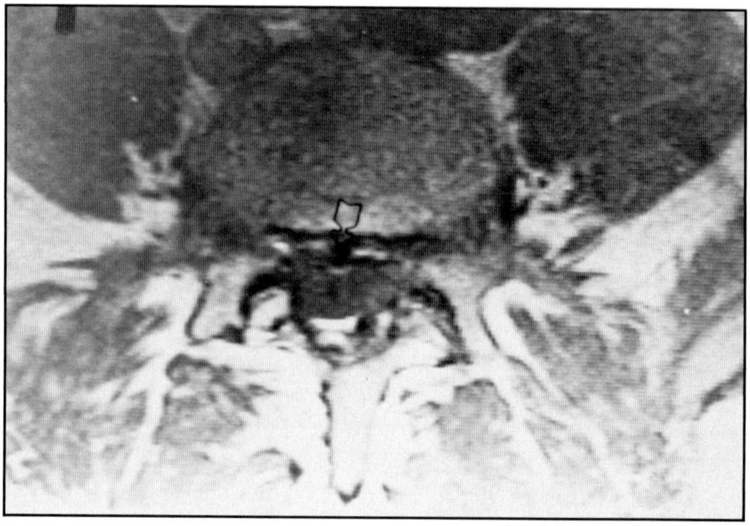

Figure 10-7: Spinal epidural catheter (open arrow) shown as a small rounded area of decreased signal. The adjacent thin crescent of bright signal may represent epidural fat or artifact.

Artifacts and Limitations

Residual Pantopaque and Other Foreign Body Artifacts

Foreign material in or around the spine may produce artifacts on MR images. Pantopaque when present in relatively large amounts is easily recognizable (Mamourian & Briggs, 1986). This oily contrast material has signal intensity behavior similar to fat with multiple pulse sequences, bright with respect to CSF on T1-weighted sequences and less intense than CSF on T2-weighting. This signal behavior, associated with a fat-fluid level indicating the Pantopaque-CSF interface, is diagnostic (Figure 10-5). Smaller droplets of Pantopaque scattered among the nerve roots of the cauda equina present a more confusing picture; I have seen such droplets misinterpreted as small introdural metastases. Correlation to radiographs is helpful in making this distinction.

Occasional postoperative studies (Figures 10-6a-d) demonstrate an MR artifact suggesting a metallic foreign body. However, radiographs and CT scans in these cases may demonstrate no metallic foreign material. Microscopic particles of metal resulting from wear and/or contact of orthopedic instruments, particularly drill bits, have recently been demonstrated to explain this appearance (Heindel et al., 1986).

A spinal epidural catheter (Figure 10-7) produces a small rounded area of decreased signal intensity within the spinal canal; the diagnosis is confirmed by the clinical history and radiographs.

Surgical clips within the spinal canal cause local artifact related to perturbation of the magnetic field. Larger surgical implants such as Harrington or other orthopedic rods, cause more pronounced artifact, but do not preclude MR imaging (Figure 6-14).

Miscellaneous Artifacts

Post-myelographic artifacts may be demonstrated by MR imaging. Figure 10-8a is a metrizamide myelogram performed via L3-4 injection following initial unsuccessful bloody spinal tap at L2-3. No L2-3 defect is visible myelographically, and clinically the patient demonstrated no evidence of abnormality at this level. MR study several hours later shows a very definite anterior extradural defect at the L2-3 disc level (Figure 10-8b), despite the presence of normal hydration signal at the L2-3 disc. Although unproven, this is presumed to represent a post-myelographic defect, either a small hematoma or perhaps even a small amount of nuclear material extruded through a needle puncture in the annulus.

Sections through the lower lumbar levels occasionally show a prominent pattern of epidural veins (Figure 10-9); these are easily identifiable when surrounded by epidural fat but could become more problematic when directly adjacent to the disc margin.

An appearance of alternating light and dark stripes in the image is occasionally seen (Figure 10-10); this artifact is related to a combination of effects of motion and numerical rounding on the image reconstruction algorithm utilizing the Fourier transform. This appearance, most prominently seen on late echoes of a multi-echo sequence, must not be confused with nerve roots or other actual anatomic structures.

A variety of other miscellaneous artifacts related to system malfunction have been described (Cahill, 1985). A discussion of these system artifacts is beyond the scope of this chapter; although the causes of these artifacts may be complex, varied, and difficult to ascertain, the artifactual nature of the images produced is generally obvious.

Partial volume effects unrelated to scoliosis include sections through a congenitally asymmetric lamina (Figure 10-3) simulating the appearance of a partial laminectomy.

Figure 10-8: Post-myelographic artifact.

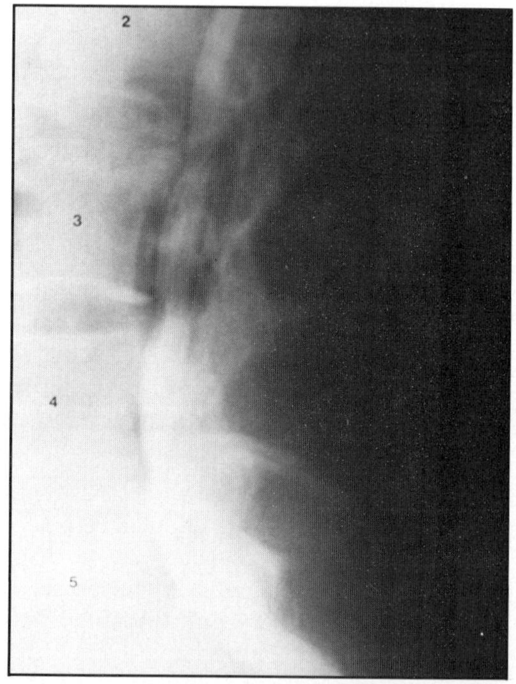

Figure 10-8A: Lateral myelographic view shows no abnormality at L2-3. Initial L2-3 tap was traumatic.

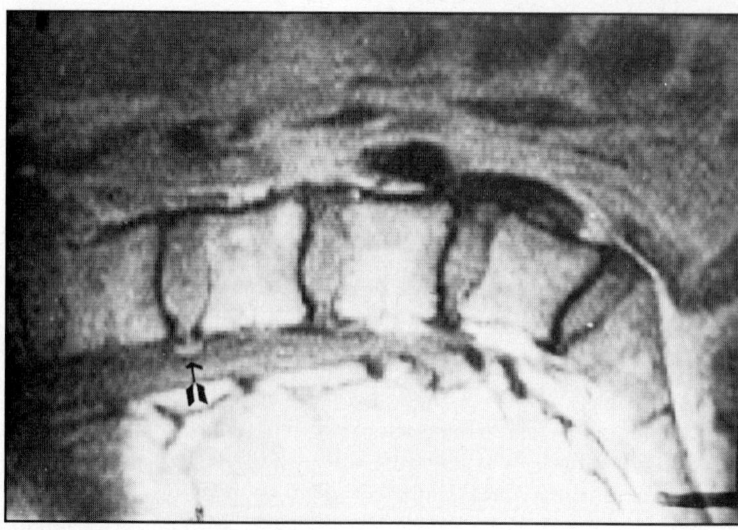

Figure 10-8B: Sagittal MR demonstrating apparent L2-3 anterior extradural defect iso-intense with disc (arrow).

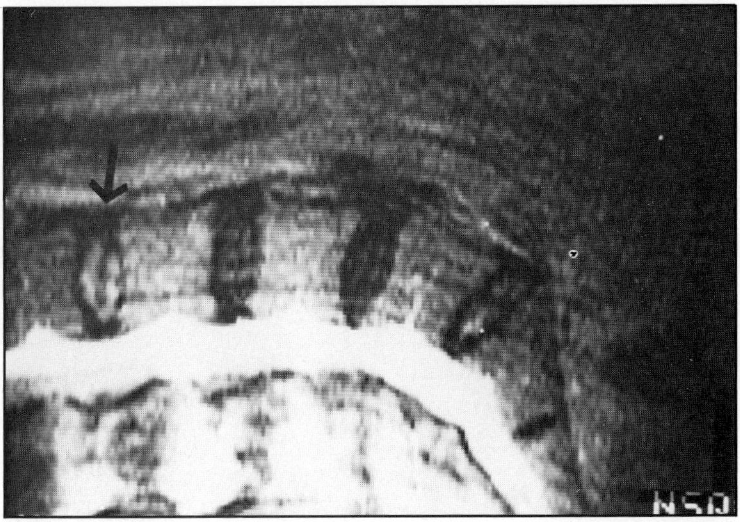

Figure 10-8C: The L2-3 disc (arrow) has normal hydration signal. The anterior extradural defect is iso-intense with CSF. No clinical evidence of L2 abnormality. Finding presumably represents post-myelographic artifact from either small hematoma or small iatrogenic extrusion of disc material.

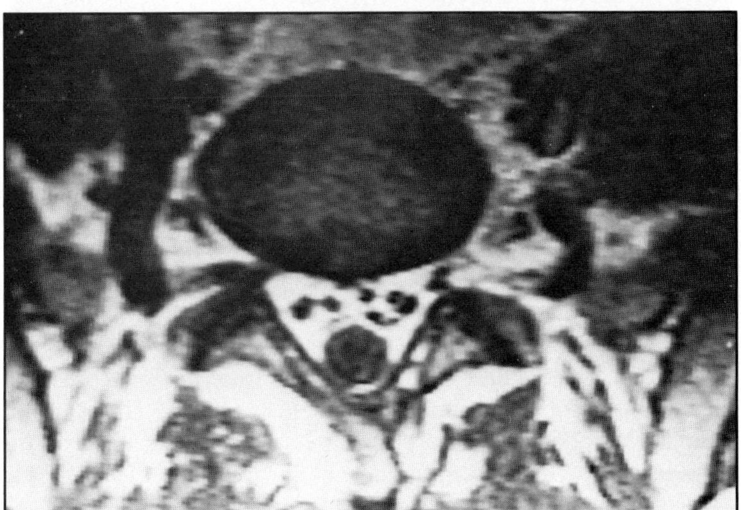

Figure 10-9: Multiple epidural veins seen as small rounded low intensity structures within the abundant epidural fat.

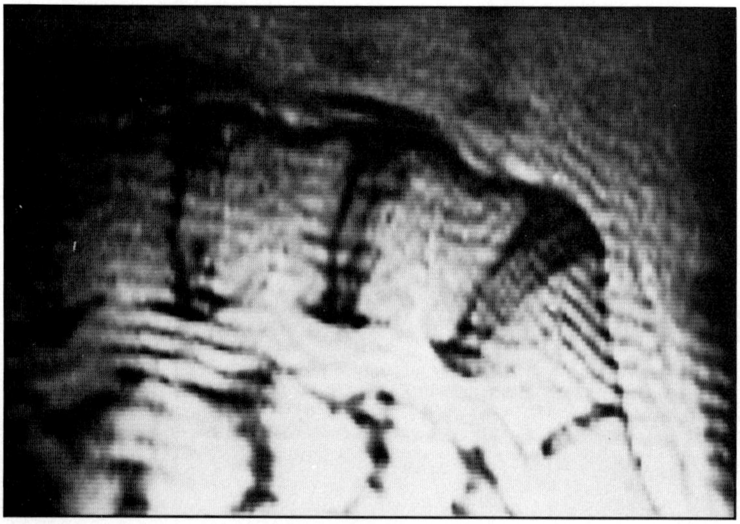

Figure 10-10: Pattern of stripes is obviously artifactual and is related to motion and truncation (rounding) error.

Limitations of Lumbar Spine MRI

A small percentage of patients are unable to undergo MR studies because of pacemakers or other contraindications. An additional small percentage of the population will be unable to complete the examination because of claustrophobia or other factors preventing cooperation for the time period involved.

Because of the time and expense involved in an MR study, any practical imaging protocol of necessity represents a compromise. Not all pulse sequences, in all planes of interest, can be obtained for every patient.

Although MR presents a very detailed anatomic map, earlier hopes of specific tissue characterization have not yet been realized. In particular, although the normal nucleus pulposus differs markedly from the annulus fibrosis, the degenerating nucleus pulposus often produces a signal very similar to the annulus. Herniated disc fragments show quite a bit of variation in their signal intensity depending upon their hydration, and are iso-intense with the theca utilizing certain sequences. In practice, this has not proven to be a serious limitation.

Perhaps the most serious limitation of MR imaging is its inability to fully assess the clinical significance of lesions demonstrated (Figure 10-11). Of course, this limitation is not unique to MR but

Figure 10-11: Small central disc protrusion.

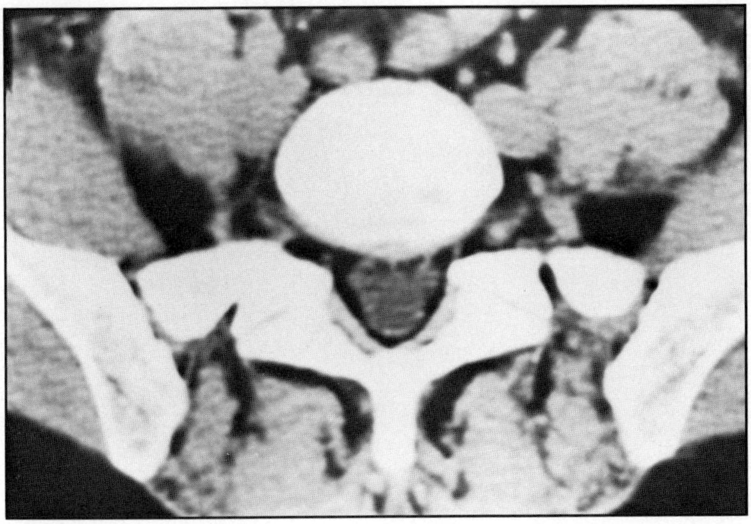

Figure 10-11A: CT Scan.

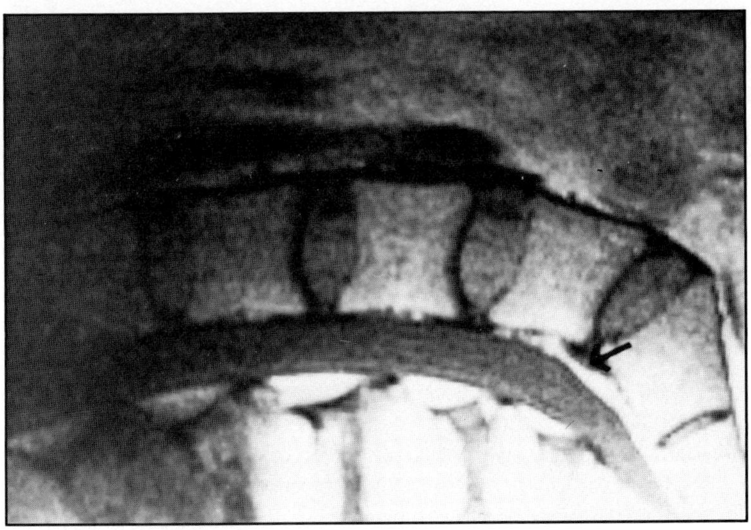

Figure 10-11B: Sagittal MR. The small protrusion (arrow) is separated from the theca by epidural fat.

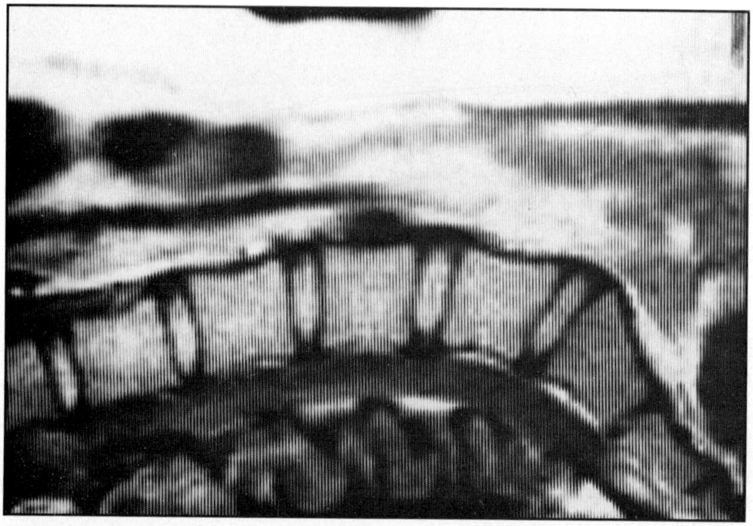

Figure 10-11C: Transverse MR again shows the small central protrusion. Theca and S1 roots separated from the protrusion by epidural fat.

applies to all imaging modalities. There is, however, a danger that the greater sensitivity of MRI will lead to the detection of an increasing number of abnormalities of uncertain clinical significance.

At this time, the static nature of MR images may represent a limitation in the evaluation of patients whose symptomatology is related to activity; the importance of this potential limitation is unknown (Chapter 8-2G).

Legal Implications of Spinal MRI

A substantial fraction of patients referred for spinal MR study will have a history of injury related to motor vehicle accident, work-related injury, or other injury involving potential litigation. The legal profession is becoming increasingly aware of the potential role of MR in providing objective evidence of spinal injury; indeed, MR has become a topic of popular interest not only at medical but also at legal continuing education programs.

Although orthopedists, neurosurgeons, and other physicians caring for patients with back injuries have come to expect frequent depositions and occasional courtroom appearances as routine, radiologists have only occasionally been required to become

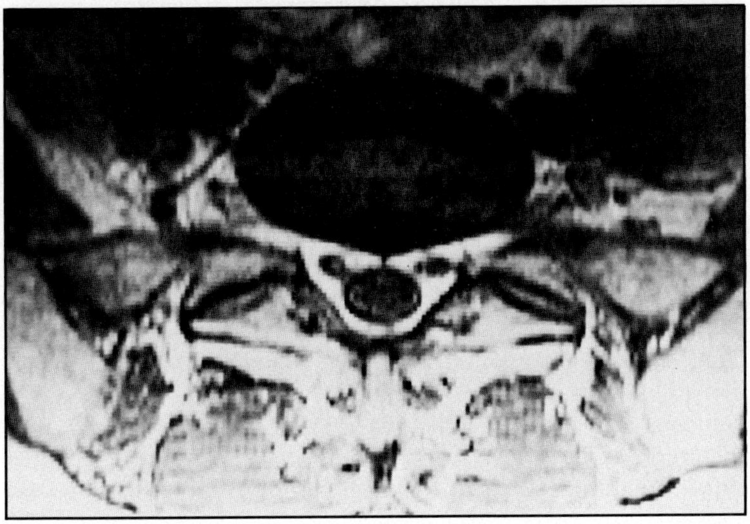

Figure 10-12: Normal study, **not** intradiscal herniations. The bright disc signal representing nucleus pulposus and transition of nucleus to annulus is normally located eccentrically within the disc space, closer to the posterior margin.

involved in the legal process. However, because of the novelty of MR imaging, lack of familiarity of clinicians with the techniques involved, and potential legal importance of the findings of MR studies, radiologists interpreting spinal MRI will frequently be asked for their testimony.

For those unfamiliar with the deposition process, Appendix E presents some simple suggestions which in my experience lead to a shorter, more pleasant, and more efficient deposition for all parties concerned. In most instances, the nature of the findings present on an MR examination can be easily described. Assessment of the age, etiology, significance, and prognostic importance of these findings is much more difficult. At this time, there is no adequate database describing the normal appearance of the lumbar spine at various ages, and particularly describing the relative frequency of diminished disc hydration at differing ages. Similarly, the exact time course of loss of hydration of the nucleus pulposus following an injury is not known precisely, and the prognostic importance of a desiccated disc is unclear. Although certain types of pathology, such as severe disc degeneration with osteophyte spurring, are clearly chronic, the sensitivity of MR scanning in identifying acute injury superimposed on chronic underlying pathology may be limited.

Under these circumstances, the best approach for the radiologist is to describe the findings present, but to be very cautious in relating these findings to a particular incident. Assessment of significance of a particular finding is often best left to the treating clinician (Figure 10-11).

The precise terminology used to describe the findings present may have implications to an attorney not intended by the reporting radiologist. For example, the normal circumference of an intervertebral disc is slightly greater than that of the adjacent vertebrae, so that in a certain sense there is a normal anatomic bulge of the disc relative to the vertebra. Despite this, it is very difficult to convince an attorney that a "bulging" disc is normal. Similarly, I have seen the normal eccentric position of the nucleus pulposus within the annulus described as intradiscal herniation (Figure 10-12). If MR is to retain credibility in both the medical and legal communities, these types of misinterpretations must be avoided.

Future Directions

Over the next several years continuing evolution of MR systems, including both hardware and software modifications, will permit the acquisition of better and better images in reasonable acquisition times. These improvements, along with an enlarging database and availability of MR contrast agents, should further increase the role of magnetic resonance imaging in the evaluation of the lumbar spine.

Hardware improvements will include magnets of increasing field uniformity. Computerized automatic shim programs now permit attainment of field uniformity of only a few parts per million over reasonable imaging volumes. Newly designed magnets which produce a local magnetic field in front of the magnet, creating in essence a surface scanner, may be possible. These would permit imaging in various postures, permitting dynamic assessment of the spine.

Surface coils of improved geometry and efficiency are on the horizon. These coils, coupled with steeper magnetic field gradients, will permit scans of increased spatial resolution.

A variety of pulse sequences including those with partial tip angles and gradient reversal will allow scans in shorter time. Chemical shift imaging allows separation of the fat and water components of the tissues. The use of pulse sequences with short

TR and short TE will provide true T1 weighted images.

Improved software including more accurate localizer scans, multiple angled obliques, and faster image processing will permit increased patient throughput. Improved RF electronics will permit thinner contiguous slices with more accurate slice profiles. These may take the form of either multislice, multi-echo imaging or of three dimensional acquisitions. Images having any desired orientation, including curved planes such as the curved coronal images will be available either by direct acquisition or as reformatted images from three dimensional acquisitions.

Improved display methods will evolve to handle the tremendous amount of data generated. These may take the form of planar displays, or of three dimensional presentations including holograms.

Magnetic contrast agents such as gadolinium DTPA are likely to prove useful, particularly in postoperative cases where the role may be similar to that of radiographic contrast agents for CT scanning.

At surgical exploration, significantly compressed nerves are often noted to have a characteristic pale appearance, often associated with edema of the nerve distal to the compression. Measurements of the relaxation parameters of nerve roots, or spectroscopic analysis of the nerve roots, have the potential to help answer the question of whether an abnormality is causing significant nerve compression.

As experience with lumbar MR scanning increases, our knowledge of the normal variation in the MR appearance will increase. This expanding database, especially as regards the incidence and natural history of disc desiccation, will permit more meaningful interpretation of lumbar MR studies. The significance and prognosis of an asymptomatic desiccated disc demonstrated on an MR study is not yet known. Should such a finding turn out to correlate with subsequent back related disability, some employers may require pre-employment lumbar spine MR screening.

Finally, and highly speculative, is the possibility that the new insights into the lumbar spine provided by MR imaging may be coupled with the evolving technologies of percutaneous discectomy, chemonucleolysis or other disc injection therapy, and robotic surgery to provide an entirely new approach to the treatment of lumbar disc disease. Surgical discectomy as now practiced produces an accelerated degeneration of the intervertebral disc, frequently leading to late degeneration of the zygapophyseal joints. These complications might be prevented by replacing the damaged nucleus pulposus with a synthetic nucleus, either surgically or percutaneously. Such a synthetic nucleus might take the form of a polymerizing gel injected through a needle, of a detachable balloon placed through a cannula, or of a biologic replacement prepared with tissue culture techniques.

In summary, magnetic resonance imaging is likely to play an increasingly important role in the evaluation of the lumbar spine. Technical refinements already under development are certain to provide images of even better quality than those available today. Images will be obtained in less time, and improved display techniques will make them easier to interpret. The use of new pulse sequences, spectroscopic imaging, and contrast enhancement will permit more precise tissue identification. New types of scanner geometry are under development; if successful, these will permit dynamic evaluation of functional abnormalities. Finally, MR scanning coupled with other emerging technologies promises a new, more rational approach to the treatment of lumbar disc disease.

Appendices

Appendix A

MR PATIENT SCREENING FORM

DATE: ______________

NAME: ______________________________

ADDRESS: ______________________________

CITY STATE ZIP

DATE OF BIRTH: __________ AGE ____ PHONE NUMBER: __________

REFERRING PHYSICIAN: ______________________________

WHAT IS YOUR PRESENT COMPLAINT? ______________________________

HAVE YOU EVER HAD SURGERY IN THE PAST? YES ______ NO ______

IF YES, WHAT PART OF THE BODY? ______________________________

IS THERE ANY KNOWN HISTORY OF CEREBRAL ANEURYSM? ______________

DO YOU HAVE A PACEMAKER? YES ________ NO ________

IS THERE ANY POSSIBILITY YOU MAY BE PREGNANT? YES ___ NO ___

HAVE YOU EVER HAD CANCER? YES _____ NO _____ IF YES, WHAT PART OF THE BODY? ______________________________

DID YOU RECEIVE RADIATION OR CHEMOTHERAPY? YES _____ NO _____

HAVE YOU EVER HAD ANY PREVIOUS DIAGNOSTIC TESTS? (CT SCANS, ULTRASOUND, NUCLEAR MEDICINE SCANS? YES ______ NO _____ IF YES, WHERE DID YOU HAVE THE SCAN? ______________________________

** PLEASE MAKE SURE ALL FERROMAGNETIC OBJECTS INCLUDING WATCHES, JEWELRY, KEYS, BANK AND CREDIT CARDS HAVE BEEN REMOVED.

SPINE MR PATIENT HISTORY

NAME ______________________________

AGE: ____________ DATE ____________

1. WHY DID YOU VISIT YOUR DOCTOR? ______________________________

2. WhAT DO YOU THINK CAUSED THE PROBLEM? ______________________________

3. DESCRIBE YOUR PAIN (SHARP, BURNING, ETC.) ______________________________

4. DOES THE PAIN GO DOWN YOUR ARM OR LEG? IN THE BACK OR FRONT? RIGHT, LEFT OR BOTH? ______________________________

5. WHAT IF ANYTHING MAKES IT WORSE? (STANDING, SITTING, LYING DOWN, ETC.) ______________________________

6. DO YOU HAVE ANY WEAKNESS? __________ WHERE? ______________________________

7. DO YOU HAVE ANY NUMBNESS? __________ WHERE? ______________________________

8. HAVE YOU HAD ANY BOWEL OR BLADDER CHANGES? DESCRIBE: ______________________________

9.

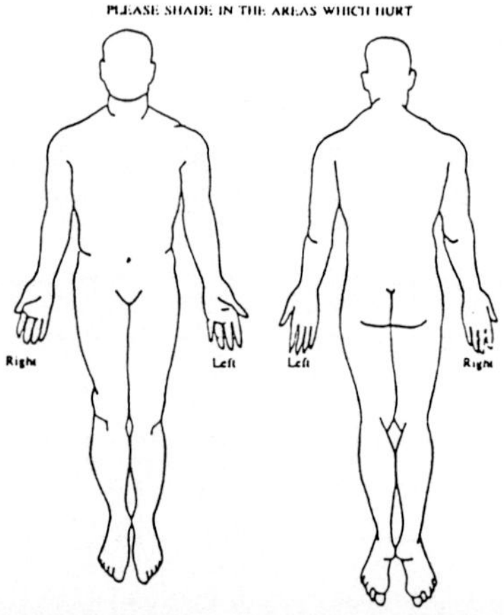

10. HAVE YOU HAD SURGERY ON YOUR BACK OR NECK? ____________

WHEN? ____________

WHERE? ____________

WHAT WAS DONE? ____________

____

____

Appendix B

M. R. PATIENT PROTOCOL

DATE: ____________________

PATIENT NAME: ____

I.D. NUMBER: ____

EXAM ORDERED: ____

DIAGNOSIS: ____

____

PROTOCOL NAME: ____

ADDITIONAL ACQUISITION: ____________________________

____

M. R. PROTOCOL

PROTOCOL NAME: ______________________________

ACQUISITION NAME	ACQUISITION #	ACQUISITION TIME
______________________________	_________	____________
______________________________	_________	____________
______________________________	_________	____________
______________________________	_________	____________
______________________________	_________	____________
______________________________	_________	____________

TOTAL ACQUISITION TIME: ____________

M. R. ACQUISITION

ACQUISITION: NAME: ____________________ # ______ TIME: _____

COIL: HEAD ________ BODY ________ SURFACE ______________

POSITIONING: HEAD FIRST ___ FEET FIRST ___ OTHER ____________

CENTERING ______________________________

PLANE: AXIAL ___ CORONAL ___ SAGITTAL ___ OTHER ____________

SLICES: SINGLE ______ MULTI _______ 3DI _______ 3DA ________

THICKNESS ____ GAP ____ NUMBER (TR/TE+15)) _______

PULSE SEQUENCE: SE: _______ ISE: _______ OT1: ______ CS: ______

N_y: _______ TR: ________ TI: _______ TE: ______

N_{Ex}: ______ ZOOM: ___________ ECHOES: ________

AT (TR x N_y x N_{Ex}): _____________

GATING: CARDIAC: ____ RESPIRATORY: ____ BOTH: _____ OTHER: ____

CONTRAST: ORAL: ___________ RECTAL: ____________ IV: __________

PHOTO FORMAT: 2 X 1: ______ 4 X 1: ______ 6 X 1: ______

9 X 1: _______ 15 X 1: _____

COMMENTS: ____

____

____

____

____

M. R. PATIENT PROTOCOL

DATE: 17 AUG 86

PATIENT NAME: John Doe

I.D. NUMBER: 123456

EXAM ORDERED: Lumbar Spine

DIAGNOSIS: ? HNP. Right Sided Sciatica

Scoliosis

PROTOCOL NAME: Routine Lumbar

ADDITIONAL ACQUISITION: Coronal T1W

M. R. PROTOCOL

PROTOCOL NAME: Routine Lumbar

ACQUISITION NAME	ACQUISITION #	ACQUISITION TIME
Spine Scout	4	2
Spine Sagittal T1W	5	5
Spine Sagittal ME	6	13
Spine Axial	7	12

TOTAL ACQUISITION TIME: 32 min.

M. R. ACQUISITION

ACQUISITION: NAME: Spine Scout # 4 TIME: 2

COIL: HEAD ____ BODY X SURFACE ____

POSITIONING: HEAD FIRST X FEET FIRST ____ OTHER ____

CENTERING Midline

PLANE: AXIAL ____ CORONAL ____ SAGITTAL X OTHER ____

SLICES: SINGLE ____ MULTI X 3DI ____ 3DA ____

THICKNESS 5mm GAP 1mm NUMBER (TR/TE+15)) 9

PULSE SEQUENCE: SE: X ISE: ____ OT1: ____ CS: ____

N_y: 128 TR: 500 TI: ____ TE: 40

N_{Ex}: 2 ZOOM: ____ ECHOES: 1

AT (TR x N_y x N_{Ex}): 2

GATING: CARDIAC: ____ RESPIRATORY: ____ BOTH: ____ OTHER: ____

CONTRAST: ORAL: ____ RECTAL: ____ IV: ____

PHOTO FORMAT: 2 X 1: ____ 4 X 1: ____ 6 X 1: ____

9 X 1: X 15 X 1: ____

COMMENTS: ____

M. R. ACQUISITION

ACQUISITION: NAME: Spine Sagittal T1W # 5 TIME: 5

COIL: HEAD ____ BODY ____ SURFACE X

POSITIONING: HEAD FIRST X FEET FIRST ____ OTHER ____

CENTERING Midline

PLANE: AXIAL ____ CORONAL ____ SAGITTAL X OTHER ____

SLICES: SINGLE ____ MULTI X 3DI ____ 3DA ____

THICKNESS 5 GAP 1 NUMBER (TR/TE+15)) 9

PULSE SEQUENCE: SE: X ISE: ____ OT1: ____ CS: ____

N_y: 160 TR: 500 TI: ____ TE: 40

N_{Ex}: 4 ZOOM: - ECHOES: 1

AT (TR x N_y x N_{Ex}): 5

GATING: CARDIAC: ____ RESPIRATORY: ____ BOTH: ____ OTHER: ____

CONTRAST: ORAL: ____ RECTAL: ____ IV: ____

PHOTO FORMAT: 2 X 1: ____ 4 X 1: ____ 6 X 1: ____

9 X 1: X 15 X 1: ____

COMMENTS: ____

M. R. ACQUISITION

ACQUISITION: NAME: Spine Sagittal ME # 6 TIME: 13

COIL: HEAD ____ BODY ____ SURFACE X

POSITIONING: HEAD FIRST X FEET FIRST ___ OTHER ____

CENTERING Midline

PLANE: AXIAL ___ CORONAL ___ SAGITTAL X OTHER ____

SLICES: SINGLE X MULTI ____ 3DI ____ 3DA ____

THICKNESS 1cm GAP ___ NUMBER (TR/TE+15)) 1

PULSE SEQUENCE: SE: X ISE: ____ OTI: ____ CS: ____

N_y: 128 TR: 2000 TI: ____ TE: 32

N_{Ex}: 3 ZOOM: – ECHOES: 8

AT (TR x N_y x N_{Ex}): 13

GATING: CARDIAC: ___ RESPIRATORY: ___ BOTH: ___ OTHER: ___

CONTRAST: ORAL: ____ RECTAL: ____ IV: ____

PHOTO FORMAT: 2 X 1: ____ 4 X 1: ____ 6 X 1: ____

9 X 1: X 15 X 1: ____

COMMENTS: 1. Select midline section from sagittal T1W

2. On large patient use N_{ex} = 4

M. R. ACQUISITION

ACQUISITION: NAME: Spine Axial # 7 TIME: 12

COIL: HEAD ____ BODY ____ SURFACE X

POSITIONING: HEAD FIRST X FEET FIRST ___ OTHER ____

CENTERING Mid L5

PLANE: AXIAL ___ CORONAL ___ SAGITTAL ___ OTHER Angled Axial

SLICES: SINGLE ____ MULTI X 3DI ____ 3DA ____

THICKNESS 4 GAP 1 NUMBER (TR/TE+15)) 17

PULSE SEQUENCE: SE: X ISE: ____ OT1: ____ CS: ____

N_y: 128 TR: 950 TI: ____ TE: 40

N_{Ex}: 6 ZOOM: 25% ECHOES: 1

AT (TR x N_y x N_{Ex}): 12

GATING: CARDIAC: ___ RESPIRATORY: ___ BOTH: ___ OTHER: ___

CONTRAST: ORAL: ____ RECTAL: ____ IV: ____

PHOTO FORMAT: 2 X 1: ____ 4 X 1: ____ 6 X 1: ____

9 X 1: X 15 X 1: ____

COMMENTS: 1. Angle axials parallel to disc

2. Obtain additional axial acquisition through any suspicious level on sagittal

3. Use N_y = 160 on large patient

Appendix C

SPINE EXAMINATION WORKSHEET

PATIENT NAME ____________________ DATE ____________

LUMBAR SEGMENTS ________ TRANSITIONAL VERTEBRA ________

VERTEBRAE: ALIGNMENT ______ HEIGHT ______ SIGNAL ______

		TRI JOINT COMPLEX				CANAL				OTHER
	RIGHT NEURAL CANAL	RIGHT FACET	DISC	DISC SIGNAL	LEFT FACET	RT. LAT. RECESS	CENTRAL CANAL	LT.LAT. RECESS	LT. NEURAL CANAL	
L1-L2										
L2-L3										
L3-L4										
L4-L5										
L5-S1										

MISCELLANEOUS FINDINGS ____

____

GRADING		ABBREVIATIONS		
1= Normal	* = Soft Tissue	LAM = Laminectomy	NF = Not Fused	R = Right
2= Slight	OR = Osteophytic Ridging	HL = Hemilaminectomy	IJ = Irregular Joint	L = Left
3= Mild	PD = Pars Defect	FP = Focal Protrusion	DN = Degenerative Narrowing	F = Fused
4 = Moderate	FH = Flavum Hypertrophy	EX = Extrusion	PRL= Pseudoretrolisthesis	C = Central
5 = Severe	DS = Decreased Signal	SPL= Spondylolisthesis	RL = Retrolisthesis	SL = Sublux
	IS = Increased Signal	DH = Decreased Height	DAB = Diffuse Annular Bulge	SP = Spur

KEY IMAGES		EXAM QUALITY	
Axial	____	Excellent	____
Sag T1W	____	Good	____
Sag T2W	____	Fair	____
Other	____	Poor	____

____

RADIOLOGIST

Appendix D

SAMPLE NORMAL REPORT

MAGNETIC RESONANCE IMAGING OF THE LUMBAR SPINE

DATE: ________

Indications:

Technique: Imaging on the 0.6T superconducting scanner. Acquisitions include multi-slice T1 weighted sagittal, multi-slice T1 weighted transaxial, and mid-line sagittal multi-echo with TR2000 for proton density and T2 weighting, including the use of closely coupled coils, where appropriate.

Findings: Alignment of the visualized lumbar vertebral bodies appears normal. The lumbar vertebral bodies demonstrate normal heights and normal signal intensities for the pulse sequences utilized.

Intervertebral discs visualized show normal heights and normal signal patterns for the pulse sequences utilized.

On the sagittal T2 weighted images producing the "MR myelogram" effect there is no significant intradural or extra-dural abnormality.

Cross-sections through the lower lumbar levels show normal bony dimensions of the central spinal canal. No focal disc herniations are evident. No significant central or lateral spinal stenosis is seen.

The visualized paralumbar musculature appears unremarkable.

IMPRESSION: NEGATIVE

Thank you for referring this patient.

Appendix E

Conduct of Depositions

Many spinal MR cases are related to litigation in some way. The following suggestions are offered to those physicians, particularly radiologists, who are called to testify.

1. The deposition is a formal legal process involving sworn testimony. An attorney may request a deposition in order to obtain *information* about a case (discovery process), or to obtain *testimony* which is later to be read to a jury. Frequently, in order to protect the interests of his client, an attorney will issue a subpoena to all physicians involved in a case. The initial response to the subpoena should be a telephone call to the attorney requesting the subpoena. Sometimes an informal telephone conversation is all that is required to answer the attorney's questions, and a formal deposition can be avoided.

2. A *subpoena duces tecum* is an order to bring or send the documents or other materials requested. The dates on a *trial* subpoena often indicate the broad time period (docket) during which a case is scheduled, and not a specific time to appear.

3. A material witness has direct knowledge of the facts of a particular case. He may be questioned about these facts, but not about his expert opinion. An expert witness is called for his expert knowledge. A physician testifying about his own patient often fills both rolls. A material witness is entitled only to a nominal witness fee, whereas an expert witness is entitled to fair compensation for his time. Define your roll in advance. It is appropriate for an expert witness to charge for his time portal to portal, that is for the total time he is away from his practice. The local medical society, or local orthopedic surgeons or neurosurgeons, are good sources of information about expert witness fees in your locality.

4. Attorneys are usually willing to hold depositions in your office or hospital. Most depositions involve a minimum of two attorneys plus a court reporter; some may be videotaped. Courtesy dictates that you be on time, and sche-

dule the deposition when you are not likely to be interrupted by emergencies.

5. A brief predeposition conference with the requesting attorney, either in person or by telephone, is a great time saver. This is standard, acceptable practice.
6. Often a written curriculum vitae can be submitted for the record, replacing lengthy testimony.
7. *Going off the record* is useful during the course of the deposition to indicate to the attorneys the general direction of your testimony.
8. Before the deposition it is helpful to select the key images from the MR study, and be prepared to discuss the case from them. Remember that your testimony (transcribed or videotaped) is directed at a jury with very limited knowledge of the subject.
9. Diagnose only what is on the films—no more and no less.
10. Assessment of the clinical significance of findings present on the MR study is often best left to the physician who has actually examined the patient.
11. Choose your words carefully. Don't be afraid to say "I don't know."
12. An occasional misguided attorney, dissatisfied by the content of your testimony, may try to discredit you as a witness by provoking your temper. Remain cool. Fortunately this tactic, more common at trial, is rare during depositions.
13. As an expert witness at deposition, you are paid for your *time*, not for your *testimony*. Remember this, and answer accordingly should an attorney ask "how much are you being paid for this testimony?"
14. At the conclusion of the deposition, you may be asked "read or waive?" In most instances, it is safe to waive reading of the transcript if you are not a party to the action.

Bibliography

Adams, M., Hutton, W.: Gradual Disc Prolapse. Spine, 10:524-531, 1985.

Aguilla, L.A., Piraino, D.W., Modic, M.T., et al: The Intranuclear Cleft of the Intervertebral Disk: Magnetic Resonance Imaging. Radiology 155:155-158, 1985.

Banna, M.: Clinical Radiology of the Spine and the Spinal Cord. Rockville, Md.: Aspen Systems Corporation, 1985.

Barnes, P.D., Lester, P.D., et al.: Magnetic Resonance Imaging in Infants and Children with Spinal Dysraphism. AJNR 7:465-472, 1985.

Berger, P., Atkinson, D. et al; High Resolution Surface Coil Magnetic Resonance Imaging of the Spine: Normal and Pathologic Anatomy. RadioGraphics 6:4 573-602, July 1986.

Berquist, T.H., Ehman, R. L.: MRI Evaluates Diseases of Musculoskeletal System. Diagnostic Imaging, 7:88 - 91, 1985.

Bradley, W., Adey, W., et al;: Magnetic Resonance Imaging of the Brain, Head and Neck: Fundamentals of Magnetic Resonance Imaging Interpretation. Rockville, Md.: Aspen Systems Corporation, 1985. p. 1 - 16.

Brinckmann, P.: Injury of the Annulus Fibrosus and Disc Protrusions: An In Vitro Investigation on Human Lumbar Discs. Spine, 149-531, 1986.

Brown, M.D.: The Pathophysiology of Disc Disease. Orthopedic Clinics of North America 2: 359-370, 1971.

Burnett, K.R., Levine, J., Sieger, L.: MRI Evaluation of the Cervical Spine of High Field Strength. Applied Radiology, Nov/Dec 1985. p.47-55.

Burton, C.: Conservative Management of Lumbar Disc Disease. Genant, H., (ed.) Spine Update 1984.

Burton, C.: Diagnosis and Treatment of Lateal Spin Stenosis: Implications Regarding the "Failed Back Surgery Syndrome". 20:235. In Genant, H. (ed.) Spine Update 1984, 235-241, San Francisco, California, Radiology Research and Education Foundation.

Byrd, S., Cohn, M., et al: The Radiographic Evaluation of the Symptomatic Postoperative Lumbar Spine Patient. Spine 10: 652-661, 1985.

Cahill, P., Quality Assurance and Image Artifacts in MRI, presented at Palm Beach MRI Update, West Palm Beach, Florida, 1985.

Chafetz, N., Computed Tomography of Lumbar Disc Disease. Genant, H., et al (eds.), Computed Tomography of the Lumbar Spine, San Francisco, University of California Printing Department. 1982.

Chafetz, N., Genant, H., et al: Computed Tomography of The Spine. Chapter 10, p. 427.

Chafetz, N., Genant, H.K., Moon, K.L.: Recognition of Lumbar Disk Herniation with NMR. AJR 141:1154-1156, 1983.

Cohen, M.D., Klatte, E.C., Baehner, R., et al: Magnetic Resonance Imaging of Bone Marrow Disease in Children. Radiology 151: 715-718, 1984. p. 715.

Cohen, M.D.: Pediatric Magnetic Resonance Imaging. Philadelphia, Pennsylvania: W. B. Saunders, Co., 1986.

Daffner, R.H., Lupetin, A.R., Dash, N., et al: MRI in the Detection of Malignant Infiltration of Bone Marrow. AJR 146:353-358, 1986.

Dall, B., Rowe, D.: Degenerative Spondylolisthesis: Its Surgical Management. Spine 10: 668, 1985.

Di Chiro, G., Doppman, J.L., Dwyer, A.J.: Tumors and Arteriovenous Malformations of the Spinal Cord: Assessment Using MR. Radiology 156: 689-697, 1985.

Dihlman, W,: Die lumbosakrale Rethrolisthesis und Pseudoretrolisthesis. Fortschr. Rontgenstr. 104 (1966) 264.

Dooms, G.C., Fisher, M.R., Hricak, H., et al: Bone Marrow Imaging: Magnetic Resonance Studies Related to Age And Sex. Radiology 155:429-432, 1985.

Dorwart, R.: Fundamentals of Computed Tomographic Evaluation of Lumbar Disc Disease. 8:67. In Genant, H.K., Spine Update, 1984 67-78.

Dorwart, R.: Fundamentals of the Computed

In Genant, H.K., Spine Update, 1984 67-78.

Dorwart, R.: Fundamentals of the Computed Tomographic Assessment of Spinal Stenosis. 18:181. In Genant, H., (ed.) Spine Update 1984, San Francisco, California. Radiology Research and Education Foundation. 181-189.

Dupuis, P., Yong-Hing, K., Cassidy, J.D., et al: Radiologic Diagnosis of Degenerative Lumbar Spinal Instability. Spine, Vol. 10, No. 3, 1985.

Easton, E.J., Powers, J.A.: Musculoskeletal Magnetic Resonance Imaging. Thorofare, New Jersey: Charles B. Slack, Inc, 1986.

Epstein, B.S.: The Spine, A Radiological Text and Atlas. Philadelphia: Lea & Febiger, 1976.

Feffer, H. L., Wiesel, S.W., et al: Degenerative Spondylolisthesis. Spine, Vol. 10, No. 3, 1985.

Finneson, B.E.: Low Back Pain. Philadelphia, Pennsylvania: J.B. Lippincott Co., 1981.

Frymoyer, J.W., Selby, D.K.: Segmental Instability. Spine, Vol. 10, No. 3, 1985.

Gehweiler, J.A., Osborne, R.L., et al: The Radiology of Vertebral Trauma. Philadelphia, Pa., W. B. Saunders, 1980.

Genant, H.K., Chafetz, N., Helms, C.A.: Computed Tomography of the Lumbar Spine. San Francisco, California: University of California, 1982.

Genant, H.K., Spine Update 1984. San Francisco, CA., Radiology Research and Education Foundation, 1983.

Gertzbein, S.D., Seligman, J., Holtby, R. et al: Centrode Patterns and Segmental Instability in Degenerative Disc Disease. Spine, 10:3, 1985.

Gibson, M., Buckley, J., Mawhinney, R. et al; Magnetic Resonance Imaging and Discography in the Diagnosis of Disc Degeneration. Nottingham, England: Journal of Bone and Joint Surgery 68-B:3 369-373.

Gonzalez, C.F., Grossman, C.B., Masdeu, J.C.: Head and Spine Imaging. New York: John Wiley and Sons, 1985.

Han, J.S., Benson, J.E., Kaufman, B., et al,: Demonstration of Diastematomyelia and Associated Abnormalities with MR Imaging. AJNR 6:215-219.

Han, J.S., Kaufman, B., El Yousef, S.J., et al: NMR Imaging of the Spine. AJNR 141:1137-1145, 1983.

Haughton, V.M., Williams, A.L.: Computed Tomography of the Spine. St. Louis: C. V. Mosby Co., 1982.

Heindel, W., Freidmann, G., et al; Artifacts in MR Imaging After Surgical Intervention. JCAT 10: 596-599, 1986.

Heithoff, K., Ray, C.: Principles of the Computed Tomographic Assessment of Lateral Spinal Stenosis. In Genant, H., (ed.) Spine Update 1984, p 191-233, San Francisco, California. Radiology and Research Education Foundation 1983.

Hyman, R., Edwards, J., Vacirca, et al.: 0.6T MR Imaging of the Cervical Spine: Multislice and Multiecho Techniques. AJNR 6:229-236 1985.

Kelly, W., Paglen, P., Pearson, J. et al; Ferromagnetism of Intraocular Foreign Body Causes Unilateral Blindness after MR Study. AJNR 7:243-245, March/April 1986.

Kirkaldy-Willis, W. H., Yong-Hing, K.: Pathology and Pathogenesis of Lumbar Spondylosis and Stenosis. 17:169. Genant, H.K., Spine Update 1984, 169-180.

Kirkaldy-Willis, W.H.: Presidential Symposium on Instability of the Lumbar Spine. Spine 10: 254, 1985.

Kraemer, J., Kolditz, J. et al: Water and Electrolyte Content of Human Intervertebral Discs Under Variable Load. Spine 10: 69-71, 1985.

Larsen, J.L., The Posterior Surface of the Lumbar Vertebral Bodies. Part 2: An Anatomic Investigation Concerning the Curvatures in the Horizontal Plane. Spine 10: 901-906, 1985.

Lee, B., Kazam, E., and Newman, A.: Computed Tomography of the Spine and Spinal Cord. Radiology 128: 95, 1978.

Lombardi, J., Wiltse, L., et al: Treatment of Degenerative Spondylolisthesis. Spine 10: 821-827, 1985.

Mani, J.R.: Pitfalls in the Computed Tomographic Diagnosis of Herniated Discs. In Genant, H. (ed.): Spine Update 1984. San Francisco, California, Radiology Research and Education Foundation, 1983.

Maravilla, K., Lesh, P., Weinreb, J., et al: Magnetic Resonance Imaging of the Lumbar Spine with CT Correlation. AJNR 6:237-245, 1985.

Marmourian AC; Briggs RW: Appearance of Pantopaque on MR Images. Radiology 1986 Feb; 158 (2):457-60.

Margulis, A.R., Higgins, C.B., Kaufman, L.: Clinical Magnetic Resonance Imaging. 1983. San Francisco, California, Radiology Research and Education Foundation, 1983.

McCullouch, J., An Approach to the Patient With Sciatica. Genant, H., Spine Update 1984, 19-22.

Mikhael, M.A., Ciric, I.S., Kudrna, J.C.: Recognition of Lumbar Disc Disease With Magnetic Resonance Imaging. Computerized Radiology 9:213-222, 1985.

Mixter, WJ, Barr JS: Rupture of the Intervertebral Disc With Involvement of the Spinal Canal. New England Surgical Society, Boston, Sept 30, 1933.

Modic, M.T., Masaryk, T. et al; Lumbar Herniated Disk Disease and Canal Stenosis: Prospective Evaluation by Surface Coil MR, CT and Myelography. AJNR 7:709-717, July/August 1986.

Modic, M.T., Weinstein, M.A., Pavlicek, W.: Magnetic Resonance Imaging of the Cervical Technical and Clinical Observations. AJR 141: 1129-1136, 1983.

Modic, M., Pavlicek, W., et al: Magnetic Resonance Imaging of Intervertebral Disk Disease. Radiology 152:102 - 111, 1984.

Modic, M., Masaryk, T. et al: Magnetic Resonance Imaging of the Spine. Radiologic Clinics of North America 24:2, June 1986.

Modic, M., Weinstein, M.A., Pavlicek, W.:

Nuclear Magnetic Resonance Imaging of the Spine. Radiology 148:757-762, 1983.

Moon, K.L., Genant, H.K., Helms, N.I.: Musculoskeletal Applications of Nuclear Magnetic Resonance. Radiology 147:161-171, 1983.

Morris, J., Surgical Management of Lumbar Disc Disease: An Orthopedic Perspective. Genant, H., et al; (eds.), Computed Tomography of the Lumbar Spine. 139-145. San Francisco, Ca., University of California Printing Department. 1982.

Nachesmons, A.: Lumbar Spine Instability, A Critical Update and Symposium Summary. Spine, Vol. 10, No. 3, 1985.

Naylor, A.: The Biochemical Changes in the Human Intervertebral Disc in Degeneration and Nuclear Prolapse. Orthopedic Clinics of North America, 2:2, July 1971.

Norman, D., Mills, C.M., Brant-Zawadski, M., et al: Magnetic Resonance Imaging of the Spinal Cord and Canal: Potentials and Limitations. AJR 141: 1147-1152, 1983.

Parks, W., Schiff, D.C.M.: The Applied Anatomy of the Intervertebral Disc: Orthopedic Clinics of North America 2:2 : 309-324, 1971.

Pech, P., Haughton, V.M.: Lumbar Intervertebral Disk: Correlative MR and Anatomic Study. Radiology 156:699-701, 1985.

Pope, M.H., Panjabi, M.: Biomechanical Definitions of Spinal Instability. Spine, Vol 10, No. 3 1985.

Post, M.J.D.: Radiographic Evaluation of the Spine. New York: Masson Publishing USA, Inc., 1980.

Ramsey, R., Zacharia, C.: MR Imaging of the Spine after Radiation Therapy: Easily Recognizable Effects. AJNR 6:247-251, 1985.

Ramsey, R., Zacharia, C.: MR Imaging of the Spine after Radiation Therapy: Easily Recognizable Effects. AJNR 6:247-251, March/April 1985.

Ramsey, R.: MR of the Spine: Showing Defects Without Artifacts. Diagnostic Imaging, 8:74-79.

Rauschning, W., Detailed Sectional Anatomy of the Spine. Rothman, S., Glenn, W. Multiplanar CT of the Spine. p. 33 - 85. Baltimore, Maryland: University Park Press, 1985.

Reis, N., Lanir, A., et al: Magnetic Resonance Imaging in Orthopaedic Surgery: A glimpse into the future. The Journal of Bone and Joint Surgery 67B: 659-664, 1985.

Rothman, R.H., Simeone, F.A.: The Orthoped Clinics of North America. 2:2 July 1971. Diseases of the Intervertebral Disc. Philadelphia, Pennsylvania: W.B. Saunders Co., 1971.

Rothman, R.H., Simeone, F.A.: The Spine, Second Edition. 1: 1982. Philadelphia, Pennsylvania: W.B. Saunders Co. 1982.

Sackett, J.F., Strother, C.M.: New Techniques in

Myelography. Hagerstown, Md., Harper & Row, 1979.

Schmorl, G., Junghanns, H.: The Human Spine in Health and Disease. New York: Grune & Stratton, 1971.

Shapiro, R.: Myelography, Third Edition. Chicago: Year Book Medical Publishers, Inc., 1975.

Sundaram, M., A wwad, E.E.: Magnetic Resonance Imaging of Arachnoid Cysts Destroying the Sacrum. AJR 146:359-360, 1986.

Teplick, J.G., Laffey, P.A., Berman, A., et al,: Diagnosis and Evaluation of Spondylolisthesis and/or Spondylolysis on Axial CT. AJNR 7:479-491, May/June 1986.

Teplick, J.G., Laffey, P.A., Berman, A., et al,: Diagnosis and Evaluation of Spondylolisthesis and/or Spondylolysis on Axial CT. AJNR 7:479-491, 1986.

Thoen, D., Halversen, G., et al; Interpretation of Lumbar Spine CT Scans. Salt Lake City, Utah: Western Neurological Associates, 1982.

Tibrewal, S., Pearcy, M.: Lumbar Intervertebral Disc Heights in Normal Subjects and Patients with Disc Herniation. Spine 10: 452-454, 1985.

Tsuji, H., Yoshioka, T., et al: Developmental Balloon Disc of the Lumbar Spine in Healthy Subjects. Spine 10: 907-911, 1985.

Vanharanta, H., Korpi, J., et al: Radiographic Measurements of Lumbar Spinal Canal Size and Their Relation to Back Mobility. Spine 10: 461-466, 1985.

Von Einsiedel, H.: Nuclear Magnetic Resonance of The Spine. In Gonazalez, see, et al; (eds.), Head and Spine Imaging. New York, John Wiley and Sons, 1985. p 917 - 931.

Weatherley, C., Prickett, C., et al: Discogenic Pain Persisting Despite Solid Posterior Fusion. The Journal of Bone and Joint Surgery 68-B: 142-143, 1986.

Weintreb, J.C., Cohen, J.M., et al: Iliopsoas Muscles: MR Study of Normal Anatomy and DisRadiology 156: 435-440, 1985.

Wolf, G., Popp, C., NMR, A Primer for Medical Imaging. Thorofare, New Jersey: Charles B. Slack, Inc. 1984.

Index

Note: Numbers in *italics* refer to illustrations; numbers followed by (t) refer to tables.

Abnormalities, 57
  grading system for. See Grading system.
  See also Congenital abnormalities.
Acquisition time, 26, 26(t)
Agenesis of sacral spine, *112*
Anatomy. See names of specific structures.
Aneurysm, 8, 30
Annulus fibrosis, 54(t)
  anatomy of, 117-118, 124
  degeneration of, 124-125
  diagnosis of, 122(t)
  diagram of, *74*
  pathology of, *121*, 122-124
  rupture of, 122-123
  sagittal view of, *69*
  signal intensity of, 71
Arachnoiditis, 6, 62
Articular process(es), inferior hypertrophy of, *162, 163*
Articular process(es), superior, *165-167*
  hypertrophy of, *171, 172, 174*
Artifact, *224, 225, 230*
  catheter, *226,* 222
  chemical shift, *69,* 71, *74*
  foreign bodies, 226-227
  myelographic, *223, 229*
  partial volume effects, 215, 227
  postoperative, 226-227
  system, 227
  with Harrington rod, *111*
  with metallic implant, *204*
Axial plane, 83-87
  transaxial images, 86-87

Back pain, 3-11
  costs of, 3, 4(t)
  diagnosis of, 3-4, 5
  history taking, 5, 244
  levels differentiated, 6(t)
  MR imaging for, 4-5
  onset sudden of, 124
  surgery for, 4
  tests for, 4. See also individual tests.
  x-ray with, 5
Blood, flow effects of, 29, *29*
Bone scans, 7, *192*
Bone tissue, signal intensity of, 23, 23(t)
Brightness, 22-23. See also Gray scale and Signal intensity.

Canal, intervertebral, 54(t), *73,* 76
  anatomy of, 155, *155*
  impingement of, *143, 144*
  narrowing of, *175*
  parasagittal view of, 75, 77
  sagittal view of, *77,* 153
  stenosis of, *141,* 161, 166, 168. See also Stenosis, intervertebral canal.
Canal, nerve exit. See Canal, intervertebral.
Canal, spinal, 54(t)
  anatomy of, 154-156
  AP diameter stenosis, 157
  epidural space of, 71, 75
  narrowing of, 157, *160, 161*
    interpretation of, 178-179
  normal size of, 153-154
  parasagittal view of, 76
  sagittal view of, 8, *69*
  size, 153-154
    significance of, 152-153
  subarticular recess of, 154-155
Cartilage, signal intensity of, 23, 71
Cauda equina syndrome, 157
Cerebral spinal fluid, signal intensity of, *100*
  structures iso-intense with, *106, 107*
Chemonucleolysis, 150, 235
Chordoma, *203*
Claustrophobia, 10-11, 10(t), 230

Coils, 17
  body, 17, 27
    acquisition with, *45*
  surface, 17, 27
    acquisition with, *45*
    sensitivity pattern, *27, 202*
Computed tomography, 6, 7-8, 15, 60, 62
Computer, 8
Congenital abnormalities, 89-114
  of cord, *108, 109*
  of vertebrae, 93, *94-98,* 98-99
  sacral agenesis, *112*
Contraindications, 8-9, 8(t), 29-30, 230
Cord, tethered, *108, 109*
Coronal plane, *86,* 87-88
  diagram of, *87*
Cysts, signal intensity of, 23

Diastematomyelia, 110
Disc herniation, 4, 34, 99, *231*
  asymmetrical, *127*
  central subligamentous, *128*
  MRI sensitivity for, *60,* 61
  posterolateral, *126*
  recurrent, *133, 148*
  signal intensity of, 230
  studies for, 62
  vectors of, 124
  views of, 54, *58, 126-129, 134-136*
Disc, intravertebral
  alignment of, 71
  anatomy of, 117-120, *118*
  coronal view of, *86*
  degeneration of, 120, 124-125, *146, 175, 197*
    in spinal stenosis, 156-157, *175, 185*
  dehydration of, 124-125, 156
  dimensions of, 71, 119(t)
  disease of, 115-150
  impingement of, *143, 144*
  injury to, 120, *187*
  nutrition of, 119-120
  pathophysiology of, 117-120, *121*
  postoperative, 125, *133*
  terminology for, 120, 122
Disc space calcification, 113

Discitis, 7, *191, 195,* 194, *195, 196, 198*
Dysraphism, spinal, 104, 110. See also
  Myelodysplasia.

Edema, signal intensity of, 23
Electrodiagnostic studies, 62
End plate(s), 54(t), *82*
  abnormality of, *96,* 98-99
  destruction of, *195, 196*
  hypertrophy of, 156
  osteophytosis of, *171*
  sagittal view of, 68, *69*
  signal intensity of, 201
Epidural veins. See Veins, epidural.
Extradural defect, *135, 137*

Facetectomy, medial, 157, 161, *166*
Facet(s), articular, 54(t)
  hypertrophy of, 155, 156, 161
Facet joint(s), 54(t), *82*
  hypertrophy of, *170*
Fat, epidural, 54(t), 125
  in image analysis, 125, *147*
  signal intensity of, 23, *70, 100,* 125
Fat graph, *148*
Fat wedge sign, *96, 99, 136, 138, 139*
Fibrosis, epidural, 125
  postsurgical formation of, 125
Films, 18
  storage, 18
Flow effects, 29, *29*
Foremen, neural. See Canal, intervertebral.
Foramenal stenosis. See Stenosis, intervertebral
  canal.
Fourier transform, 24, 227
Fracture(s), compression, *186, 188*
Fragment(s), free, 123, *130*
  views of, *129-132, 140-142, 145, 146*
Future developments, 234-236
  chemical shift imaging, 234
  of hardware, 234
  of software, 235
  surgery and, 235

Gallium scans, 7

Gradient zoom, 27
Grading system, *55*, 57
Gray scale, 22-23, 22(t)

Hemangioma, of vertebral bodies, 205, *206, 207*
  signal intensity of, 205, *206*
Hematoma, signal intensity of, 23
Hemilaminectomy, *148, 149*
Hemivertebra, congenital, 88, 91, *93*
  coronal view of, 91, *93*

Image directions, *46*
  horizontal, *45*
  transverse, *46*
  vertebral, *46*
Image interpretation, 49-64
  axial images, *56, 58*
  background needed, 51
  compared to other studies, 59(t)
  coronal images, *57*
  correlation of images, *58*
  sagittal images, *56, 58*
  viewing angles, 51, *56, 57*
Image quality, 47
Image weighting, 21, 21(t), 40, 47
  CSF key with, 47
Implants, electronic, 8-9, 8(t), 29-30
Implants, metallic, 9
  Harrington rod, *110, 111*
Infection, of lumbar spine, 186, 191, 194
  signal intensity of, *197*
Inflammation, signal intensity of, 23
Intranuclear cleft, *190*, 191

Lamina(e), congenital asymmetry, *218, 219*, 227
Laminectomy, 157, *164*
Legal implications, 232-234
  deposition process, 233, 251-252
  terminology used, 234
Leukemia, *210*, 211
Ligamenta flava, 54(t), 157
  hypertrophied, *158, 169*
  ligament, ilio-lumbar, *176*
Ligament, longitudinal, *74*
  anatomy of, 120, 124
  elevated, *128, 133*
  signal intensity of, 23, 71
Lipoma, *109*
Longitudinal relaxation time, 18. See also T1.
Low back pain. See Back pain and Sciatica.
Lumbar spine, anatomy of, 65-88
Lumbar spine examination, 31-47
  acquisition definition, 33
  sample study, *51, 52*
  structures evaluated, 54(t)
  technique of, 33
  See also names of specific structures.
Magnets utilized, 16-17, 16(t)
Marrow, leukemia in, *210*, 211
  signal intensity of, 23
Matrix size, *44*
Meningioma, *209*
Metastases, 205. See also Neoplasm.
MR imaging, advantages, 4-5
  bone scan compared with, 7
  certainty of, 60
  computed tomography compared with, 7-8, 15, 24, 54, 59(t), 62, 153
  follow-up for, 63-65
  gallium scan compared with, 7
  gradient system of, 17, 27
  interpretation of, 176, 178-179
  legal implications of, 232-234
  limitations of, 230-232
  other studies with, 62
  significance of, 60-62
  surgery and, 61, 63
  system components, 16(t)
  tissue characterization with, 230
  use of atlas, 67
  washboard spine, 219
  with spinal stenosis, 153
  x-ray compared with, 5, 54, 59(t)
MR protocol. See Protocol.
Multi-echo imaging, 29, *36*
Muscle tissue, signal intensity of, 23, 23(t)
Myelodysplasia, 104, *108*, 110
Myelography, 59(t), 60, 62, 75, *135*
  artifact of, *228, 229*
Myelomeningocele, *108*, 110, *110, 111*

Neoplasm, 201, 205, 211, *202-209*
  axial image of, *202*
  coronal image of, *202*
  intradural, 205
  postsurgical image, *204*
  signal intensity of, 23, *202*
Neural foramen. See Canal, intervertebral.
Nerve(s), of intervertebral disc, 120
  signal intensity of, 78
  visualization of, 78
Nerve roots, 54(t), *61, 80, 101*
  abnormalities of, 101-104
  asymmetrical, *175*
  axial view of, 83, *84, 85*
  compression of, 62, 156-157, *159, 169, 172, 187*
  conjoined, 101, *101-103*
  cysts of, 104, *105, 107*
  dysfunction of, 157
  in intervertebral canal, 155
  irritation of, 62
  myelography of, *102*
  swelling of, *143, 145, 174*
Nucleus pulposus, 54(t)
  anatomy of, 118-120
  diagnosis of, 122(t)
  extrusion of, 123
  hydration of, 119-120
  intranuclear cleft of, 71
  pathology of, *121*
  physiology of, 119
  replacement of, 236
  sagittal view of, *69*
  saignal intensity of, 71
  T2 weighted views of, *191*
    See also Fragment(s), free.

Ochronosis, 113
Osteomyelitis, 7, 194
Osteophyte(s), *58, 130, 144, 146, 168, 175*
Osteophytosis, 156, *171*

Pantopaque, *222, 223,* 226
  signal intensity of, 226
Paradoxical enhancement, 29, *29*
Paravertebral muscle, 54(t)
Patients, contraindications, 8-9, 8(t)
  difficulties with, 10-11
  handling system, 17
  history, 244
  positioning, 9, *9*
  screening, 9, 239
  sedation for, 10
Pedicle(s), *79*
  parasagittal section of, *72*
Physics, 15-30
Pixel(s), 22, 24, 27
Planes, 15, 28-29, *28*
  angled axial, *28*
  axial, 28-29, *28, 38, 52, 53*
    reference image for, 68
  compound angled, 28
  coronal, 40, *40*
  disc, *39*
  MAVIN, *28*
  oblique, 28
  sagittal, 28, *28, 35, 36*
    compared to CT scan, 54
    midline, *53*
    of spine, 33
    reference image, *34*
    weighted, *52*
  sagittal scout, *38, 78*
  transaxial, 54
  varying angles, *28*
Prevertebral structures, 54(t), 67
Prosthesis, MRI with, 8
Protocol, 10, 33, 241, 242, 245, 246
Pseudopseudoretrolisthesis, *99*, 99
Pseudoretrolisthesis, *94-98*, 99, 101, *126, 139*
Psoas muscle, *86*, 87
Pulse, generator of, 17
  90°, 20-22
  180°, 20-22
  spin echo sequence, 20-22, *20*

Radiation effects, 184, 186, 191, 194, *189, 190*
  in marrow, 186
Recess(es), lateral, 54(t), *72, 75*, 154-155. See also under Canal, spinal.
Relaxation, 18-20

parameters of, 18-20
T1, 18-20
Report of MRI, 62-63, 250
Retrolisthesis, *94*, 99, 166

Safety, 29-30. See also Contraindications.
Sagittal plane, 67-83
key sections of, 67-68, *68*
midline, 68, 71, 75
diagram of, *74*
parasagittal, 68, *72*, 75-76
scout view, *78*
Sciatica, 3-11, 62, 124. See also Back pain.
Scoliosis, 40, 88, 215-216
asymmetry with, 215-216, *206*
coronal projection of, *216, 217*
evaluation with MRI, 216
partial volume effects with, 215
theca involvement in, *217*
Sensitivity of MRI, 60-62, 205
bone scan compared with, 7, 205
litigation use of, 233
Siderosis, 113
Signal averaging, *43*
Signal intensity, 22-23, 22(t), 71
decreased, *188, 192, 193*
diseases affecting, 110, 113
increased, 191, 194, *193, 197, 198, 199*
loss of, *131, 147*
of infection, 194, *195*
of inflammation, *199*
of marrow, *142*
of metastases, *189, 190, 200*
of T1 weighted images, *189*, 194
of T2 weighted images, *188*, 194
of tissues, 23
of vertebral bodies, *210*
See also Gray scale.
Slice(s) for MRI, multislice imaging, 24-25
optimal thickness, 7
profiles of, 25(t)
sizes used, 25
varying thickness, *41*
Specificity of MRI, disc disease, 5
inflammation, 5
neoplasm, 5
spinal stenosis, 5
Spinal stenosis. See Stenosis, spinal.
Spine. See Lumbar spine and names of particular structures.
Spin echo pulse sequence, 20-22, *20*. See also Pulse.
Spin lattice, 18. See also T1.
Spin relaxation time, 19. See also T2.
Spondylolisthesis, 93, *94, 159, 160*, 166, 183, *185*
sagittal views, 183, *184*
Stenosis, central canal, 157-161, *162*
axial image of, *158, 161*
sagittal image of, *160*
signs of, 157
surgical treatment of, 157, 161
Stenosis, dynamic spinal, 173
Stenosis, far lateral, 173, *176, 177, 178*
Stenosis, intervertebral canal, 161, 166, 168, *163, 172*
factors in, *171*
parasagittal image of, *163, 170*
Stenosis, severe concentric, *173, 174*
Stenosis, lateral, *159*. See also Stenosis, intervertebral canal and Stenosis, subarticular recess.
Stenosis, spinal, 5, 34, 151-179
acquired, 154-155
congenital, 154
diagnosis of, 154
CT scan for, 153
MRI for, 153, 176, 178-179
pathogenesis of, 156-157
types of, *156*
Stenosis, subarticular recess, 161, *170, 171*
axial view of, *168*
signs of, 161
surgical decompression of, 161, 168
Surgery, findings compared, 63-65, *64*
decompression with, *164*
failure of, *166*, 215
for lateral stenosis, 168
See also names of specific procedures.
Syrinx, *108*

TE, 20-22, 22(t)
T1, 18-20, 19(t), 40, 47
  weighted image of, *69*
    hemangioma and, *207*
    metastases and, *200*
    osteomyelitis and, 194
    signal intensity of, 71, 75, *189*
T2, 19-20, 19(t), 40, 47
  relaxation of, 20-21
  weighted image of, 21, *70*
    hemangioma and, *208*
    meningioma and, *209*
    metastases and, *200*
    osteomyelitis and, 194
    signal intensity of, 71, 75, *188*, 191, *198*
    spinal stenosis and, *160*
TR, 21, 21(t)
  varying of, *42*
Tarlov cyst(s), 104, *105*. See also Nerve roots, cysts of.
Tendon, signal intensity of, 23
Tethered cord. See Cord, tethered.
Thallassemia, 113
Theca, displacement of, *138, 141, 148*
  normal, *158*
  parasagittal view of, *72*
  sagittal view of, *162*
Thecal sac, 54(t), 75, *111*
  compression of, 156
  signal intensity of, 23
  spinal stenosis involving, 156-157
Time for imaging, 26, 26(t)
Transverse spin, 19. See also T2.
Trauma, 88, 124, *147*, 183-184, *186*
Tumor(s). See Neoplasm and names of specific tumors.

Variables, user selected, 15-30
Veins, epidural, *77, 229*
Venous plexus, 77
Vertebrae, transitional, 91, *92*, 215
Vertebral body (bodies), 54(t), *155*
  abnormalities of, 93, *94*, 98, *155*
    fat wedge sign, *96, 99*
    in AP diameter, 99, *100*, 101
    See also names of specific conditions.
  anatomy of, 91-92
  axial study of, *165*
  CT image of, *165*
  coronal view of, *86*
  hemangioma of, 205, *206, 207*. See also Hemangioma.
  hypertrophy of, 168
  sagittal view of, 68, *69*
  signal intensity of, *210, 216*
Voxel(s), 22

Washboard spine, 219

X-ray, compared to MRI, 5
  examination with, 5, 60